Management of Advanced Prostate Cancer

Choung Soo Kim
Editor

Management of Advanced Prostate Cancer

Springer

Editor
Choung Soo Kim
Department of Urology
Asan Medical Center
Seoul
Soul-t´ukpyolsi
South Korea

ISBN 978-981-10-6942-0 ISBN 978-981-10-6943-7 (eBook)
https://doi.org/10.1007/978-981-10-6943-7

Library of Congress Control Number: 2018949600

This Springer imprint is published by Springer Nature, under the registered company Springer Nature Singapore Pte Ltd.
The registered company address is: 152 Beach Road, #21-01/04 Gateway East, Singapore 189721, Singapore

Preface

Prostate cancer is the second most common cancer in men worldwide and the fifth cause of cancer-related death in men. As the economy developed, the incidence of prostate cancer increased and substantial public health burden was on the rise. Although the examination of prostate-specific antigen increased, the chance of early detection of prostate cancer and advanced prostate cancer still exists and most cancer-related deaths are caused by not-localized, but advanced prostate cancer. Until now there is no perfect solution to overcome the advanced prostate cancer. Many efforts have been made and are under way to control the disease in various fields. There are many clinical trials to treat metastatic prostate cancer whether it is hormone sensitive or castration resistant. New treatment approaches were approved after successful clinical trials. Therefore, our mission was to show the journey to overcome the advanced prostate cancer.

The contents of the book range from localized high-risk prostate cancer to metastatic castration-resistant prostate cancer. We divided the book into four parts of treatment: surgery, radiotherapy, androgen deprivation therapy, and systemic chemotherapy-immunotherapy. In addition, this book contains recent clinical trials and some basic medical science and refers to the most recent references. This book covers universal content, while some areas include the latest in-depth professional content, so this book will be valuable for clinicians, specialists in urology or radiology, and researchers who deal with prostate cancer.

I would like to thank all the authors for their thoughtful and timely contribution. Without the efforts and knowledge of the authors, this book could not be completed. I hope this book helps you with your research.

Seoul, South Korea
June 2018

Choung-Soo Kim

Contents

Part I

Surgery for Advanced Prostate Cancer

Choung Soo Kim

1 Natural History of High-Risk Prostate Cancer

Sangjun Yoo and In Gab Jeong

1.1 Introduction

Prostate cancer is the second most common cancer among men worldwidely and more than a million patients were newly diagnosed as prostate cancer [1]. Moreover, in developed countries, prostate cancer is ranked first among male cancer. In the view of mortality, prostate cancer is the fifth most common cause of death among male cancer, and approximately 307,500 patients died from prostate cancer worldwidely in 2012. Given the high incidence of prostate cancer, the number of deaths from prostate cancer is relatively small compared to other cancers. In other words, prostate cancer is relatively indolent cancer, but nevertheless, a huge number of patients die from prostate cancer due to the high incidence of the disease.

Since the usage of prostate-specific antigen (PSA) tests increased as screening purpose, early detection of prostate cancer has increased, and death from prostate cancer has been gradually reduced over time. However, in other parts, the concerns about the overdiagnosis and overtreatment have increased. As a result, in 2008, United States Prevention Services Task Force (USPSTF) concluded that there was insufficient evidence to recommend a PSA test even under men with 75 years old and UTPSTF recommended against routine PSA screening in 2012. After these recommendations, a decline in the incidence of localized prostate cancer has been reported, and these has been a raising concern for worsening of prostate cancer-specific survival, which could be a sign for increasing aggressiveness of the newly diagnosed prostate cancer. Based on some recent studies, intermediate- or high-risk prostate cancer reported to increase by 6% from 2011 to 2013 [2], which support this concern. In addition, metastatic prostate cancer has been increased from 2004 to 2013 [3].

In addition, it is known that most of these prostate cancer-related deaths are caused by high-risk prostate cancer. In this regard, the need for proper assessment and treatment for high-risk prostate cancer is growing more than ever before. Thus, in recent years, there is a continuing effort to improve survival of high-risk prostate cancer by more active and multidisciplinary treatment although active surveillance is gradually taking place in the treatment for low-risk prostate cancer. In addition, many studies on high-risk prostate are continuing, and the treatment for high-risk prostate cancer is currently undergoing change. In addition, the development of imaging studies has enabled more precise disease staging and early diagnosis of metastatic disease. Therefore,

S. Yoo, M.D., Ph.D.
Department of Urology, SMG-SNU Boramae Medical Center, Seoul, South Korea

I. G. Jeong, M.D., Ph.D. (✉)
Department of Urology, Asan Medical Center, Seoul, South Korea
e-mail: igjeong@amc.seoul.kr

C. S. Kim (ed.), *Management of Advanced Prostate Cancer*,
https://doi.org/10.1007/978-981-10-6943-7_1

clinicians should pay more attention to high-risk prostate cancer than ever before, and it is important to know the definitions, epidemiology, and natural history of high-risk prostate cancer. In this chapter, we will look at the natural history of high-risk prostate cancer, in addition to its definition and epidemiology of high-risk prostate cancer.

1.2 The Definition of High-Risk Prostate Cancer

The risk of prostate cancer has been traditionally stratified into three groups, including low-, intermediate-, and high-risk prostate cancer based on the Gleason score, PSA level at diagnosis, and clinical stage. D'Amico et al. first defined high-risk prostate cancer as follows: clinical stage of T2c or greater, Gleason score of 8–10, or PSA level greater than 20 ng/mL [4]. Since then, various definitions of high-risk prostate cancer have been introduced although most definitions of high-risk prostate cancer are made using PSA level, Gleason score, and clinical stage similar to D'Amico's definition. The widely accepted definitions for high-risk prostate cancer were summarized in Table 1.1.

However, since the risk stratification for prostate cancer generally divides all prostate cancer into three risk groups, each risk group includes prostate cancer with a wide variety of prognoses. Among each risk group, high-risk prostate cancer especially includes the most variety of disease, including localized disease with high Gleason score, locally advanced disease, lymph node invasive disease, hormone-naïve metastatic disease, and castration-resistant disease. In this regard, National Comprehensive Cancer Network (NCCN) guidelines further divided high-risk prostate cancer into high-risk and very high-risk prostate cancer [5]. In NCCN guidelines, very high-risk prostate cancer was defined as clinical stage of T3b or T4, primary Gleason pattern 5, or greater than 4 biopsy cores with Gleason score of 8–10. In addition, new grading system for prostate cancer was suggested by the 2014 International Society of Urological Pathology (ISUP) consensus conference on Gleason grading of prostatic carcinoma reflecting the results of recent studies [6]. Based on the 2014 ISUP criteria, high Gleason score, previously included Gleason score 8–10, was divided into two groups with Gleason grade group 4 (Gleason score of 8) and Gleason grade group 5 (Gleason score of 9 or 10).

However, as the increasing number of treatment options has been developed, more refined classifications of the risk of prostate cancer are clinically needed. As a result, prostate cancer nomogram and/or prostate cancer risk assessment has been suggested to individually assessed the probability and risk of prostate cancer in each patient. Moreover, in recent studies, genetics-related factors have showed promising impacts on differentiating the prognosis of high-risk prostate cancer. Therefore, more accurate and individualized risk stratification could be possible in near future if these could be applied to daily clinical practice.

Table 1.1 Definition of high-risk prostate cancer

	PSA (ng/mL)	Gleason score	Clinical stage
D'Amico	>20	≥8	≥T2c
American Urological Association	>20	≥8	≥T2c
National Comprehensive Cancer Network	>20	≥8	≥T3a
European Association of Urology	>20	≥8	≥T3a
Radiation Therapy Oncology Group	20–100	≥8	≥T2c

1.3 Risk Factors for High-Risk Prostate Cancer

Various factors are known to affect the probability of prostate cancer development. In addition, some of these factors and other factors are useful for predicting the presence of high-risk prostate cancer. For example, recently introduced Prostate Cancer Prevention Trial Risk Calculator

(PCPTRC) incorporated ethnicity and family history for differentiating high-grade prostate cancer from low-grade prostate cancer [7]. In addition, there have been a large number of studies, which reported the probability of upstaging or upgrading after surgery. These predictors, which are associated with the presence of high-risk prostate cancer, could be helpful for selecting the appropriate treatment with an accurate risk classification for each patient with prostate cancer in the current clinical situation. Here, we briefly introduce well-established factors associated with the presence of high-risk prostate cancer.

Ethnicity has been reported as one of the most well-established risk factors associated with the presence of high-risk prostate cancer, and African-Americans reported to have advanced prostate cancer compared to European American men. Conversely, Asian-American, Hispanic men, American Indian, Alaskan Native men, and Pacific Islanders with prostate cancer generally showed superior oncological outcomes compared to European American men with prostate cancer. Although the reasons for these findings are not yet sufficiently evaluated, recent genetics studies might be helpful in explaining these results. Recently, inherited gene change in prostate cancer is widely under investigation. Among these, BRCA2 (breast cancer type 2) mutation reported to confers about threefold elevated risk of high-risk prostate cancer. In addition, PTEN (phosphatase and tensin homolog) loss on chromosome 10, which reported to be common mutated genes in human cancer, regarded as worse prognostic factors for prostate cancer. Although TMPRSS2- (transmembrane protease, serine 2) ERG (estrogen-regulated gene) fusion status is a key genomic event for prostate cancer, its' prognostic value has not been proven. Similarly, a family history of lethal prostate cancer is regarded as a predictor for the development of high-risk prostate cancer. However, more studies are needed to incorporate genetic factors in daily practice with sufficient reliability although some of genetic tests commercially available. Nevertheless, these information from genetics studies are expected to provide a great boost in the diagnosis and treatment of prostate cancer in a near future.

There are several other possible factors associated with the development of high-risk prostate cancer. Recently, there has been an increasing evidence, which suggesting the association between obesity and aggressive prostate cancer. Similarly the association between metabolic syndrome and high-risk prostate cancer has been suggested although the high level of evidence is needed. The mechanisms that explain the relationship between obesity/metabolic syndrome and high-risk prostate cancer are as follows: (1) insulin/insulin-like growth factor (IGF) axis, (2) decreased level of androgen level, and (3) chronic inflammation. Based on the previous studies, prostatic inflammation and lower testosterone level are also reported as variables associated with high-grade prostate cancer. Prostate size is another variable, which is inversely associated with the high-grade and advanced prostate cancer although most of these associations are based on the retrospective observational studies.

5α-reductase inhibitors (5αRIs) has been a well-known variable associated with the high-risk prostate cancer. Previously, 5αRIs have been suggested as chemopreventive drugs for prostate cancer, in addition to selenium, vitamin E, vitamin D, nonsteroidal anti-inflammatory drugs, statin medications, and a selective estrogen receptor modulator. Up to now, no compound, including 5αRIs, showed proven ability to prevent the development of prostate cancer and/or high-risk prostate cancer. However, interestingly, two large randomized studies evaluating the chemopreventive effects of 5αRIs reported that there was an increment in prostate cancer with Gleason score 8 or greater after treating 5αRI. On the contrary, more recent study reported that 5aRI was not associated with an increment in high-grade prostate cancer although overall prostate cancer was decreased after treating 5aRI, which was in accordance with previous two large randomized studies [8]. Considering these conflicting results, the associations between the usages of 5aRIs are currently controversial and remained to be verified.

1.4 Natural History of High-Risk Prostate Cancer

Currently, 20–35% of patients among newly diagnosed prostate cancer are determined as high-risk prostate cancer, and prostate cancer classified into high-risk disease showed various stage and aggressiveness. In this regard, natural history of high-risk prostate cancer could be also varied depending on the staging and the response to the hormonal treatment. For this reason, the natural history of prostate cancer will be presented based on these characteristics as follows: localized or locally advanced high-risk prostate cancer, hormone-naïve metastatic prostate cancer, and castration-resistant prostate cancer.

1.4.1 Localized or Locally Advanced High-Risk Prostate Cancer

Traditionally, clinical stage of the prostate cancer has been determined based on the physical examinations (e.g., digital rectal examination). However, with the recent development of imaging modalities, radiologic examinations have been carried out to enable more precise preoperative staging of prostate cancer. Multiparametric magnetic resonance imaging (MRI) is currently regarded as the most reliable imaging study for evaluating the characteristics and staging or prostate cancer. For intermediate- or high-risk prostate cancer, MRI is recommended if its results change patient management. Multiparametric MRI has been reported as a useful diagnostic method for detecting locally advanced prostate cancer with sensitivity of 43–80% and specificity of 77–95%. Moreover, recent studies reported that MRI showed reliable results for predicting the local staging of prostate cancer (locally confined vs. extracapsular extensive vs. seminal vesicle invasive), which is regarded as an important variable predicting oncological outcomes. However, most of the studies on the natural history of high-risk prostate cancer were published before the application of recent imaging studies, and, as a result, there is little research on natural history according to the local staging based on the imaging studies. In this regard, the natural history of localized or locally advanced high-risk prostate cancer will be presented together.

There have been only a few studies assessing the natural history of untreated localized or locally advanced high-risk prostate cancer. A European study with three decades of follow-up duration reported that about a half of patients with poorly differentiated disease died from prostate cancer within 5 years although these patients had early and localized prostate cancer at the timing of diagnosis [9]. Moreover, all men with high Gleason score (from 8 to 10) prostate cancer died within 10 years after diagnosis. Other study also reported that patients with high-grade prostate cancer had a high-risk of dying from prostate cancer within 10 years. Based on that study, about 121 deaths expected to be occurred per 1000 person-year [10]. Unfortunately, there is no large study reporting survival after conservative management in locally advanced disease. Previous study reported that patients with locally advanced disease developed distant metastases at 10 years in 12–55% of patients. In addition, based on small series, the 5-year overall survival of untreated patients with locally advanced prostate cancer reported to be widely variable from 10% to 92%, which might affect by the different patient and tumor characteristics among studies [11]. Because most of studies in these fields are small and biased, the natural history though to be not fully understood and cannot be applied to the total population of patients with locally advanced disease.

1.4.2 Hormone-Naïve Metastatic Prostate Cancer

The traditional definition of hormone-sensitive metastatic prostate cancer is challenging after the approval of second-generation hormonal agents, including enzalutamide and abiraterone acetate. Because a considerable proportion of patients who treated with chemotherapy due to the resistant to the first-generation hormonal agents still respond to the second-generation hormonal agents, the concepts of hormone-naïve prostate cancer have recently been proposed. In this section, the natural history of hormone-naïve prostate cancer with any suspicious metastatic lesion on preoperative imaging studies will be presented.

In high-risk prostate cancer, metastatic work-ups, including pelvic computed tomography (CT) or MRI and bone scan, are recommended after considering the life expectancy and the presence of symptoms. However, unfortunately, the accuracy of the CT or MRI on detecting metastatic lymph nodes is not met for expectations. In this regard, several novel imaging studies for lymph node evaluation have been developed and introduced, such as 68 gallium- (68Ga) labeled prostate-specific membrane antigen (PSMA) positron emission tomography (PET) or 11 choline (11C) PET, which showed better accuracy compared to that of CT or MRI although these methods are not widely applied up to now. After wide spreads of these imaging studies, prognoses of lymph node invasive prostate cancer could be assessed based on the preoperative imaging studies, and these changes will be helpful for assessing the natural history of lymph node invasive prostate cancer. However, currently, there is only scanty data for the natural history of lymph node metastatic prostate cancer because most of the currently available data for these prostate cancers are from pathologically confirmed lymph node metastatic disease on surgical specimens obtained from radical prostatectomy with lymph node dissection. Based on the results from ECOG 388610 and 388611, patients with lymph node metastatic disease based on the results from lymphadenectomy without radical prostatectomy, who primarily underwent observation with delayed androgen deprivation therapy (ADT), showed a median survival of 11.3 years, which was significantly lower than patients who underwent immediate ADT (13.9 years). A median survival after radical prostatectomy reported to be about 12 years from retrospective long-term followed-up study. Although it is hard to conclude that any treatment is superior than the others, any single treatment is not thought to be satisfactory. In this regard, currently, the role of multidisciplinary treatment in patients with hormone-naïve metastatic prostate cancer is increasing, and, currently, increasing evidence has been published that radical prostatectomy and lymph node dissection performed as part of multidisciplinary treatment improve the oncological outcomes in patients with lymph node metastatic prostate cancer.

Prostate cancer most commonly spreads to the axial bone, and bone metastases eventually cause symptoms, such as bone pain, fracture, and decreased quality of life. Radionuclide bone scan is most widely used diagnostic examination to detect bone metastases in patients with prostate cancer. Although the specificity is not met for the expectance, the sensitivities of bone scan are between 62% and 89%, which thought to be acceptable. A median survival of patients with metastatic prostate cancer reported to be about 30–42 months [12]. A median survival of patients with metastatic disease after radical prostatectomy was about 6.6 years [13]. However, because some of these patients received a short course of hormonal therapy or salvage radiation therapy, interpretation of these results requires cautions. In these patients with metastasis, the burden of disease has been regarded as one of the most important predictors for oncological outcomes after treatment. The median survival of entire patients with bone metastasis who receive hormonal therapy reported to be about 30–35 months. However, in patients with solitary bone metastasis, the median survival was about 50 months. In this regard, the oligometastatic prostate cancer has been proposed based on the metastatic tumor burden. The oligometastasis was first defined by Hellman and Weichselbaum at 1995 as the state of metastases with five or less with untreated primary tumor. Recent advances in radiologic imaging have led to an increase in the diagnosis of oligometastatic prostate cancer. Due to the low specificity of bone scan, several imaging strategies, including single-photon emission computerized tomography (SPECT), PET, and skeletal MRI, for detecting bone metastasis have emerged, and some of these showed reliable results. The natural history of patients diagnosed as having oligometastatic prostate cancer on advanced imaging studies needs to be assessed in the future.

1.4.3 Castration-Resistant Prostate Cancer

Castration-resistant prostate cancer is defined in the European Association of Urology (EAU)—European Society for Radiotherapy and Oncology (ESTRO)—International Society of Geriatric Oncology (SIOG) guidelines as follows: castrate serum testosterone level <50 ng/mL or 1.7 nmol/L plus one of following (1) biochemical progression (three consecutive rises of PSA, 1 week apart, resulting in two 50% increases over the nadir, with PSA > 2 ng/mL (2) radiologic progression (the appearance of new lesions: either two or more new bone lesions on bone scan or enlargement of a soft tissue lesion using Response Evaluation Criteria in Solid Tumors (RECIST) criteria. In American Urological Association (AUA) guidelines, castration-resistant prostate cancer is defined as prostate cancer with a rising PSA level and/or radiographic evidence of prostate cancer progression despite medical or surgical castration.

Castration-resistant prostate cancer could be further divided according to the presence of metastasis (nonmetastatic vs. metastatic castration-resistant prostate cancer). Currently, nonmetastatic castration-resistant prostate cancer is now seen in increasing proportions in the clinic because an increasing number of patients now begin hormonal treatment at very early stages. However, at present, there is no consensus regarding the most appropriate management for patients with nonmetastatic castration-resistant prostate cancer, and, moreover, the natural history of these patients remained to be assessed. In the current clinical guidelines, clinical trial is suggested as the most preferred treatment for these patients. In addition, more data are needed to characterize the natural history of nonmetastatic castration-resistant prostate cancer, and further study in these fields is needed.

Metastatic castration-resistant prostate cancer most commonly involves the bone and resulted in bone pain and pathologic fracture, similar to hormone-naïve metastatic prostate cancer. Most of the treatments for castration-resistant prostate cancer are performed on these patients. Although there have been only a few studies reporting the natural history of castration-resistant prostate cancer, survival in these patients is progressively improving with development of therapeutic drugs. A median survival in patients with castration-resistant prostate cancer after docetaxel was approximately 18.9 months, but a median survival after using enzalutamide and abiraterone acetate was 18.4 and 15.8 months in postchemotherapy setting and 35.3 and 34.7 months in prechemotherapy setting, respectively, although these data cannot be directly compared. Recently, more drugs and an increasing number of novel therapeutic targets for the treatment of castration-resistant prostate cancer have been under development than ever before, and some of currently developing drugs are likely to further expand our therapeutic arsenal in the near future. In addition, the site of metastases confers a prognostic impact in patients with prostate cancer. Although visceral metastasis in patients with prostate cancer reported to be relatively uncommon, it has been reported to be associated with poor survival. A median survival from diagnosis of visceral metastasis in men with castration-resistant prostate cancer was about 7 months [14]. Among visceral metastases, a median survival in patients with liver metastases is about 10 months and lung metastasis is about 14.4 months although patients with bone metastasis is about 15.7–19.0 months [15]. There are several prognostic biomarkers for castration-resistant prostate cancer including age, Gleason score, PSA, PSA kinetics, performance status, and pain. In addition, laboratory findings, including hemoglobin level, alkaline phosphatase, lactate dehydrogenase, and albumin, are also regarded as a prognostic factor for castration-resistant prostate cancer. Recently, novel methods for predicting the prognosis of castration-resistant prostate cancer, including the number of circulating tumor cells, have been proposed.

1.5 Summary

- Traditionally, high-risk prostate cancer is defined as follows: biopsy Gleason score 8–10, PSA level at diagnosis greater than 20 ng/mL, and clinical stage T2c/T3 or greater.

- However, the definition of high-risk prostate cancer is evolving, and a more individualized risk stratification model is expected to be presented in near future.
- There have been several factors related to the presence of high-risk prostate cancer although most of these need to be further validated.
- The natural history of high-risk prostate cancer is diverse because high-risk prostate cancer is consisted of wide variety of disease, in terms of the staging and the response to the hormonal treatment.
- Nonetheless, most high-risk prostate cancer has a detrimental effect on survival, and multidisciplinary treatment should be considered.

References

1. Torre LA, Bray F, Siegel RL, Ferlay J, Lortet-Tieulent J, Jemal A. Global cancer statistics, 2012. CA Cancer J Clin. 2015;65(2):87–108.
2. Hall MD, Schultheiss TE, Farino G, Wong JY. Increase in higher risk prostate cancer cases following new screening recommendation by the US Preventive Services Task Force (USPSTF). Am Soc Clin Oncol. 2015;33:143.
3. Weiner A, Matulewicz R, Eggener S, Schaeffer E. Increasing incidence of metastatic prostate cancer in the United States (2004–2013). Prostate Cancer Prostatic Dis. 2016;19(4):395.
4. Boorjian SA, Karnes RJ, Rangel LJ, Bergstralh EJ, Blute ML. Mayo Clinic validation of the D'amico risk group classification for predicting survival following radical prostatectomy. J Urol. 2008;179(4):1354–60. discussion 60-1
5. Mohler JL, Armstrong AJ, Bahnson RR, D'Amico AV, Davis BJ, Eastham JA, et al. Prostate cancer, version 1.2016. J Natl Compr Cancer Netw. 2016;14(1):19–30.
6. Epstein JI, Egevad L, Amin MB, Delahunt B, Srigley JR, Humphrey PA. The 2014 International Society of Urological Pathology (ISUP) consensus conference on gleason grading of prostatic carcinoma: definition of grading patterns and proposal for a new grading system. Am J Surg Pathol. 2016;40(2):244–52.
7. Ankerst DP, Hoefler J, Bock S, Goodman PJ, Vickers A, Hernandez J, et al. Prostate cancer prevention trial risk calculator 2.0 for the prediction of low- versus high-grade prostate cancer. Urology. 2014;83(6):1362–8.
8. Preston MA, Wilson KM, Markt SC, Ge R, Morash C, Stampfer MJ, et al. 5α-Reductase inhibitors and risk of high-grade or lethal prostate cancer. JAMA Intern Med. 2014;174(8):1301–7.
9. Popiolek M, Rider JR, Andrén O, Andersson S-O, Holmberg L, Adami H-O, et al. Natural history of early, localized prostate cancer: a final report from three decades of follow-up. Eur Urol. 2013;63(3):428–35.
10. Albertsen PC, Hanley JA, Fine J. 20-year outcomes following conservative management of clinically localized prostate cancer. JAMA. 2005;293(17):2095–101.
11. van den Ouden D, Schroder FH. Management of locally advanced prostate cancer. 1. Staging, natural history, and results of radical surgery. World J Urol. 2000;18(3):194–203.
12. James ND, Spears MR, Clarke NW, Dearnaley DP, De Bono JS, Gale J, et al. Survival with newly diagnosed metastatic prostate cancer in the "Docetaxel Era": data from 917 patients in the control arm of the STAMPEDE trial (MRC PR08, CRUK/06/019). Eur Urol. 2015;67(6):1028–38.
13. Yossepowitch O, Bianco FJ Jr, Eggener SE, Eastham JA, Scher HI, Scardino PT. The natural history of noncastrate metastatic prostate cancer after radical prostatectomy. Eur Urol. 2007;51(4):940–7. discussion 7-8
14. Pezaro CJ, Omlin A, Lorente D, Nava Rodrigues D, Ferraldeschi R, Bianchini D, et al. Visceral disease in castration-resistant prostate cancer. Eur Urol. 2014;65(2) 270–3.
15. Pond GR, Sonpavde G, de Wit R, Eisenberger MA, Tannock IF Armstrong AJ. The prognostic importance of metastatic site in men with metastatic castration-resistant prostate cancer. Eur Urol. 2014;65(1):3–6.

Identifying the Best Candidate for Radical Prostatectomy in High-Risk Prostate Cancer

2

Jung Jun Kim and Sung Kyu Hong

2.1 Introduction

Radical prostatectomy (RP) has been regarded as one of the gold standard therapeutic option for localized or locally advanced prostate cancer patients. However, the surgery for localized low-risk prostate cancer may not be the standard anymore due to the concern of overtreatment recently. On the other hand, regarding the treatment of high-risk or locally advanced prostate cancer, the role of surgery started to extend their territory.

The optimal purpose or outcome of the RP is the complete removal of the malignant tissue, inside or outside of the prostate. Therefore, the surgery for $T_xN_0M_0$ should be the best, and the surgery for $T_xN_1M_0$ could be also considered with concomitant lymph node dissection. But, the preoperative nodal (N) staging based on conventional computed tomogram (CT), magnetic resonance imaging (MRI), or positron emission tomography (PET) has limitation of sensitivity and specificity, and the routine standard or extended pelvic lymph node dissection has their own limitation because extra pelvic lymph node should be missed during procedure. With current standard imaging protocol, preoperative clinical staging cannot precisely rule out nodal or metastatic disease. False-positive outcome of current imaging protocol also has another obstacle for precise classification of RP candidate. We should agree that many patients classified as high-risk preoperatively pathologically diagnosed as organ-confined cancer from RP specimen and could be cured by RP alone [1].

Anyway, patients with locally advanced, clinical nodal/metastatic disease, or high-grade/high-risk cancer have been demonstrated more possibility of pathological nodal disease consequently poor survival after RP historically [2, 3]. Therefore, clinical risk classification tool considering three prognostic parameters—PSA, Gleason score (GS), and clinical stage—has been classically utilized to estimate the suitability of surgical treatment of prostate cancer [4]. Nomograms [5, 6] and classification based on image-based biopsy information are one of the efforts to improve the predictive performance to classify proper surgical candidate [7].

The recent guideline of the European Association of Urology (EAU) recommends the best surgical candidate as <20 ng/mL, with a clinical stage ≤cT3a, and a biopsy GS ≤8. However, we cannot conclude that patients excluded from that criteria are not the candidate for surgery, because

J. J. Kim
Seoul National University Bundang Hospital, Seongnam, South Korea

S. K. Hong (✉)
Seoul National University Bundang Hospital, Seongnam, South Korea

Seoul National University, Seoul, South Korea
e-mail: skhong@snubh.org

C. S. Kim (ed.), *Management of Advanced Prostate Cancer*,
https://doi.org/10.1007/978-981-10-6943-7_2

some of those patients such as more advanced/poorly differentiated tumor could be beneficial after surgery [8]. Hypothetically, locally advanced disease or pelvic nodal disease could be surgically remove by conventional surgical technique including extend lymph node dissection [9, 10]. The rate of nodal disease of cT3 cases is between 11% and 41% [11, 12]. And the positive biopsy core is one of the parameter to predict nodal disease [13].

The nerve-sparing technique improves surgical complication profile including incontinence and erectile dysfunction. However, the nerve-sparing technique could induce the positive margin especially among T3 disease; the more precise preoperative clinical T staging is required for precision medicine. However, more surgical experience itself seems not only improve positive margin but also functional outcome [9].

2.2 RP for High-Grade Cancer

The GS of pathological specimen, which is high-grade disease, is related with nodal disease and worse survival outcome. However, there is no solid evidence supports survival benefit of radical prostatectomy for high-grade cancer, even if the cure rate after surgery only could less than not high-grade cancer. There could be discrepancy between the biopsy and pathological grade. Downgrade incidence is not negligible, and the biochemical progression-free survival (BPFS) could be increased after downgrading [14–17]. The outcome of this study suggests the possibility of downgrading up to one-third. And the exclusion of surgical option could be incorrect. Literatures also have been reported the decent oncological outcome of RP for high-grade cancer. Five-year biochemical recurrence-free survival was reported from 32% to 78%, and nodal disease was 6% to 20% [14, 17–22]. Manoharan et al. [15] recommended RP as a reasonable treatment option for high-risk cancer if T1/2, especially if PSA ≤20 ng/mL. The high grade is related to extracapsular extension of tumor. But if the high-grade cancer is confined at prostate, the patients tend to demonstrate better oncological prognosis [23]. In conclusion, high-grade patients do not necessarily have the poor prognosis after RP. This outcome indicates the importance of screening and early treatment before metastasis for high-grade disease.

The screening method to predict the organ-confined disease among high-grade cancer is important. More precise classification of organ-confined high-grade cancer could improve the surgical prognosis. Because organ-confined high-risk disease definitely induces better prognosis after RP than not organ-confined disease, [17–19] found higher 5- and 10-year estimated biochemical recurrence-free survival among men with organ-confined disease and negative.

2.3 RP for T3/4 N0 M0 Disease

Compare to classic RP series, recent RP series with modern technique demonstrates better surgical outcome for locally advanced disease consisting pT3a (extracapsular extension or bladder neck invasion), pT3 (seminal vesicle invasion), and pT4 (adjacent organ invasion).

A single-center retrospective study, which analyzed the cancer-free state of 842 cT3 patients disease demonstrated 85%, 73%, and 67% at 5, 10, and 15 years. The cancer-specific survival (CSS) rates were 95%, 90%, and 79%, respectively. The meantime for adjuvant therapy after surgery was similar between cT2 and cT3 disease (4.3 vs. 4.0 years). Another RP series of 235 patients (10.3%) with unilateral cT3a [24] demonstrated 10-year CSS, and overall survival (OS) rates were 91.6% and 77.0%, respectively.

The OS and CSS rates at 10 years reported by Joniau et al. analyzing the 51 patients with cT3b–T4 were 72.5% and 70.7%, respectively. The positive margin rate was up to 62.7% [25]. Another long-term period more than 20 years of follow-up study analyzed the CSS rates, and the local recurrence-free of 843 cT3 patients reported 81% and 76%, respectively [26].

The US National Cancer Institute's Surveillance, Epidemiology, and End Results (SEER) database analysis is one of the largest studies that demonstrated the oncological prognosis of cT4 disease. From the analysis of 1093 cT4 patients, both of the relative and observed survival of RP patients were better than non-RP patients, such as hormone therapy (alone or with radiotherapy) [27]. Another population-based study, which analyzed 3000 nonmetastatic cT3 or cT4 patients demonstrated the ratio of RP has been increased over time, started exceeding 10% at 2005. The outcome of these population-based studies suggests that the role of RP among cT3 or cT4 disease has been extended from traditional prostate cancer series to contemporary series.

The studies described comparable oncological outcome between RP alone and radiotherapy, and the less need for long-term adjuvant ADT among RP than radiotherapy supports the benefit of RP than other treatment strategy without RP [28, 29].

In summary, these outcomes suggest that RP (with or without adjuvant or salvage treatment when needed) could control locally advanced cancer and consequently achieved long-term survival.

2.4 RP for Node-Positive Disease

Standard or extended pelvic lymph node dissection with RP should be the best option for localized prostate cancer with nodal disease within pelvic lymph node. However, until now, to our best knowledge, there is no standard preoperative evaluation tool to detect the location of lymph node with both of high sensitivity and specificity. The routine CT scan has low sensitivity because it could miss lymph node less than 1 cm, the diagnostic performance of PET-CT is variable according to the ligand, and the protocol or guideline is not standardized yet.

Even though, we have to agree that some portion of nodal disease, such as patients with limited nodal tumor burden could be cured by RP with pelvic lymph node dissection, the expected survival could be increased after RP [30]. However, we should also agree that there is no reliable evidence exists to support the partial lymph node removal could increase oncological outcome. Therefore, the issue should be how to properly select the patients could have more chance to be cured.

Few retrospective studies demonstrated the decent oncological prognosis of RP group among clinical or pathological nodal disease [31, 32]. Moschini et al. also recently reported clinical nodal disease did not significantly worsen cancer-specific survival according to 17 years of median follow-up [33]. However, most of them do not have properly controlled non-RP comparison group. One study demonstrated the prognosis, most of them (~90%) were treated adjuvant hormonal therapy, and the 10-year CSS and BCR for pathological nodal disease were 85.8% and 56%, respectively [32].

The data from the Munich cancer registry (1988–2007) is interesting [34]. Some of the patients intraoperatively decided continue or abandon RP after lymph node dissection. They compared oncological prognosis of 456 abandoned RP patients with 957 RP patients pathologically nodal positive. The 10-year overall survival of RP group was 64% but 28% among abandoned RP group. RP was strong independent parameter predicting survival with HR 2.04 (95% confidence interval; 1.59–2.63). Another study which also highlights the beneficial impact of RP on survival is the systematic review investigating whether prostate local treatment in nodal disease improves the efficacy of ADT. The survival benefit was significant with HR of OS 0.69 (95% CI: 0.61–0.79) [35]. These data support the role of RP as multimodality therapeutic strategy. However, there is paucity of data RP alone cure or improve the oncological prognosis of nodal disease. Because the long-term survival with RP alone is limited for nodal disease, data vary between 10% and 14% [36]. To figure out the role of RP alone for nodal disease, the oncological outcome of contemporary RP technique should be analyzed in the future. Recent technical advance for extended lymph node dissection probably improves the oncological prognosis. Even if there is not enough evidence to support RP alone, the role as a multimodality therapeutic option is more clear and expectable currently [30].

2.5 The Efficacy of RP over External Beam Radiation Therapy (EBRT) with or Without ADT (Androgen Deprivation Therapy)

As the classic scheme of locally advanced prostate or nodal prostate cancer avoids surgery, the data supporting RP is relatively limited than the one supporting EBRT. According to the deviation of the previous literatures, it is natural that most of the guideline focuses on EBRT rather than RP.

Regardless of the therapeutic efficacy of the surgery, the benefit of surgery over EBRT should start with more precise staging. The surgical specimen allows pathological staging, more accurate than clinical staging. Better risk assessment could induce proper adjuvant treatment at proper time point.

Regarding the therapeutic efficacy, oncological prognosis of RP with high-risk prostate cancer has been comparable with EBRT outcomes [37–39]. The other few series demonstrated diverse outcome, but the oncological prognosis was similar. Recent study demonstrated slightly increased risk of distant metastasis among EBRT than RP cohort [40]. Another retrospective study by Aizer et al. [41] reported that the efficacy of EBRT with ADT for high-risk disease is better than RP with respect to BFS. Ellis et al. [42] reported the worse outcome of RP among GS 5 dominant cancers, but it seems improper to conclude that RP is not proper therapeutic option for GS 5 because the outcome is far worse than the outcome of other contemporary database, such as Kattan nomogram.

The other majority of reports demonstrated the superiority of RP over EBRT with respect to OS and/or CSS [43–47]. However, all of them are retrospective, not only poorly controlled but also biased. The rate of adjuvant of salvage treatment could not be controlled when the outcome is compared between RP and RT (radiation therapy). Furthermore, comorbidities influencing the decision of the surgical methodology could not be controlled. Another critical bias is staging. The pathological staging is only possible for RP patients, so the precise stage matching is not even possible. The discrepancy of clinical and pathological staging among high-risk cancer was well described in large RP series ($n = 1366$) [48]. The upstaging and downstaging were 29% and 11% among clinical high-risk cancers.

The profile of adjuvant or salvage treatment is different between RP and EBRT. Among RP group, the salvage treatment such as RP or ADT was 76%, higher than 43% of RP [40]. The median time to salvage was much shorter for the RP patients as well (13 month vs. 69 month). Another studies reported the rate of adjuvant treatment after RP for high-risk prostate from 41% to 48% [38, 48].

In summary, the RP is a considerable option for high-risk cancers classically indicating EBRT in terms of efficacy. However, there is not well-designed comparative study that draws the efficacy superiority of one methodology for high-risk prostate cancer developed yet.

2.6 Safety of RP Compare to EBRT (with or Without ADT)

The studies published based on PROSTQA database demonstrated the safety of RP and RT (EBRT/Brachytherapy) in detail. The database prospectively developed and evaluated quality-of-life study of both modality of pain with 5-year follow-up [49–51]. RP is definitely related with better sexual function and continence. And the additional ADT after primary treatment worsen these functional outcomes. The most significant finding was that the rate of ADT was higher than RT group than RP group, so the functional outcome is consequently worse in ADT group. The negative influence of ADT on functional outcome is not surprising considering the role of testosterone on male patient. And even short-term neoadjuvant ADT also worsen sexual and vitality/hormonal quality of life [52].

Another concern of ADT is cardiovascular morbidities. Although one of the recent meta-analysis found not significant increase of cardiovascular deaths among ADT patients than normal control [53], a joint consensus meetings stated that ADT is associated with excessive cardiovascular event, particularly patients with preexisting cardiovascular comorbidities [54]. The cardiovascular risk elevation seems to be due to obesity, dyslipidemia, and decreased insulin sensitivity.

RP for cancer control also improved the urinary functional symptoms such as obstructive or irrigative urinary symptom, which was not significant among RT group. Besides, bowel dysfunction was more definite among RT group than RP. Among dose-escalated EBRT group, the dysfunction was more significant, up to 11% of moderate/significant bowel problem patients [55]. Regarding the toxicity of primary cancer control therapeutic option, a comparative toxicity study of RT vs. RP has recently published, comparable in 15-year toxicity. In the older age, more comorbidities and higher grade should be considered for interpretation of the outcome [56].

2.7 RP in Elderly Patients

Even if the general efficacy and safety of RP is better than other therapeutic options, the surgical decision-making could be prudential and differ according to patients' characteristics, especially for patients with severe morbidity or relative short life expectancy. Old age generally represents relatively short life expectancy and higher surgical morbidities. However, the 10-year competing mortality rate after RP with two or higher Charlson comorbidity score and older than 65 years old was reported down to 26% (95% CI 17–35) [57]. These outcomes suggest that the RP is relatively safe surgical option for elderly patients. Especially patients with higher oncological risk factor, the delay of surgery may not justified because of old age or medical comorbidities [58]. The benefit and risk of surgery should be estimated and calculated for each patient; the individual decision-making is always required. The benefit of surgery should be the priority decision key factor for urooncologist.

However, to our best knowledge, we do not have enough clinical evidence or decision-making tools whether RP should be preferred or not especially when the patient is both oncological high-risk and old age. The curative effect and predicted morbidity should be compared for each patient. The surgery should more preferred high oncological risk elderly than low oncological risk elderly. For low-risk elderly, nonsurgical treatment could be recommended.

2.8 Recent Efforts for Identifying the Better Candidate for RP Among Patients with High-Risk Prostate Cancer

The most general and classic rule to choose proper candidate for RP should be to consider RP as first-line treatment with localized prostate cancer for patients of more than 10-year life expectancy [8]. However, the potential benefit of RP in high-risk disease patients is less than non-high-risk patients and sometimes controversial, as we described [38, 43, 59–61]. Historically, the very purpose of RP is curative, less recommended for individuals with less possibility of cure. Otherwise, RT or ADT has been recommended for high-risk patients [62]. This is because the best virtue of radical surgery is the whole eradication of cancer cells form patient's body and consequently complete cure.

However, several recent literatures reported the role of RP for high-risk patients and could induce better oncological prognosis, even if sometimes adjuvant modalities could be required [1, 14, 28, 38, 43, 59, 63–65]. Unfortunately, we do not have enough information to the exact reason why the survival benefit induced at this time point. Of course, some (22–63%) of the patients are clinically misclassified preoperatively as high-risk definition [1, 14, 64, 65]. And the extraprostatic local invasion and pelvic nodal disease could be cured by improved surgical technique. However, we could not conclude that the survival benefit is significant and is even significant when partial resection of tumor burden is performed because all evidences are just circumferential. Therefore, the guideline to select proper indication for RP among high-risk cancer patients cannot but be unavailable currently [8, 66].

Even though, most of urooncologist should agree that if the metastatic focus including lymph node could be detected with high sensitivity and specificity, the surgical indication would be more widen up to nodal or metastatic disease. Recently, series of nuclear medicine imaging methodology are suggested for more accurate clinical imaging staging for prostate cancer patients, which demonstrates higher sensitivity and specificity than conventional staging tools. The prostate-specific membrane antigen (PSMA) is one of the specific ligand bind poorly differentiated or metastatic prostate cancer cell, which could bind also radioisotope for visualization and/or eradication of cancer cell. Ga-PSMA, F-PSMA, and Lu-PSMA are one of the small molecules binded to isotope [67–71]. PET-CT scan combined to these novel isotopes enables the detection of nodal disease even before surgery with high sensitivity and specificity, consequently inducing better clinical staging.

The effort to develop clinical calculator/nomogram to predict the specimen-confined cancer among high-risk patients is also ongoing [48]. This literature also analyzed the positive impact of specimen-confined disease on the cancer-specific mortality. However, the nomogram is not externally validated, and the performance is limited, and the pathological staged organ-confined disease may not be precise especially when the extrapelvic node exists. No preoperative tool to predict the survival benefit of RP directly in high-risk prostate cancer has been published.

2.9 Summary

Although subject to biases, several retrospective studies support the role of surgery and potential benefit versus radiation in patients with high-risk prostate cancer. Matched cohort and multivariable analyses attempting to control for biases have demonstrated associations with RP and biochemical recurrence-free, overall, and prostate cancer-specific survival.

As more survival is expected for organ-confined, non-nodal disease by radical surgery, the best way to select better candidate of RP is to predict non-nodal, nonmetastatic organ-confined diseases and resect the possibly metastatic nodes if it exists. Novel preoperative imaging modalities such as PSMA CT/PET scan would provide more precise clinical N or M staging and better selection of surgical candidate. And nomograms and calculators to evaluate the survival benefit of each individual started to develop and would help with the decision of the radical surgery compare with other therapeutic options.

References

1. Yossepowitch O, Eggener SE, Bianco FJ, Carver BS, Serio A, Scardino PT, et al. Radical prostatectomy for clinically localized, high risk prostate cancer: critical analysis of risk assessment methods. J Urol. 2007;178(2):493–9.
2. Khan MA, Mangold LA, Epstein JI, Boitnott JK, Walsh PC, Partin AW. Impact of surgical delay on long-term cancer control for clinically localized prostate cancer. J Urol. 2004;172(5):1835–9.
3. Gerber G, Thisted R, Chodak G, Schroder F, Frohmuller H, Scardino P, et al. Results of radical prostatectomy in men with locally advanced prostate cancer: multi-institutional pooled analysis. Eur Urol. 1997;32(4):385–90.
4. Joniau S, Briganti A, Gontero P, Gandaglia G, Tosco L, Fieuws S, et al. Stratification of high-risk prostate cancer into prognostic categories: a European multi-institutional study. Eur Urol. 2015;67(1):157–64.
5. Gallina A, Chun FK-H, Briganti A, Shariat SF, Montorsi F, Salonia A, et al. Development and split-sample validation of a nomogram predicting the probability of seminal vesicle invasion at radical prostatectomy. Eur Urol. 2007;52(1):98–105.
6. Joniau S, Hsu C-Y, Lerut E, Van Baelen A, Haustermans K, Roskams T, et al. A pretreatment table for the prediction of final histopathology after radical prostatectomy in clinical unilateral T3a prostate cancer. Eur Urol. 2007;51(2):388–96.
7. Van Poppel H, Ameye F, Oyen R, Van De Voorde W, Baert L. Accuracy of combined computerized tomography and fine needle aspiration cytology in lymph node staging of localized prostatic carcinoma. J Urol. 1994;151(5):1310–4.
8. Mottet N, Bellmunt J, Bolla M, Briers E, Cumberbatch MG, De Santis M, et al. EAU-ESTRO-SIOG guidelines on prostate cancer. Part 1: screening, diagnosis, and local treatment with curative intent. Eur Urol. 2017;71(4):618–29.
9. Van Poppel H, Vekemans K, Da Pozzo L, Bono A, Kliment J, Montironi R, et al. Radical prostatectomy for locally advanced prostate cancer: results of a feasibility study (EORTC 30001). Eur J Cancer. 2006;42(8):1062–7.
10. Van Poppel H. Surgery for clinical T3 prostate cancer. Eur Urol Suppl. 2005;4(4):12–4.
11. Van Poppel H, Goethuys H, Callewaert P, Vanuytsel L, Van de Voorde W, Baert L. Radical prostatectomy can provide a cure for well-selected clinical stage T3 prostate cancer. Eur Urol. 2000;38(4):372–9.
12. Ward JF, Slezak JM, Blute ML, Bergstralh EJ, Zincke H. Radical prostatectomy for clinically advanced (cT3) prostate cancer since the advent of prostate-specific antigen testing: 15-year outcome. BJU Int. 2005;95(6):751–6.
13. Briganti A, Karakiewicz PI, Chun FK-H, Gallina A, Salonia A, Zanni G, et al. Percentage of positive biopsy cores can improve the ability to predict lymph

node invasion in patients undergoing radical prostatectomy and extended pelvic lymph node dissection. Eur Urol. 2007;51(6):1573–81.
14. Donohue JF, Bianco FJ, Kuroiwa K, Vickers AJ, Wheeler TM, Scardino PT, et al. Poorly differentiated prostate cancer treated with radical prostatectomy: long-term outcome and incidence of pathological downgrading. J Urol. 2006;176(3):991–5.
15. Manoharan M, Bird V, Kim S, Civantos F, Soloway M. Outcome after radical prostatectomy with a pretreatment prostate biopsy Gleason score of≥8. BJU Int. 2003;92(6):539–44.
16. Grossfeld GD, Latini DM, Lubeck DP, Mehta SS, Carroll PR. Predicting recurrence after radical prostatectomy for patients with high risk prostate cancer. J Urol. 2003;169(1):157–63.
17. Bastian PJ, Gonzalgo ML, Aronson WJ, Terris MK, Kane CJ, Amling CL, et al. Clinical and pathologic outcome after radical prostatectomy for prostate cancer patients with a preoperative Gleason sum of 8 to 10. Cancer. 2006;107(6):1265–72.
18. Mian BM, Troncoso P, Okihara K, Bhadkamkar V, Johnston D, Reyes AO, et al. Outcome of patients with Gleason score 8 or higher prostate cancer following radical prostatectomy alone. J Urol. 2002;167(4):1675–80.
19. Lau WK, Bergstralh EJ, Blute ML, Slezak JM, Zincke H. Radical prostatectomy for pathological Gleason 8 or greater prostate cancer: influence of concomitant pathological variables. J Urol. 2002;167(1):117–22.
20. Thompson IM. Survival after radical retropubic prostatectomy of men and clinically localized high grade carcinoma of the prostate. Cancer. 1996;78(1):181.
21. Tefilli MV, Gheiler EL, Tiguert R, Banerjee M, Sakr W, Grignon D, et al. Role of radical prostatectomy in patients with prostate cancer of high Gleason score. Prostate. 1999;39(1):60–6.
22. Serni S, Masieri L, Minervini A, Lapini A, Nesi G, Carini M. Cancer progression after anterograde radical prostatectomy for pathologic Gleason score 8 to 10 and influence of concomitant variables. Urology. 2006;67(2):373–8.
23. Ohori M, Goad JR, Wheeler TM, Eastham JA, Thompson TC, Scardino PT. Can radical prostatectomy alter the progression of poorly differentiated prostate cancer? J Urol. 1994;152(5):1843–9.
24. Hsu C-Y, Joniau S, Oyen R, Roskams T, Van Poppel H. Outcome of surgery for clinical unilateral T3a prostate cancer: a single-institution experience. Eur Urol. 2007;51(1):121–9.
25. Joniau S, Hsu C-Y, Gontero P, Spahn M, Van Poppel H. Radical prostatectomy in very high-risk localized prostate cancer: long-term outcomes and outcome predictors. Scand J Urol Nephrol. 2012;46(3):164–71.
26. Mitchell CR, Boorjian SA, Umbreit EC, Rangel LJ, Carlson RE, Karnes RJ. 20-Year survival after radical prostatectomy as initial treatment for cT3 prostate cancer. BJU Int. 2012;110(11):1709–13.
27. Johnstone PA, Ward KC, Goodman M, Assikis V, Petros JA. Radical prostatectomy for clinical T4 prostate cancer. Cancer. 2006;106(12):2603–9.
28. Spahn M, Joniau S, Gontero P, Fieuws S, Marchioro G, Tombal B, et al. Outcome predictors of radical prostatectomy in patients with prostate-specific antigen greater than 20 ng/ml: a European multi-institutional study of 712 patients. Eur Urol. 2010;58(1):1–7.
29. Edge SB, Compton CC. The American Joint Committee on Cancer: the 7th edition of the AJCC cancer staging manual and the future of TNM. Ann Surg Oncol. 2010;17(6):1471–4.
30. Gakis G, Boorjian SA, Briganti A, Joniau S, Karazanashvili G, Karnes RJ, et al. The role of radical prostatectomy and lymph node dissection in lymph node–positive prostate cancer: a systematic review of the literature. Eur Urol. 2014;66(2):191–9.
31. Frohmüller H, Theiss M, Manseck A, Wirth M. Survival and quality of life of patients with stage D1 (T1-3 pN1-2 MO) prostate cancer. Eur Urol. 1995;27:202–6.
32. Boorjian SA, Thompson RH, Siddiqui S, Bagniewski S, Bergstralh EJ, Karnes RJ, et al. Long-term outcome after radical prostatectomy for patients with lymph node positive prostate cancer in the prostate specific antigen era. J Urol. 2007;178(3):864–71.
33. Moschini M, Briganti A, Murphy CR, Bianchi M, Gandaglia G, Montorsi F, et al. Outcomes for patients with clinical lymphadenopathy treated with radical prostatectomy. Eur Urol. 2016;69(2):193–6.
34. Engel J, Bastian PJ, Baur H, Beer V, Chaussy C, Gschwend JE, et al. Survival benefit of radical prostatectomy in lymph node–positive patients with prostate cancer. Eur Urol. 2010;57(5):754–61.
35. Verhagen PC, Schröder FH, Collette L, Bangma CH. Does local treatment of the prostate in advanced and/or lymph node metastatic disease improve efficacy of androgen-deprivation therapy? A systematic review. Eur Urol. 2010;58(2):261–9.
36. Bader P, Burkhard FC, Markwalder R, Studer UE. Disease progression and survival of patients with positive lymph nodes after radical prostatectomy. Is there a chance of cure? J Urol. 2003;169(3):849–54.
37. Kupelian PA, Potters L, Khuntia D, Ciezki JP, Reddy CA, Reuther AM, et al. Radical prostatectomy, external beam radiotherapy<72 Gy, external beam radiotherapy ≥72 Gy, permanent seed implantation, or combined seeds/external beam radiotherapy for stage T1–T2 prostate cancer. Int J Radiat Oncol Biol Phys. 2004;58(1):25–33.
38. Boorjian SA, Karnes RJ, Viterbo R, Rangel LJ, Bergstralh EJ, Horwitz EM, et al. Long-term survival after radical prostatectomy versus external-beam radiotherapy for patients with high-risk prostate cancer. Cancer. 2011;117(13):2883–91.
39. Westover K, Chen MH, Moul J, Robertson C, Polascik T, Dosoretz D, et al. Radical prostatectomy vs radiation therapy and androgen-suppression therapy in high-risk prostate cancer. BJU Int. 2012;110(8):1116–21.

40. Zelefsky MJ, Eastham JA, Cronin AM, Fuks Z, Zhang Z, Yamada Y, et al. Metastasis after radical prostatectomy or external beam radiotherapy for patients with clinically localized prostate cancer: a comparison of clinical cohorts adjusted for case mix. J Clin Oncol. 2010;28(9):1508–13.
41. Aizer AA, James BY, Colberg JW, McKeon AM, Decker RH, Peschel RE. Radical prostatectomy vs. intensity-modulated radiation therapy in the management of localized prostate adenocarcinoma. Radiother Oncol. 2009;93(2):185–91.
42. Ellis CL, Partin AW, Han M, Epstein JI. Adenocarcinoma of the prostate with Gleason score 9-10 on core biopsy: correlation with findings at radical prostatectomy and prognosis. J Urol. 2013;190(6):2068–73.
43. Cooperberg MR, Vickers AJ, Broering JM, Carroll PR. Comparative risk-adjusted mortality outcomes after primary surgery, radiotherapy, or androgen-deprivation therapy for localized prostate cancer. Cancer. 2010;116(22):5226–34.
44. Hoffman RM, Koyama T, Fan K-H, Albertsen PC, Barry MJ, Goodman M, et al. Mortality after radical prostatectomy or external beam radiotherapy for localized prostate cancer. J Natl Cancer Inst. 2013;105(10):711–8.
45. Kibel AS, Ciezki JP, Klein EA, Reddy CA, Lubahn JD, Haslag-Minoff J, et al. Survival among men with clinically localized prostate cancer treated with radical prostatectomy or radiation therapy in the prostate specific antigen era. J Urol. 2012;187(4):1259–65.
46. Nepple KG, Stephenson AJ, Kallogjeri D, Michalski J, Grubb RL, Strope SA, et al. Mortality after prostate cancer treatment with radical prostatectomy, external-beam radiation therapy, or brachytherapy in men without comorbidity. Eur Urol. 2013;64(3):372–8.
47. Sooriakumaran P, Nyberg T, Akre O, Haendler L, Heus I, Olsson M, et al. Comparative effectiveness of radical prostatectomy and radiotherapy in prostate cancer: observational study of mortality outcomes. BMJ. 2014;348:g1502.
48. Briganti A, Joniau S, Gontero P, Abdollah F, Passoni NM, Tombal B, et al. Identifying the best candidate for radical prostatectomy among patients with high-risk prostate cancer. Eur Urol. 2012;61(3):584–92.
49. Pardo Y, Guedea F, Aguiló F, Fernández P, Macías V, Mariño A, et al. Quality-of-life impact of primary treatments for localized prostate cancer in patients without hormonal treatment. J Clin Oncol. 2010;28(31):4687–96.
50. Sanda MG, Dunn RL, Michalski J, Sandler HM, Northouse L, Hembroff L, et al. Quality of life and satisfaction with outcome among prostate-cancer survivors. N Engl J Med. 2008;358(12):1250–61.
51. Ferrer M, Guedea F, Suárez JF, de Paula B, Macías V, Mariño A, et al. Quality of life impact of treatments for localized prostate cancer: Cohort study with a 5year follow-up. Radiother Oncol. 2013;108(2):306–13.
52. Gay HA, Michalski JM, Hamstra DA, Wei JT, Dunn RL, Klein EA, et al. Neoadjuvant androgen deprivation therapy leads to immediate impairment of vitality/hormonal and sexual quality of life: results of a multicenter prospective study. Urology. 2013;82(6):1363–9.
53. Nguyen PL, Je Y, Schutz FA, Hoffman KE, Hu JC, Parekh A, et al. Association of androgen deprivation therapy with cardiovascular death in patients with prostate cancer: a meta-analysis of randomized trials. JAMA. 2011;306(21):2359–66.
54. Levine GN, D'amico AV, Berger P, Clark PE, Eckel RH, Keating NL, et al. Androgen-deprivation therapy in prostate cancer and cardiovascular risk: a science advisory from the American Heart Association, American Cancer Society, and American Urological Association: endorsed by the American Society for Radiation Oncology. CA Cancer J Clin. 2010;60(3):194–201.
55. Hamstra DA, Conlon AS, Daignault S, Dunn RL, Sandler HM, Hembroff AL, et al. Multi-institutional prospective evaluation of bowel quality of life after prostate external beam radiation therapy identifies patient and treatment factors associated with patient-reported outcomes: the PROSTQA experience. Int J Radiat Oncol Biol Phys. 2013;86(3):546–53.
56. Resnick MJ, Koyama T, Fan K-H, Albertsen PC, Goodman M, Hamilton AS, et al. Long-term functional outcomes after treatment for localized prostate cancer. N Engl J Med. 2013;368(5):436–45.
57. Froehner M, Koch R, Litz RJ, Hakenberg OW, Wirth MP. Which patients are at the highest risk of dying from competing causes ≤0 years after radical prostatectomy? BJU Int. 2012;110(2):206–10.
58. Albertsen PC, Moore DF, Shih W, Lin Y, Li H, Lu-Yao GL. Impact of comorbidity on survival among men with localized prostate cancer. J Clin Oncol. 2011;29(10):1335–41.
59. Abdollah F, Sun M, Thuret R, Jeldres C, Tian Z, Briganti A, et al. A competing-risks analysis of survival after alternative treatment modalities for prostate cancer patients: 1988–2006. Eur Urol. 2011;59(1):88–95.
60. Eastham JA, Evans CP, Zietman A. What is the optimal management of high risk, clinically localized prostate cancer? Urol Oncol. 2010;28:557–67. Elsevier.
61. Yossepowitch O, Eastham JA. Role of radical prostatectomy in the treatment of high-risk prostate cancer. Curr Prostate Rep. 2008;6(3):107–14.
62. Hamilton AS, Albertsen PC, Johnson TK, Hoffman R, Morrell D, Deapen D, et al. Trends in the treatment of localized prostate cancer using supplemented cancer registry data. BJU Int. 2011;107(4):576–84.
63. Miocinovic R, Berglund RK, Stephenson AJ, Jones JS, Fergany A, Kaouk J, et al. Avoiding androgen deprivation therapy in men with high-risk prostate cancer: the role of radical prostatectomy as initial treatment. Urology. 2011;77(4):946–50.
64. Walz J, Joniau S, Chun FK, Isbarn H, Jeldres C, Yossepowitch O, et al. Pathological results and rates of treatment failure in high-risk prostate can-

cer patients after radical prostatectomy. BJU Int. 2011;107(5):765–70.
65. Loeb S, Schaeffer EM, Trock BJ, Epstein JI, Humphreys EB, Walsh PC. What are the outcomes of radical prostatectomy for high-risk prostate cancer? Urology. 2010;76(3):710–4.
66. Mohler JL, Armstrong AJ, Bahnson RR, D'Amico AV, Davis BJ, Eastham JA, et al. Prostate cancer, version 1.2016. J Natl Compr Canc Netw. 2016;14(1):19–30.
67. Öbek C, Doğanca T, Demirci E, Ocak M, Kural AR, Yıldırım A, et al. The accuracy of 68Ga-PSMA PET/CT in primary lymph node staging in high-risk prostate cancer. Eur J Nucl Med Mol Imaging. 2017;44:1–7.
68. Budäus L, Leyh-Bannurah S-R, Salomon G, Michl U, Heinzer H, Huland H, et al. Initial experience of 68 Ga-PSMA PET/CT imaging in high-risk prostate cancer patients prior to radical prostatectomy. Eur Urol. 2016;69(3):393–6.
69. Herlemann A, Wenter V, Kretschmer A, Thierfelder KM, Bartenstein P, Faber C, et al. 68 Ga-PSMA positron emission tomography/computed tomography provides accurate staging of lymph node regions prior to lymph node dissection in patients with prostate cancer. Eur Urol. 2016;70(4):553–7.
70. Maurer T, Gschwend JE, Rauscher I, Souvatzoglou M, Haller B, Weirich G, et al. Diagnostic efficacy of 68 gallium-PSMA positron emission tomography compared to conventional imaging for lymph node staging of 130 consecutive patients with intermediate to high risk prostate cancer. J Urol. 2016;195(5):1436–43.
71. Leeuwen PJ, Emmett L, Ho B, Delprado W, Ting F, Nguyen Q, et al. Prospective evaluation of 68Gallium-prostate-specific membrane antigen positron emission tomography/computed tomography for preoperative lymph node staging in prostate cancer. BJU Int. 2017;119(2):209–15.

Neoadjuvant Therapy Prior to Radical Prostatectomy

3

Se Young Choi and Choung Soo Kim

3.1 Introduction

The terminology "neoadjuvant" stemmed from Greek "neos" that means new or before and the Latin language "adjuvāre" that means help or aid. Neoadjuvant therapy is the application of systemic care before operation or radiotherapy. Neoadjuvant therapy has some benefits in several tumors such as the bladder, testis, breast, colon, and lung. Conceptually, neoadjuvant therapy may decrease the size of the tumor before surgery or eliminate concealed micrometastases. In cases of neoadjuvant therapy before radiation therapy, shrinkage of the tumor is able to localize the site of the target with optimal doses while decreasing radiation exposure to surrounding normal tissue.

The concept of neoadjuvant therapy was first reported in 1944, and before radical perineal prostatectomy, bilateral orchiectomy was performed [1]. After the 1970s, the invention of pharmacological medicine about controlling hormone helped to choose medical castration as an option instead of surgical orchiectomy. There is an early report about the use of estrogen and sequential radiotherapy in 1984 [2]. Although the study was a small size (n = 25), patients who treated with estrogens before radiotherapy had superior disease-free survival than radiation therapy alone (55% vs. 47%, respectively). Since then, there were many studies about radiotherapy combined with neoadjuvant therapy. RTOG8610 was the early phase III study that compared neoadjuvant androgen deprivation therapy (ADT) with external beam radiotherapy (EBRT) and EBRT alone in localized prostate cancer [3]. Patients in the neoadjuvant treatment group were treated with both goserelin 3.6 mg every 4 weeks and flutamide 250 mg for 2 months before EBRT. The neoadjuvant treatment group showed improvement in 10-year biochemical failure (65% vs. 80%, p < 0.001) and recurrence-free survival (11% vs. 3%, p < 0.001) than only EBRT group. D'Amico et al. performed another randomized controlled trial comparing radiation therapy alone to radiation therapy with ADT including 2 months of neoadjuvant therapy [4]. The patients included more than PSA 10 ng/mL, more than Gleason score 7, or more than T3a. The ADT plus radiation showed superior overall survival (88% vs. 78%, p = 0.04) and cancer-specific death (0 vs. 6 cases, p = 0.02). The European Organization for Research and Treatment of Cancer (EORTC) group performed randomized phase III study comparing EBRT alone and EBRT with ADT for 3 years including 1 month neoadjuvant therapy of cyproterone acetate (50 mg daily three times) [5]. The combined treatment reduces risk in 10-year disease-free

S. Y. Choi · C. S. Kim (✉)
Department of Urology, Asan Medical Center, University of Ulsan College of Medicine, Seoul, South Korea
e-mail: cskim@amc.seoul.kr

C. S. Kim (ed.), *Management of Advanced Prostate Cancer*,
https://doi.org/10.1007/978-981-10-6943-7_3

survival (hazard ratio 0.42, $p < 0.0001$) than radiation alone. The ADT plus EBRT showed better 10-year recurrence-free survival (22.7% vs. 47.7%, $p < 0.0001$) and overall survival (39.8% vs. 58.1%, $p = 0.0004$). In addition, there was no significant difference between two groups in cardiovascular mortalities. Like these reports, radiation therapies combined with ADT including neoadjuvant therapy have been established in locally advanced prostate cancer.

Contrastively, neoadjuvant therapy before radical prostatectomy has still studied the clinical and oncological outcomes. Several trials did not prove the improvement in progression-free and overall survival. Nevertheless, the interest about neoadjuvant therapy before an operation is increasing in advanced or oligometastatic prostate cancer as one method of multimodal therapy. Although the development of prostate-specific antigen (PSA) screening increased early detection of prostate cancer, there are still many patients who are diagnose as high-risk prostate cancer. At initial diagnosis, 17–31% patients have high-risk prostate cancer [6]. The rate of biochemical recurrence after radical prostatectomy for high-risk prostate cancer is about 55–70% [7]. Among them, 13% progresses to metastatic prostate cancer, and 6% died because of prostate cancer [8]. The ideal treatment guidelines for these high-risk prostate cancer patients have not yet been established [9], but standard cares about high-risk prostate cancer in international guidelines are suggested as EBRT with ADT or EBRT plus brachytherapy with/without ADT or radical prostatectomy with lymph node dissection. In spite of these treatments, 10-year overall mortality was about 30–40% in locally advanced high-risk prostate cancer. Therefore, neoadjuvant therapy has been considered as a possible way out for better survival. In this article, we focus recent studies about neoadjuvant therapies before radical prostatectomy in patients with localized prostate cancer.

3.2 Neoadjuvant Hormonal Therapy

Randomized controlled trials about neoadjuvant ADT were performed during two decades (Table 3.1). There were many different conditions of the tumor including clinical stage, used medicines, and primary end points. Then, usually the trials showed increased organ-confined disease and decreased positive surgical margins. However, until recent, oncological gain in biochemical recurrence or overall survival was not proved.

For the first time at Memorial Sloan-Kettering Center (MSKCC), Fair et al. reported biochemical recurrence after surgery [10]. Fifty-two (70%) patients who received neoadjuvant therapy and 39 (59%) patients of the only prostatectomy had organ-confined and margin negative disease ($p = 0.17$), but the neoadjuvant group (19%) had lower positive margin rate than only prostatectomy group (37%) ($p = 0.023$). Their median follow-up duration was 35 months. The neoadjuvant hormonal therapy did not make significant differences in biochemical recurrence ($p = 0.73$). They suggested that neoadjuvant therapy could reduce positive surgical margin, and further follow-up was required to confirm the survival gain.

Overall survival was firstly evaluated by Schulman and colleagues [11]. This trial researched 402 patients including 192 patients who received neoadjuvant goserelin with flutamide. Pathologic downstaging was observed in 7% of only prostatectomy group and 15% of the neoadjuvant group ($p < 0.01$). Neoadjuvant group (26.3%) showed lower positive surgical margin rates than only prostatectomy group (47.5%) ($p < 0.05$). However, neoadjuvant group could not show superior biochemical recurrence-free survival (67% vs. 76%, $p = 0.18$) and overall survival (95% vs. 94%, $p = 0.64$) than only prostatectomy group. They admitted that this trial was not yet mature enough to show significant results, and at the present time, neoadjuvant therapy did not have any base to use.

Meta-analysis of neoadjuvant hormonal therapy evaluated ten randomized clinical trials [12]. Neoadjuvant hormonal therapy could reduce the positive surgical margin (odd ratio [OR] 0.34, $p < 0.0001$). However, the treatment did not show improvement in overall survival (OR 1.11, $p = 0.69$). And neoadjuvant therapy showed borderline significance in cancer recurrence rate (OR 0.74, $p = 0.05$). Kumar and colleagues suggested that neoadjuvant therapy may improve local control, but did not improve overall survival.

Table 3.1 Clinical trials of neoadjuvant hormonal therapy before radical prostatectomy

Trials	Neoadjuvant regimen	Neoadjuvant duration	Patients	Clinical stage	Positive margin rate (%)	BCR-free rate (%)	OS (%)	Median follow-up (mo)
Goldenberg et al. (1996) [24]	Cyproterone vs. only prostatectomy	3 months	112 vs. 101	T1b–T2c	64.8 vs. 27.7 ($p = 0.001$)	NR	NR	NR
Labrie et al. (1997) [25]	Leuprolide + flutamide vs. only prostatectomy	3 months	90 vs. 71	T2–T3	7.8 vs. 33.8 ($p < 0.001$)	NR	NR	NR
Fair et al. (1999) [10]	Leuprolide + flutamide vs. only prostatectomy	3 months	69 vs. 72	T1–T3	19 vs. 37 ($p = 0.023$)	No difference ($p = 0.73$)	NR	35
Schulman et al. (2000) [11]	Goserelin + flutamide vs. only prostatectomy	3 months	192 vs. 210	T2–T3	T2; 13 vs. 37 ($p < 0.01$) T3; 42 vs. 61 ($p = 0.01$)	74 vs. 67 ($p = 0.18$)	93 vs. 95 ($p = 0.64$)	48
Soloway et al. (2002) [26]	Leuprolide + flutamide vs. only prostatectomy	3 months	138 vs. 144	T2b	18 vs. 48 ($p < 0.001$)	64.8 vs. 67.6 ($p = 0.663$)	NR	60
Selli et al. (2002) [27]	Goserelin + bicalutamide vs. only prostatectomy	12 weeks or 24 weeks	143 (12 weeks), 122 (24 weeks) vs. 128	T2–T3	25.9 (12 weeks, $p = 0.003$), 18.7 (24 weeks, $p < 0.001$) vs. 46.5	NR	NR	NR
Aus et al. (2002) [28]	Triptorelin + cyproterone vs. only prostatectomy	3 months	63 vs. 63	T1b–T3a	23.6 vs. 45.5 ($p = 0.016$)	49.8 vs. 51.5 ($p = 0.588$)	No difference ($p = 0.513$)	82
Klotz et al. (2003) [29]	Cyproterone vs. only prostatectomy	3 months	42 vs. 34	T1b–T2c	NR	37.5 vs. 33.6 ($p = 0.924$)	5 years; 88.4 vs. 93.9 ($p = 0.38$)	69
Prezioso et al. (2004) [30]	Leuprolide + cyproterone vs. only prostatectomy	3 months	91 vs. 92	T1a–T2b	39 vs. 60 ($p = 0.01$)	NR	NR	6
Gravina et al. (2007) [31]	Bicalutamide vs. only prostatectomy	120 days	61 vs. 58	T2–T3a	13.1 vs. 34.5 ($p = 0.011$)	NR	NR	NR
Yee et al. (2010) [32]	Goserelin + flutamide vs. only prostatectomy	3 months	72 vs. 64	T1b–T3	19.4 vs. 37.5 ($p = 0.022$)	76.4 vs. 79.7 ($p = 0.7$)	NR	96
Sayyid et al. (2017) [33]	Degarelix vs. degarelix/bicalutamide vs. LHRH agonist/bicalutamide	3 months	13 vs. 14 vs. 12	≥T2	No difference	No difference	NR	NR

NR not reported, *BCR* biochemical recurrence, *OS* overall survival, *LHRH* luteinizing hormone-releasing hormone

In view of the results so far achieved, neoadjuvant hormonal therapy need not be recommended as basic treatment.

The disharmony between pathologic advantage and lack of survival gain may result from various factors. One reason for failure to gain survival outcomes may be from the short duration of 3 months that most of the trials choose. In cases of radiotherapy, long period (3 years) of ADT made survival gain [5]. Longer duration (8 months; 12%) of neoadjuvant therapy reduced positive surgical margin compared to 3 months (23%, $p = 0.011$) [13]. In addition, previous trials included heterogeneous patients who consisted in low- to high-risk groups. Longer durations of follow-up may be needed to achieve the significant survival gain, because the prognosis of localized prostate cancer is relatively favorable.

3.3 Neoadjuvant Chemotherapy with or Without ADT

Neoadjuvant chemotherapy gets the limelight in bladder or breast cancer, which improved oncologic outcomes. However, in advanced prostate cancer, neoadjuvant chemotherapy showed limited rationale, lacking phase III trials. Using chemotherapy like docetaxel has a rationale that randomized trials showed improved oncologic outcomes in metastatic castration-resistant prostate cancer (CRPC). We summarized neoadjuvant chemotherapy in Table 3.2 and neoadjuvant chemo-hormonal therapy in Table 3.3.

Phase I/II trials showed acceptable toxicity of neoadjuvant chemotherapy. Chi et al. conducted the largest phase II study of 72 patients with high-risk prostate cancer [14]. Four patients stopped the neoadjuvant chemotherapy because

Table 3.2 Clinical studies of neoadjuvant chemotherapy

Trials	Neoadjuvant regimen	Neoadjuvant duration	Patients	Selection criteria	Positive margin rate (%)	BCR-free rate (%)	OS (%)	Median follow-up (mo)
Dreicer et al. (2004) [34]	Docetaxel 40 mg/m²	Weekly for 6 weeks	29	cT2b–T3, Gleason ≥8, or PSA > 15 ng/mL	4	71	NR	23
Friedman et al. (2008) [35]	Docetaxel 36 mg/m² Capecitabine 1250 mg/m²	(Weekly docetaxel for 3 weeks + capecitabine for 2 weeks in 4 week cycle) × 3–6 cycles	15	>cT2, Gleason ≥8, or PSA > 15 ng/mL	54.5	NR	NR	NR
Shepard et al. (2009) [36]	Paclitaxel 150 mg/m²	(Weekly for 3 weeks in 4 week cycle) × 2 cycles	19	≥ cT2b, Gleason ≥8, or PSA ≥ 15 ng/mL	55	NR	NR	NR
Garzotto et al. (2010) [37]	Docetaxel 35 mg/m² Mitoxantrone 4 mg/m²	(Weekly for 3 weeks in 4 week cycle) × 4 cycles	57	cT2c, surgically resectable cT3a, or Gleason ≥4+3	33	2 years; 65.5 5 years; 49.8	NR	63
Nosov et al. (2016) [38]	Docetaxel 36 mg/m² vs. only prostatectomy	3 weekly × 6 cycles	21 vs. 23	≥cT2c, Gleason ≥7, or PSA > 10 ng/mL	52.2 vs. 52.4 ($p > 0.05$)	57.1% vs. 39.1% ($p = 0.25$)	CSS; 90.5 vs. 60.9 ($p = 0.042$) OS; 75.5 vs. 54.6 ($p = 0.09$)	141.6 vs. 128.4

NR not reported, *BCR* biochemical recurrence, *OS* overall survival, *CSS* cancer-specific survival

Table 3.3 Clinical studies of neoadjuvant chemo-hormonal therapy

Trials	Neoadjuvant regimen	Neoadjuvant duration	Patients	Selection criteria	Positive margin rate (%)	BCR-free rate (%)	OS (%)	Median follow-up (mo)
Clark et al. (2001) [39]	Etoposide 50 mg/m^2/day Estramustine 10 mg/kg/day	(3 weeks in 4 week cycle) × 3 cycles	33	cT2b–T3, Gleason ≥8, or PSA >15 ng/mL	13	88	NR	14
Hussain et al. (2003) [40]	Docetaxel 70 mg/m^2 Estramustine 280 mg	Docetaxel; once for 3 weeks Estramustine; 3 days for 3 weeks 3–6 cycles	21	≥cT2b, Gleason ≥8, or PSA ≥15 ng/mL	30	71	NR	15.1
Prayer-Galetti et al. (2007) [41]	Docetaxel 70 mg/m^2 Estramustine 600 mg/m^2 Triptorelin 3.75 mg	Docetaxel; once for 4 weeks Estramustine; daily for 3 weeks Triptorelin; 4 weeks (in 4 weeks cycle) × 3 cycles	22	≥cT3, Gleason ≥8, or PSA ≥15 ng/ml	26.3	53	NR	53
Chi et al. (2008) [14]	Docetaxel 35 mg/m^2 Buserelin 6.6 mg Nilutamide 150 mg (or flutamide 250 mg, bicalutamide 50 mg)	Docetaxel; weekly for 6 weeks Buserelin; every 8 weeks Antiandrogens daily for first 4 weeks (in 8-week cycle) × 3 cycles	72	≥2 positive biopsies, cT3, Gleason ≥7, or PSA ≥20 ng/mL	27	70	NR	42.7
Mellado et al. (2009) [42]	Docetaxel 36 mg/m^2 Goserelin 10.8 mg Flutamide 250 mg Dexamethasone 8 mg	Docetaxel; weekly for 3 weeks Goserelin; once Flutamide; daily Dexamethasone; every before docetaxel (in 4-week cycle) × 3 cycles	57	cT3, Gleason ≥7 (4 + 3), or PSA >20 ng/mL	35.3	31.6	NR	35
Narita et al. (2012) [43]	Docetaxel 30 mg/m^2 Leuprorelin 11.25 mg Bicalutamide 81 mg Estramustine 560 mg	Docetaxel; weekly for 6 weeks Leuprorelin; once every 3 months Bicalutamide; first 12 weeks Estramustine; daily for 6 weeks	18	cT3, Gleason 10, or PSA ≥15 ng/mL	0	16.7	NR	18

(continued)

Table 3.3 (continued)

Trials	Neoadjuvant regimen	Neoadjuvant duration	Patients	Selection criteria	Positive margin rate (%)	BCR-free rate (%)	OS (%)	Median follow-up (mo)
Thalgott et al. (2015) [15]	Docetaxel 75 mg/m^2 Buserelin 9.45 mg Bicalutamide 50 mg Prednisolone 10 mg	Docetaxel; once for 3 week Buserelin; once Bicalutamide; daily Prednisolone; daily (in 3-week cycle) × 3 cycles	15	non-metastatic locally advanced adenocarcinoma of the prostate with a biochemical 5-year recurrence risk of >40%	36.4 (including lymph node metastases)	53.3	100	44.3
Siberstein et al. (2015) [44]	Goserelin NR Paclitaxel NR Carboplatin NR Estramustine NR	Goserelin; every 3 months (Estramustine, Paclitaxel, Carboplatin) × 4–6 cycles	34 vs. 123 (only prostatectomy)	≥cT3, Gleason≥8, or PSA>20 ng/mL	24 vs. 38	30.9 vs. 63.8 ($p < 0.0001$)	NR	31

NR not reported, *BCR* biochemical recurrence, *OS* overall survival of toxicity. The others completed the protocol, and two showed the pathologic complete response. Seventeen patients had positive surgical margins. After median 42.7-month follow-up, 19 patients had biochemical recurrences. Recent phase II trial about neoadjuvant chemotherapy was published in 2015 by Thalgott et al. [15]. There was no pathologic complete response. By the Kattan nomogram, the biochemical recurrence rate of patients was predicted as 90%. However, 55% was confirmed as biochemical recurrence after 48.6 months, so the authors indicated that neoadjuvant therapy may improve the biochemical recurrence.

A phase III study is carried out by the Cancer and Leukemia Group B (CALGB) to confirm the effect of neoadjuvant docetaxel with ADT [16]. They enrolled 788 patients who had cT1–T3, Gleason score 8–10, and PSA < 100 ng/mL. Neoadjuvant therapy regimens are docetaxel (75 mg/m^2, every 21 days) every 3 weeks of 6 cycles and ADT (leuprolide or goserelin) for 18–24 weeks. And then, radical prostatectomy with staging pelvic lymphadenectomy would be conducted within 2 months. They will compare only prostatectomy group after randomization, and their primary end point will be 3-year biochemical recurrence. The estimated primary completion date would be June 2018. Table 3.4 shows ongoing trials of neoadjuvant chemo-hormonal therapy (at www.clinicaltrials.gov).

Neoadjuvant chemo-hormonal therapy reduced tumor burden and was confirmed feasibility and safety in previous phase II studies, but phase III trials should confirm that these results are associated with survival gain. Still now there are no long-term oncologic outcomes of neoadjuvant chemo-hormonal therapy except nonrandomized phase I or II trials without a control group. Current guidelines do not recommend neoadjuvant chemotherapy before prostatectomy.

3.4 Neoadjuvant Therapy Using Novel Medicines

After confirming the survival gain of new medicines such as abiraterone and enzalutamide, neoadjuvant therapies of those medicines have been investigated. A neoadjuvant phase II trial of leuprolide with abiraterone was performed in localized prostate cancer patients (n = 58) [17]. Leuprolide with abiraterone for 24 weeks before prostatectomy was compared with leuprolide with abiraterone for 12 weeks after randomization. This study showed extremely low levels of prostate tissue androgens and pathologic complete response, and minimal residual disease was observed more in the group of leuprolide with abiraterone for 24 weeks (62% vs. 48%). This suggested that abiraterone may improve the potency of ADT and give a rationale to the combination setting with abiraterone.

Table 3.4 Recruiting phase I/II trials of neoadjuvant chemo-hormonal therapy (www.clinicaltrials.gov [Accessed 2017 Aug])

Identifier	Study title	Interventions	Estimated enrollment	Estimated primary completion date
NCT02543255	Antiandrogens and cabazitaxel in defining complete response in prostatectomy (ACDC trial)	Abiraterone acetate with prednisone, leuprolide, cabazitaxel with pegfilgrastim	76	October 2018
NCT02494713	Hormonal therapy and chemotherapy followed by prostatectomy in patients with prostate cancer	Degarelix, doxorubicin, ketoconazole, docetaxel, estramustine	24	February 2019
NCT02716974	A study of definitive therapy to treat prostate cancer (oligo-mets)	Leuprolide acetate, bicalutamide, docetaxel	33	March 2019

There was phase II study about neoadjuvant therapy with enzalutamide [18]. Intermediate- or high-risk localized prostate cancer patients ($n = 52$) received neoadjuvant enzalutamide or enzalutamide plus dutasteride plus leuprolide for 6 months. Pathologic complete response or minimal residual disease was observed more in the combination group (17.3% vs. 0%). Median residual cancer burden was also smaller in the combination group (0.06 cm^3 vs. 0.41 cm^3). They suggested that more effective blocking of androgen receptor can be correlated to antitumor effects.

There are various medicines targeting molecular mechanisms to kill tumor cells under investigations (Table 3.5). Imatinib that was known

Table 3.5 Clinical studies of neoadjuvant therapy with targeted agents

Trials	Neoadjuvant regimen	Neoadjuvant duration	Patients	Selection criteria	Positive margin rate (%)	BCR-free rate (%)	OS (%)	Median follow-up (mo)
Febbo et al. (2006) [45]	Imatinib 200 or 300 mg	Orally twice a day for 6 weeks	11	Localized intermediate or high-risk	NR	NR	NR	NR
Vuky et al. (2009) [20]	Docetaxel 36 mg/m² Gefitinib 250 mg	Docetaxel; every 3 weeks for 2 cycles Gefitinib; daily for 56 days	31	PSA ≧20, Gleason ≧8, or cT2b–3	33	67	NR	28
Mathew et al. (2009) [19]	Docetaxel 30 mg/m² Imatinib 600 mg Bicalutamide 50 mg LHRH agonist NR	Docetaxel; weekly for first 4 weeks Imatinib; daily Bicalutamide; daily LHRH agonist; NR (in 6 week cycle) × 3 cycles	36	≧cT2c, Gleason ≧8 or PSA >20 ng/mL or cT2b Gleason 7 with PSA >10 ng/mL	18	53	94	39
Ross et al. (2012) [21]	Docetaxel 70 mg/m² Bevacizumab 15 mg/m²	Docetaxel; every 3 weeks for 6 cycles Bevacizumab; every 3 weeks for 5 cycles	41	PSA >20 ng/mL, PSA velocity >2 ng/mL/y, cT3 disease, any biopsy Gleason ≧8, or Gleason 7 with T3 or Gleason 7, PSA >10 ng/mL, or cT2	32	51	NR	13.0 (to recurrence)
Vuky et al. (2013) [46]	Docetaxel 75 mg/m² GVAX 5 × 10⁸ cells (First dose) 3 × 10⁸ cells (Boost dose)	Docetaxel; every 3 weeks for 4 cycles CVAX; 2–3 days after docetaxel for four courses	6	NR	NR	NR	NR	NR

Table 3.5 (continued)

Trials	Neoadjuvant regimen	Neoadjuvant duration	Patients	Selection criteria	Positive margin rate (%)	BCR-free rate (%)	OS (%)	Median follow-up (mo)
Kumon et al. (2016) [47]	Adenovirus vector carrying the human REIC/Dkk-3 gene 1.0×10^{10}, 1.0×10^{11} and 1.0×10^{12} viral particles in 1.0–1.2 mL	Two ultrasound-guided intratumoral injections at 2-week intervals	18	T2a–T3a Kattan's nomogram score of ≧115	NR	44	NR	NR

NR not reported, *BCR* biochemical recurrence, *OS* overall survival, *LHRH* luteinizing hormone-releasing hormone

as Gleevec inhibits platelet-derived growth factor receptor (PDGFR). Mathew et al. used docetaxel plus imatinib with ADT as neoadjuvant therapy in 36 patients [19]. There was no pathologic complete response, and 2-year progression-free survival rate was 57% with median 39-month follow-up. The authors mentioned the efficacy of imatinib with docetaxel, and ADT as neoadjuvant therapy was not obtained. Gefitinib interrupts signaling through the epidermal growth factor receptor (EGFR). Vuky et al. assessed the effect of gefitinib with docetaxel as neoadjuvant therapy [20]. Among 30 high-risk prostate cancer patients, there was no pathologic complete response, and positive margin rate was 33%. That was comparable to the rates of other former trials about neoadjuvant chemohormonal therapy. The authors concluded that gefitinib did not have an additional role in neoadjuvant setting as a single use or combination with chemotherapy. Vascular endothelial growth factor (VEGF) plays an important part in oncologic angiogenesis. Ross et al. used docetaxel with bevacizumab in high-risk prostate cancer before radical prostatectomy [21]. There was no pathologic complete response, and positive margin rate was 32%. Neoadjuvant docetaxel with bevacizumab showed tolerable toxicity, and reduced tumor burden and serum PSA, but the oncologic effect of bevacizumab was not confirmed as neoadjuvant therapy. In spite of these studies, an interest of VEGF and other targeted agents is still ongoing as clinical trials (Table 3.6).

Sipuleucel-T was approved by FDA as a treatment option for prostate cancer. That might trigger T cell immune response to the prostate. Some trials used immunotherapy as the neoadjuvant setting. Sandler et al. used sipuleucel-T to localized prostate cancer patients (n = 42) before radical prostatectomy [22]. They found that T cell infiltrated at the tumor boundary, but control group did not have any infiltration. The authors suggested their study gave a rationale for combination with sipuleucel-T, and other treatment and neoadjuvant trials with immunotherapy could provide a chance for prostate cancer. Cytotoxic T lymphocyte-associated antigen 4 (CTL4) is known as the immune checkpoint. Blocking CTLA4 can promote antitumor immunity by ipilimumab. The study about neoadjuvant ipilimumab in prostate cancer showed increased immune cell infiltration into the tumor [23]. They suggested that these immunologic changes in the tumor microenvironment can help antitumor responses. These researches using novel agents pile up the data about mechanisms and that may make a chance for clinical oncologic outcomes.

Table 3.6 Ongoing active clinical trials of neoadjuvant therapy using novel medicines (www.clinicaltrials.gov [Accessed 2017 Aug])

Identifier	Study title	Interventions	Target/mechanism	Estimated enrollment	Estimated primary completion date	Primary outcome
NCT02153918	Vaccine plus booster shots in men with prostate cancer undergoing treatment with radical prostatectomy	PROSTVAC-V/TRICOM PROSTVAC-F/TRICOM	Recombinant virus vector vaccines	27	October 2017	CD4 and CD8 cell infiltrates
NCT01695473	Neoadjuvant BKM120 in high-risk prostate cancer	BKM120	PI3K	24	December 2017	PI3K inhibition in prostate tumor tissue
NCT01385059	Axitinib before surgery in treating patients with high-risk prostate cancer	Axitinib	VEGFR	60	January 2018	Changes in pre-metastatic niche density
NCT01696877	A neoadjuvant study of androgen ablation combined with cyclophosphamide and GVAX vaccine for localized prostate cancer	GVAX	Prostate cancer cell-based vaccines	29	April 2018	Intraprostatic CD8+ T cell infiltration, adverse events
NCT01804712	Rituximab neoadjuvant therapy in patients with prostate cancer scheduled to undergo radical prostatectomy	rituximab	CD 20	18	April 2018	Histologic response rate
NCT02324998	Studying the effects of olaparib (± degarelix) given to men with intermediate-/high-risk prostate cancer before radical prostatectomy (CaNCaP03)	Olaparib	PARP	20	June 2018	Determination of PARP inhibition
NCT01832259	A study of VEGF tyrosine kinase inhibitor (pazopanib) in men with high-risk prostate cancer followed by radical prostatectomy and pelvic lymph node dissection	Pazopanib	VEGFR	30	August 2018	Decrease in pre-metastatic niche formation (lymph nodes)
NCT01990196	Neoadjuvant phase II study comparing the effects of AR inhibition with/without SRC or MEK inhibition in prostate cancer	Trametinib Dasatinib	MEK SRC	45	September 2018	N-cadherin and vimentin expression
NCT00329043	Sunitinib malate with hormonal ablation for patients who will have prostatectomy	Sunitinib	VEGFR	64	December 2018	Pathological complete response
NCT01409200	Neoadjuvant axitinib in prostate cancer	Axitinib	VEGFR	72	March 2019	Progression-free 12 months after surgery
NCT02506114	Neoadjuvant PROSTVAC-VF with or without ipilimumab for prostate cancer	PROSTVAC-V/F Ipilimumab	Virus vaccines and anti-CTLA4 antibody	75	December 2019	CD3+ T cell immune response

3.5 Summary

There were several phase II trials for neoadjuvant therapy before radical prostatectomy using ADT or chemotherapy. Most trials showed reduced positive surgical margin rates and tumor burden but failed to improve biochemical recurrence or overall survival. Neoadjuvant therapy has not been a guideline before radical prostatectomy due to lacking of phase III trials and the oncologic outcomes of phase II trials. Nevertheless, neoadjuvant trials still challenge to get a favorable outcome by understanding the biology of prostate cancer. Novel hormonal, targeted, and immunologic agents are applied to neoadjuvant settings. In near future, the results of phase III trial and ongoing trials help us to confirm the appropriate role of neoadjuvant therapy before radical prostatectomy.

References

1. Vallet B. Radical perineal prostatectomy subsequent to bilateral orchidectomy. Del Me J. 1944;16:18–20.
2. Green N, Bodner H, Broth E, Chiang C, Garrett J, Goldstein A, et al. Improved control of bulky prostate carcinoma with sequential estrogen and radiation therapy. Int J Radiat Oncol Biol Phys. 1984;10(7):971–6.
3. Roach M 3rd, Bae K, Speight J, Wolkov HB, Rubin P, Lee RJ, et al. Short-term neoadjuvant androgen deprivation therapy and external-beam radiotherapy for locally advanced prostate cancer: long-term results of RTOG 8610. J Clin Oncol. 2008;26(4):585–91.
4. D'Amico AV, Manola J, Loffredo M, Renshaw AA, DellaCroce A, Kantoff PW. 6-Month androgen suppression plus radiation therapy vs radiation therapy alone for patients with clinically localized prostate cancer: a randomized controlled trial. JAMA. 2004;292(7):821–7.
5. Bolla M, Van Tienhoven G, Warde P, Dubois JB, Mirimanoff RO, Storme G, et al. External irradiation with or without long-term androgen suppression for prostate cancer with high metastatic risk: 10-year results of an EORTC randomised study. Lancet Oncol. 2010;11(11):1066–73.
6. Bach C, Pisipati S, Daneshwar D, Wright M, Rowe E, Gillatt D, et al. The status of surgery in the management of high-risk prostate cancer. Nat Rev Urol. 2014;11(6):342–51.
7. Yuh B, Artibani W, Heidenreich A, Kimm S, Menon M, Novara G, et al. The role of robot-assisted radical prostatectomy and pelvic lymph node dissection in the management of high-risk prostate cancer: a systematic review. Eur Urol. 2014;65(5):918–27.
8. Loeb S, Schaeffer EM, Trock BJ, Epstein JI, Humphreys EB, Walsh PC. What are the outcomes of radical prostatectomy for high-risk prostate cancer? Urology. 2010;76(3):710–4.
9. Heidenreich A, Bastian PJ, Bellmunt J, Bolla M, Joniau S, van der Kwast T, et al. EAU guidelines on prostate cancer. Part II: treatment of advanced, relapsing, and castration-resistant prostate cancer. Eur Urol. 2014;65(2):467–79.
10. Fair WR, Rabbani F, Bastar A, Betancourt J. Neoadjuvant hormone therapy before radical prostatectomy: update on the Memorial Sloan-Kettering Cancer Center Trials. Mol Urol. 1999;3(3):253–60.
11. Schulman CC, Debruyne FM, Forster G, Selvaggi FP, Zlotta AR, Witjes WP. 4-Year follow-up results of a European prospective randomized study on neoadjuvant hormonal therapy prior to radical prostatectomy in T2-3N0M0 prostate cancer. European Study Group on Neoadjuvant Treatment of Prostate Cancer. Eur Urol. 2000;38(6):706–13.
12. Kumar S, Shelley M, Harrison C, Coles B, Wilt TJ, Mason MD. Neo-adjuvant and adjuvant hormone therapy for localised and locally advanced prostate cancer. Cochrane Database Syst Rev. 2006;4:CD006019.
13. Gleave ME, Goldenberg SL, Chin JL, Warner J, Saad F, Klotz LH, et al. Randomized comparative study of 3 versus 8-month neoadjuvant hormonal therapy before radical prostatectomy: biochemical and pathological effects. J Urol. 2001;166(2):500–6; discussion 6–7.
14. Chi KN, Chin JL, Winquist E, Klotz L, Saad F, Gleave ME. Multicenter phase II study of combined neoadjuvant docetaxel and hormone therapy before radical prostatectomy for patients with high risk localized prostate cancer. J Urol. 2008;180(2):565–70; discussion 70.
15. Thalgott M, Rack B, Horn T, Heck MM, Eiber M, Kubler H, et al. Detection of circulating tumor cells in locally advanced high-risk prostate cancer during neoadjuvant chemotherapy and radical prostatectomy. Anticancer Res. 2015;35(10):5679–85.
16. Chang AJ, Autio KA, Roach M 3rd, Scher HI. High-risk prostate cancer-classification and therapy. Nat Rev Clin Oncol. 2014;11(6):308–23.
17. Taplin ME, Montgomery B, Logothetis CJ, Bubley GJ, Richie JP, Dalkin BL, et al. Intense androgen-deprivation therapy with abiraterone acetate plus leuprolide acetate in patients with localized high-risk prostate cancer: results of a randomized phase II neoadjuvant study. J Clin Oncol Off J Am Soc Clin Oncol. 2014;32(33):3705–15.
18. Montgomery B, Tretiakova MS, Joshua AM, Gleave ME, Fleshner N, Bubley GJ, et al. Neoadjuvant enzalutamide prior to prostatectomy. Clin Cancer Res. 2017;23(9):2169–76.
19. Mathew P, Pisters LL, Wood CG, Papadopoulos JN, Williams DL, Thall PF, et al. Neoadjuvant platelet derived growth factor receptor inhibitor therapy combined with docetaxel and androgen ablation for high risk localized prostate cancer. J Urol. 2009;181(1):81–7; discussion 7.

20. Vuky J, Porter C, Isacson C, Vaughan M, Kozlowski P, Picozzi V, et al. Phase II trial of neoadjuvant docetaxel and gefitinib followed by radical prostatectomy in patients with high-risk, locally advanced prostate cancer. Cancer. 2009;115(4):784–91.
21. Ross RW, Galsky MD, Febbo P, Barry M, Richie JP, Xie W, et al. Phase 2 study of neoadjuvant docetaxel plus bevacizumab in patients with high-risk localized prostate cancer: a Prostate Cancer Clinical Trials Consortium trial. Cancer. 2012;118(19):4777–84.
22. Fong L, Carroll P, Weinberg V, Chan S, Lewis J, Corman J, et al. Activated lymphocyte recruitment into the tumor microenvironment following preoperative sipuleucel-T for localized prostate cancer. J Natl Cancer Inst. 2014;106(11):pii: dju268.
23. Gao J, Ward JF, Pettaway CA, Shi LZ, Subudhi SK, Vence LM, et al. VISTA is an inhibitory immune checkpoint that is increased after ipilimumab therapy in patients with prostate cancer. Nat Med. 2017;23(5):551–5.
24. Goldenberg SL, Klotz LH, Srigley J, Jewett MA, Mador D, Fradet Y, et al. Randomized, prospective, controlled study comparing radical prostatectomy alone and neoadjuvant androgen withdrawal in the treatment of localized prostate cancer. Canadian Urologic Oncology Group. J Urol. 1996;156(3):873–7.
25. Labrie F, Cusan L, Gomez JL, Diamond P, Suburu R, Lemay M, et al. Neoadjuvant hormonal therapy: the Canadian experience. Urology. 1997;49(3A Suppl):56–64.
26. Soloway MS, Pareek K, Sharifi R, Wajsman Z, McLeod D, Wood DP Jr, et al. Neoadjuvant androgen ablation before radical prostatectomy in cT2bNxMo prostate cancer: 5-year results. J Urol. 2002;167(1):112–6.
27. Selli C, Montironi R, Bono A, Pagano F, Zattoni F, Manganelli A, et al. Effects of complete androgen blockade for 12 and 24 weeks on the pathological stage and resection margin status of prostate cancer. J Clin Pathol. 2002;55(7):508–13.
28. Aus G, Abrahamsson PA, Ahlgren G, Hugosson J, Lundberg S, Schain M, et al. Three-month neoadjuvant hormonal therapy before radical prostatectomy: a 7-year follow-up of a randomized controlled trial. BJU Int. 2002;90(6):561–6.
29. Klotz LH, Goldenberg SL, Jewett MA, Fradet Y, Nam R, Barkin J, et al. Long-term followup of a randomized trial of 0 versus 3 months of neoadjuvant androgen ablation before radical prostatectomy. J Urol. 2003;170(3):791–4.
30. Prezioso D, Lotti T, Polito M, Montironi R. Neoadjuvant hormone treatment with leuprolide acetate depot 3.75 mg and cyproterone acetate, before radical prostatectomy: a randomized study. Urol Int. 2004;72(3):189–95.
31. Gravina GL, Festuccia C, Galatioto GP, Muzi P, Angelucci A, Ronchi P, et al. Surgical and biologic outcomes after neoadjuvant bicalutamide treatment in prostate cancer. Urology. 2007;70(4):728–33.
32. Yee DS, Lowrance WT, Eastham JA, Maschino AC, Cronin AM, Rabbani F. Long-term follow-up of 3-month neoadjuvant hormone therapy before radical prostatectomy in a randomized trial. BJU Int. 2010;105(2):185–90.
33. Sayyid RK, Evans A, Hersey K, Maloni R, Hurtado-Coll A, Kulkarni G, et al. A phase II, randomized, open-label study of neoadjuvant degarelix versus LHRH agonist in prostate cancer patients prior to radical prostatectomy. Clin Cancer Res. 2017;23(8):1974–80.
34. Dreicer R, Magi-Galluzzi C, Zhou M, Rothaermel J, Reuther A, Ulchaker J, et al. Phase II trial of neoadjuvant docetaxel before radical prostatectomy for locally advanced prostate cancer. Urology. 2004;63(6):1138–42.
35. Friedman J, Dunn RL, Wood D, Vaishampayan U, Wu A, Bradley D, et al. Neoadjuvant docetaxel and capecitabine in patients with high risk prostate cancer. J Urol. 2008;179(3):911–5; discussion 5–6.
36. Shepard DR, Dreicer R, Garcia J, Elson P, Magi-Galluzzi C, Raghavan D, et al. Phase II trial of neoadjuvant nab-paclitaxel in high risk patients with prostate cancer undergoing radical prostatectomy. J Urol. 2009;181(4):1672–7; discussion 7.
37. Garzotto M, Higano CS, O'Brien C, Rademacher BL, Janeba N, Fazli L, et al. Phase 1/2 study of preoperative docetaxel and mitoxantrone for high-risk prostate cancer. Cancer. 2010;116(7):1699–708.
38. Nosov A, Reva S, Petrov S, Mamijev E, Novikov R, Veliev E, et al. Neoadjuvant chemotherapy using reduced-dose docetaxel followed by radical prostatectomy for patients with intermediate and high-risk prostate cancer: a single-center study. Prostate. 2016;76(15):1345–52.
39. Clark PE, Peereboom DM, Dreicer R, Levin HS, Clark SB, Klein EA. Phase II trial of neoadjuvant estramustine and etoposide plus radical prostatectomy for locally advanced prostate cancer. Urology. 2001;57(2):281–5.
40. Hussain M, Smith DC, El-Rayes BF, Du W, Vaishampayan U, Fontana J, et al. Neoadjuvant docetaxel and estramustine chemotherapy in high-risk/locallyadvanced prostate cancer. Urology. 2003;61(4):774–80.
41. Prayer-Galetti T, Sacco E, Pagano F, Gardiman M, Cisternino A, Betto G, et al. Long-term follow-up of a neoadjuvant chemohormonal taxane-based phase II trial before radical prostatectomy in patients with non-metastatic high-risk prostate cancer. BJU Int. 2007;100(2):274–80.
42. Mellado B, Font A, Alcaraz A, Aparicio LA, Veiga FJ, Areal J, et al. Phase II trial of short-term neoadjuvant docetaxel and complete androgen blockade in high-risk prostate cancer. Br J Cancer. 2009;101(8):1248–52.
43. Narita S, Tsuchiya N, Kumazawa T, Maita S, Numakura K, Obara T, et al. Short-term clinicopathological outcome of neoadjuvant chemohormonal

therapy comprising complete androgen blockade, followed by treatment with docetaxel and estramustine phosphate before radical prostatectomy in Japanese patients with high-risk localized prostate cancer. World J Surg Oncol. 2012;10:1.
44. Silberstein JL, Poon SA, Sjoberg DD, Maschino AC, Vickers AJ, Bernie A, et al. Long-term oncological outcomes of a phase II trial of neoadjuvant chemohormonal therapy followed by radical prostatectomy for patients with clinically localised, high-risk prostate cancer. BJU Int. 2015;116(1):50–6.
45. Febbo PG, Thorner A, Rubin MA, Loda M, Kantoff PW, Oh WK, et al. Application of oligonucleotide microarrays to assess the biological effects of neoadjuvant imatinib mesylate treatment for localized prostate cancer. Clin Cancer Res. 2006;12(1):152–8.
46. Vuky J, Corman JM, Porter C, Olgac S, Auerbach E, Dahl K. Phase II trial of neoadjuvant docetaxel and CG1940/CG8711 followed by radical prostatectomy in patients with high-risk clinically localized prostate cancer. Oncologist. 2013;18(6):687–8.
47. Kumon H, Ariyoshi Y, Sasaki K, Sadahira T, Araki M, Ebara S, et al. Adenovirus vector carrying REIC/DKK-3 gene: neoadjuvant intraprostatic injection for high-risk localized prostate cancer undergoing radical prostatectomy. Cancer Gene Ther. 2016;23(11):400–9.

Robot-Assisted Radical Prostatectomy for High-Risk Prostate Cancer

4

Taekmin Kwon and Jun Hyuk Hong

4.1 Introduction

Owing to the profound stage migration that has been attributed to PSA screening, the proportion of high-risk prostate cancer (PCa) is decreasing. Up to the early 1990s, about a third of patients with PCa were in the high-risk category. But in recent series, its prevalence was 8–18% [1–3]. Nevertheless, treatment of high-risk PCa is a subject of continuous discussion due to poor prognosis of this patient's subset. In patients with high-risk compared with low-risk PCa, the biochemical recurrence (BCR) risk and the cancer-specific mortality rate are 3 times and 11 times higher, respectively [1]. Therefore, high-risk patients are treated with multimodal approaches, including surgery. But, evidences supporting surgery as a monotherapy and showing optimal results have emerged recently [4, 5].

Since the entry of new century, robot-assisted radical prostatectomy (RARP) was introduced and has become more prevalent due to its oncologic and functional outcomes which are not less than similar to open radical prostatectomy (RP) in organ-confined disease [6, 7]. Although RP is an important treatment option for selected patients with high-risk PCa, the role of RARP has not been fully studied. A large series of RARP in high-risk patients or randomized trials comparing RARP and other treatments has not been reported. In the past decade, RARP has been rapidly adopted for clinical practice, but recently there was only a result of evaluating high-risk disease in particular. In a recent review comparing RARP and open RP, similar positive surgical margins and BCR rates, as well as reduced bleeding and the need for transfusion and potential benefits for relief and erectile function recovery, were demonstrated [8, 9]. In this chapter, we discuss the role of RARP in the setting of high-risk PCa and indication, technical aspects, and outcomes of RARP. We hope this discussion will provide useful information in RARP for high-risk PCa.

4.2 What Is High-Risk PCa?

D'Amico et al. stratified PCa into three risk categories according to oncological outcome. High-risk PCa, which was defined as serum PSA $\geq$ 20 ng/mL, biopsy Gleason score (GS) $\geq$8, and clinical stage T2c or higher, had a posttreatment chance of BCR> 50% after 5 years [10]. Other many definitions for high-risk cancer were proposed, using different values of PSA, percentage of core involvement in biopsy, and different

T. Kwon
Department of Urology, Ulsan University Hospital, Ulsan, South Korea

J. H. Hong (✉)
Department of Urology, Asan Medical Center, Seoul, South Korea
e-mail: jhhong@amc.seoul.kr

C. S. Kim (ed.), *Management of Advanced Prostate Cancer*,
https://doi.org/10.1007/978-981-10-6943-7_4

clinical stages. In Europe, about 70% of urologists adopt the National Comprehensive Cancer Network classification that differs from D'Amico's in including clinical T3 disease or greater [11]. Among the most used risk parameters, high GS proved to be the most reliable predictor of the outcome, followed by PSA rise. The 10-year BCR-free rate is 24.1%, 26.4%, and 43.8% for GS ≥8, PSA ≥20 ng/mL, and cT3 cases, respectively. If two of these risk factors are associated, the prognosis worsens further, and in 10 years the BCR-free survival rate is about 18% [3].

4.3 RARP for High-Risk PCa

4.3.1 Nerve Sparing in High-Risk PCa During RARP

In the literature, nerve sparing (NS) was highly variable in the range of 0–100%, reflecting differences in cancer characteristics, patient population, or surgeon's preference [12, 13]. Lavery et al. studied the performance of NS in high-risk patients and used visual cues to identify poorly defined planes, bulging of the capsule, or appearance of prostate tissue on the neurovascular bundle (NVB) [14]. Intraoperative frozen sections were also an option to guide NS. In this analysis, NS was performed in 73% of patients, except for seminal vesicle invasion confirmed by biopsy, extracapsular extension of endorectal coil magnetic resonance imaging (MRI), or high tumor volume, high-Gleason grade disease. Even when controlling the characteristics of pathological diseases, NS was not associated with a positive surgical margin (PSM) or a high-risk of BCR. In another analysis, Casey et al. showed that bilateral or unilateral NS was not associated with increased PSM in patients with extraprostatic (pT3) disease [15].

4.3.2 Lymph Node Dissection in High-Risk PCa During RARP

Despite staging and possible therapeutic benefits of lymph node dissection (LND), there is a paucity of reporting. Many studies did not specify anatomical templates or only performed limited LND. An extended lymph node dissection (ELND) includes removal of all node-bearing tissue from an area bound by external iliac vein anteriorly, the pelvic sidewall laterally, the bladder wall medially, the floor of the pelvis posteriorly, Cooper's ligament distally, and the internal iliac artery proximally. The median lymph node yield from these studies was 18 nodes in 4 RARP studies that reported consistent use of ELND in high-risk patients [11, 12, 16, 17]. Overall lymph node prevalence ranged from 1% to 33%, the highest rate in ELND. In addition, the robot ELND seemed to increase the operation time at three longest operation times that routinely carry out ELND [12, 16, 17]. The occurrence of symptomatic lymphocele in ELND series was 2.4–6.6%.

4.3.3 Perioperative Morbidity During RARP

Known benefits of RARP when compared to open surgery are rapid time to recovery, decreased bleeding, and decreased analgesic use. The risk of blood transfusion is seven times higher with open RP than RARP [8]. Tewari et al. conducted a systematic review comparing open RP and RARP in all risk categories and found a 7% greater risk of perioperative complications for open RP and twice as many postoperative hospitalization days [18]. Ham et al. compared the outcomes of RARP performed in organ-confined and locally advanced PCa and found no statistical difference between two groups in many perioperative features including time of surgery, blood loss amount, length of hospital stay, and intraoperative complications [12]. Rogers et al. also demonstrated similar convalescence after RARP compared with open RP in the elderly population, in which group complications were expected to be higher [19]. Thromboembolism can be more common because LND is considered mandatory in high-risk patients. A multicenter collaborative study analyzing > 3500 patients who received RP showed that LND increased the risk of deep venous thrombosis and pulmonary thromboembolism [20].

4.4 Outcomes of RARP for High-Risk PCa

4.4.1 Oncologic Outcomes of RARP for High-Risk PCa

A systematic review by Novara et al. evaluated a series of PSM comparing open RP and RARP in all risk categories and demonstrated no difference between two methods [21]. The reported PSM rate in high-risk PCa with RARP ranges from 16% to 58% [14, 22]. Wide variations of PSM rate are also observed in contemporary open RP series with 18–48% [3]. Suardi et al. recently evaluated the PSMs of patients with high-risk PCa undergoing surgical treatment and found an odd ratio (OR) of 0.69 favoring RARP over open RP ($p = 0.04$) [23]. Despite previous studies, most series comparing surgical methods among high-risk patients found no difference in the proportion of PSM. Harty et al. compared PSMs among high-risk patients who underwent open RP, RARP, and laparoscopic prostatectomy, reporting no significant difference among three methods (53%, 41%, 50%, respectively; $p = 0.13$) [24]. After a propensity score match, Lee et al. reported PSM rates of 36% and 34% ($p = 0.76$) for patients undergoing open RP and RARP, respectively [25]. Another propensity score that matched a cohort from the Surveillance, Epidemiology, and End Results (SEER) database found PSMs in 18% of open RP cases and in 22% of RARP cases ($p = 0.4$) [26].

In the current RARP studies of high-risk PCa, the BCR is reported in the range of 13–35% [6, 12, 19, 26]. Some of the published papers are mentioned that PSA cutoff is not used, but in most cases PSA is considered as a marker of disease recurrence as more than 0.2 ng/mL. However, most series lack long-term follow-up. Survival analysis comparing RARP and open RP showed comparable disease recurrence rate. In a study by Walz et al., the BCR for follow-up of 2, 5, and 10 years was 35.2%, 52.6%, and 64.3%, respectively, in 887 high-risk PCa cases [3]. In another study of the Mayo Clinic, BCR at 5 and 10 years after open RP were 32% and 45% [1]. Concerning the RARP series, Abdollah et al. assessed the biggest cohort to date including 1100 patients and found a 10-year BCR-free rate of 50.4% [27]. Still, randomized trials comparing RARP and open RP for high-risk PCa are scarce. Existing retrospective series analyzing different surgical techniques found similar BCR-free rates for open RP and RARP [5, 25]. Estimating CSS and OS is a major concern for high-risk patients. However, it was hardly reported in the current series. In two studies, 100% of CSS was detected in the high-risk PCa cohort treated with RARP [28, 29]. Busch et al. compared the OS between patients treated with RARP and open RP and found no difference between two methods (RARP 95% vs. open RP 100%; $p = 0.09$) [30]. To wrap it up, surgical methods have not affected oncological outcomes up to now.

4.4.2 Functional Outcomes of RARP for High-Risk PCa

Considering the complex anatomy of nerve innervations and pelvic muscles around the prostate, the meticulous motion and visual advantages of robot surgery were initially accepted with anticipation to improve functional outcomes. There have been many series demonstrating early recovery of continence (within 3 months) after RARP with scrupulous dissection, anterior and posterior reconstruction, and bladder neck preservation [31, 32]. On the other hand, another nonrandomized study analyzing 1-year continence rate in all risk groups reported similar results between RARP and open RP (OR: 1.08) [7]. Other results demonstrated heterogeneous continence outcomes in men with high-risk PCa after RARP. Rogers et al. reported that 82% of his patients used one or no pad daily 1 year after RARP [19]. Koo et al. had inferior results using a no-pad definition (33% of continence at 1 year) [33]. Both studies addressed the age (>70 years) as a paramount variable for continence recovery. Other series for RARP in high-risk PCa reported more satisfactory outcomes from 92% to 100% [15, 34].

It is difficult to preserve potency in high-risk patients who are more likely to sacrifice NVB during surgery. Bilateral nerve sparing can be performed in organ-confined disease, and unilateral nerve sparing is feasible in selected patients with high-risk PCa. Jayram et al. reported 80% nerve sparing during RARP in high-risk cohort. Of those, 29% were bilaterally spared. PSM was 20%, and the potency rate was 51% at 6 months after surgery [22]. Lavery et al. achieved greater rates of bilateral nerve sparing (58%), with an intraoperative frozen section of the NVB in selected cases to assure negative margins. With a median follow-up of 1 year, 56% of the patients were potent (Sexual Health Inventory for Men ≥16), and no association was found between nerve sparing and PSM [14]. Casey et al. conducted bilateral NVB preservation in 57% of pT3 or higher patients and reported 20% PSMs [15]. They gained satisfactory PSM rates in locally advanced disease. Other reports of RARP for high-risk PCa maintain potency recovery of 20%–60% [14, 22]. Functional outcome is more likely to rest on surgeon's expertise and characteristics of cancer rather than surgical method itself.

Conclusions RARP seems to be a safe and effective option for patients who have high-risk PCa or as the first step in a multimodal strategy. Preservation of NVB is feasible in the selected cases, and there is a possibility to improve functional outcome. As for LND, its therapeutic role in RARP setting is still to be elucidated. Further longitudinal study is required to assess the long-term benefit of primary RARP in men with high-risk PCa.

References

1. Boorjian SA, Karnes RJ, Rangel LJ, Bergstralh EJ, Blute ML. Mayo Clinic validation of the D'amico risk group classification for predicting survival following radical prostatectomy. J Urol. 2008;179(4):1354–60; discussion 60–1.
2. Badani KK, Kaul S, Menon M. Evolution of robotic radical prostatectomy: assessment after 2766 procedures. Cancer. 2007;110(9):1951–8.
3. Walz J, Joniau S, Chun FK, Isbarn H, Jeldres C, Yossepowitch O, et al. Pathological results and rates of treatment failure in high-risk prostate cancer patients after radical prostatectomy. BJU Int. 2011;107(5):765–70.
4. Cooperberg MR, Vickers AJ, Broering JM, Carroll PR. Comparative risk-adjusted mortality outcomes after primary surgery, radiotherapy, or androgen-deprivation therapy for localized prostate cancer. Cancer. 2010;116(22):5226–34.
5. Petrelli F, Vavassori I, Coinu A, Borgonovo K, Sarti E, Barni S. Radical prostatectomy or radiotherapy in high-risk prostate cancer: a systematic review and metaanalysis. Clin Genitourin Cancer. 2014;12(4):215–24.
6. Yaxley JW, Coughlin GD, Chambers SK, Occhipinti S, Samaratunga H, Zajdlewicz L, et al. Robot-assisted laparoscopic prostatectomy versus open radical retropubic prostatectomy: early outcomes from a randomised controlled phase 3 study. Lancet. 2016;388(10049):1057–66.
7. Haglind E, Carlsson S, Stranne J, Wallerstedt A, Wilderang U, Thorsteinsdottir T, et al. Urinary incontinence and erectile dysfunction after robotic versus open radical prostatectomy: a prospective, controlled, nonrandomised trial. Eur Urol. 2015;68(2):216–25.
8. Novara G, Ficarra V, Rosen RC, Artibani W, Costello A, Eastham JA, et al. Systematic review and meta-analysis of perioperative outcomes and complications after robot-assisted radical prostatectomy. Eur Urol. 2012;62(3):431–52.
9. Ficarra V, Novara G, Ahlering TE, Costello A, Eastham JA, Graefen M, et al. Systematic review and meta-analysis of studies reporting potency rates after robot-assisted radical prostatectomy. Eur Urol. 2012;62(3):418–30.
10. D'Amico AV, Whittington R, Malkowicz SB, Schultz D, Blank K, Broderick GA, et al. Biochemical outcome after radical prostatectomy, external beam radiation therapy, or interstitial radiation therapy for clinically localized prostate cancer. JAMA. 1998;280(11):969–74.
11. Surcel CI, Sooriakumaran P, Briganti A, De Visschere PJ, Futterer JJ, Ghadjar P, et al. Preferences in the management of high-risk prostate cancer among urologists in Europe: results of a web-based survey. BJU Int. 2015;115(4):571–9.
12. Ham WS, Park SY, Rha KH, Kim WT, Choi YD. Robotic radical prostatectomy for patients with locally advanced prostate cancer is feasible: results of a single-institution study. J Laparoendosc Adv Surg Tech A. 2009;19(3):329–32.
13. Sagalovich D, Calaway A, Srivastava A, Sooriakumaran P, Tewari AK. Assessment of required nodal yield in a high risk cohort undergoing extended pelvic lymphadenectomy in robotic-assisted radical prostatectomy and its impact on functional outcomes. BJU Int. 2013;111(1):85–94.
14. Lavery HJ, Nabizada-Pace F, Carlucci JR, Brajtbord JS, Samadi DB. Nerve-sparing robotic prostatectomy in preoperatively high-risk patients is safe and efficacious. Urol Oncol. 2012;30(1):26–32.

15. Casey JT, Meeks JJ, Greco KA, Wu SD, Nadler RB. Outcomes of locally advanced (T3 or greater) prostate cancer in men undergoing robot-assisted laparoscopic prostatectomy. J Endourol. 2009;23(9):1519–22.
16. Yuh BE, Ruel NH, Mejia R, Wilson CM, Wilson TG. Robotic extended pelvic lymphadenectomy for intermediate- and high-risk prostate cancer. Eur Urol. 2012;61(5):1004–10.
17. Jung JH, Seo JW, Lim MS, Lee JW, Chung BH, Hong SJ, et al. Extended pelvic lymph node dissection including internal iliac packet should be performed during robot-assisted laparoscopic radical prostatectomy for high-risk prostate cancer. J Laparoendosc Adv Surg Tech A. 2012;22(8):785–90.
18. Tewari A, Sooriakumaran P, Bloch DA, Seshadri-Kreaden U, Hebert AE, Wiklund P. Positive surgical margin and perioperative complication rates of primary surgical treatments for prostate cancer: a systematic review and meta-analysis comparing retropubic, laparoscopic, and robotic prostatectomy. Eur Urol. 2012;62(1):1–15.
19. Rogers CG, Sammon JD, Sukumar S, Diaz M, Peabody J, Menon M. Robot assisted radical prostatectomy for elderly patients with high risk prostate cancer. Urol Oncol. 2013;31(2):193–7.
20. Tyritzis SI, Wallerstedt A, Steineck G, Nyberg T, Hugosson J, Bjartell A, et al. Thromboembolic complications in 3,544 patients undergoing radical prostatectomy with or without lymph node dissection. J Urol. 2015;193(1):117–25.
21. Novara G, Ficarra V. Reply to Stefano C.M. Picozzi, Cristian Ricci and Luca Carmignani's letter to the editor re: Giacomo Novara, Vincenzo Ficarra, Simone Mocellin, et al. Systematic review and meta-analysis of studies reporting oncologic outcome after robot-assisted radical prostatectomy. Eur Urol 2012;62:382–404. Eur Urol. 2013;63(2):e29–31.
22. Jayram G, Decastro GJ, Large MC, Razmaria A, Zagaja GP, Shalhav AL, et al. Robotic radical prostatectomy in patients with high-risk disease: a review of short-term outcomes from a high-volume center. J Endourol. 2011;25(3):455–7.
23. Suardi N, Dell'Oglio P, Gallina A, Gandaglia G, Buffi N, Moschini M, et al. Evaluation of positive surgical margins in patients undergoing robot-assisted and open radical prostatectomy according to preoperative risk groups. Urol Oncol. 2016;34(2):57 e1–7.
24. Harty NJ, Kozinn SI, Canes D, Sorcini A, Moinzadeh A. Comparison of positive surgical margin rates in high risk prostate cancer: open versus minimally invasive radical prostatectomy. Int Braz J Urol. 2013;39(5):639–46; discussion 47–8.
25. Lee D, Choi SK, Park J, Shim M, Kim A, Lee S, et al. Comparative analysis of oncologic outcomes for open vs. robot-assisted radical prostatectomy in high-risk prostate cancer Korean J Urol. 2015;56(8):572–9.
26. Gandaglia G, Abdollah F, Hu J, Kim S, Briganti A, Sammon JD, et al. Is robot-assisted radical prostatectomy safe in men with high-risk prostate cancer? Assessment of perioperative outcomes, positive surgical margins, and use of additional cancer treatments. J Endourol. 2014;28(7):784–91.
27. Abdollah F, Sood A, Sammon JD, Hsu L, Beyer B, Moschini M, et al. Long-term cancer control outcomes in patients with clinically high-risk prostate cancer treated with robot-assisted radical prostatectomy: results from a multi-institutional study of 1100 patients. Eur Urol. 2015;68(3):497–505.
28. Pierorazio PM, Mullins JK, Eifler JB, Voth K, Hyams ES, Han M, et al. Contemporaneous comparison of open vs minimally-invasive radical prostatectomy for high-risk prostate cancer. BJU Int. 2013;112(6):751–7.
29. Connolly SS, Cathcart PJ, Gilmore P, Kerger M, Crowe H, Peters JS, et al. Robotic radical prostatectomy as the initial step in multimodal therapy for men with high-risk localised prostate cancer: initial experience of 160 men. BJU Int. 2012;109(5):752–9.
30. Busch J, Magheli A, Leva N, Hinz S, Ferrari M, Friedersdorff F, et al. Matched comparison of outcomes following open and minimally invasive radical prostatectomy for high-risk patients. World J Urol. 2014;32(6):1411–6.
31. Menon M, Muhletaler F, Campos M, Peabody JO. Assessment of early continence after reconstruction of the periprostatic tissues in patients undergoing computer assisted (robotic) prostatectomy: results of a 2 group parallel randomized controlled trial. J Urol. 2008;180(3):1018–23.
32. Takenaka A, Tewari AK, Leung RA, Bigelow K, El-Tabey N Murakami G, et al. Preservation of the puboprostatic collar and puboperineoplasty for early recovery of urinary continence after robotic prostatectomy: anatomic basis and preliminary outcomes. Eur Urol. 2007;51(2):433–40; discussion 40.
33. Koo KC, Jung DC, Lee SH, Choi YD, Chung BH, Hong SJ, et al. Feasibility of robot-assisted radical prostatectomy for very-high risk prostate cancer: surgical and oncological outcomes in men aged >/=70 years. Prostate Int. 2014;2(3):127–32.
34. Yee DS, Narula N, Amin MB, Skarecky DW, Ahlering TE. Robot-assisted radical prostatectomy: current evaluation of surgical margins in clinically low-, intermediate-, and high-risk prostate cancer. J Endourol. 2009;23(9):1461–5.

5 Pelvic Lymphadenectomy for High-Risk Prostate Cancer

Chunwoo Lee and Dalsan You

Pelvic lymphadenectomy is considered the most reliable method of diagnosing lymph node metastases and significant adverse prognostic factor in patients with prostate cancer. In the treatment of prostate cancer, however, the clinical benefit of pelvic lymphadenectomy is debatable. In the past, it was common practice not to conduct radical prostatectomy when the lymph node positive results were seen in the frozen section during surgery [1]. Despite the recent efforts to improve clinical outcomes in patients with prostate cancer, pelvic lymphadenectomy remains controversial. Abdollah et al. recently identified that removing more lymph nodes during radical prostatectomy can significantly improve cancer-specific survival in pN1 patients [2]. Therefore, more comprehensive and accurate nodal staging through extended pelvic lymphadenectomy may indirectly [3].

Although there is no doubt that the extended lymphadenectomy increases the detection rate of lymph nodes, there is a problem with applying these principles to all patients. Because of the limitations of preoperative imaging, the nomogram is the most widely used tool when considering preoperative pelvic lymphadenectomy [3–5]. Several studies have reported the benefits of pelvic lymphadenectomy in patients with intermediate- or high-risk prostate cancer [6, 7]. However, the value of the pelvic lymphadenectomy is still controversial. These are the increasing cost, operation time, extent of surgery, the amount of bleeding, morbidities, and risk of complication due to widespread lymphadenectomy. Therefore, the goal of this chapter is to summarize the current indications, extent, robotic surgery, and complications of patients undergoing pelvic lymphadenectomy for high-risk prostate cancer.

5.1 Current Indication of Pelvic Lymphadenectomy in High-Risk Prostate Cancer

Even though pelvic lymphadenectomy is the most accurate way for assessing lymph node metastasis, the benefit of pelvic lymphadenectomy remains controversial. Although there is no doubt that the extended lymphadenectomy increases the detection rate of lymph nodes, there is a difficulty with applying these principles to all patients. Several nomograms using preoperatively available parameters have been developed to evaluate the risk of lymph node metastasis.

C. Lee
Department of Urology, Gyeongsang National University Changwon Hospital, Gyeongsang National University School of Medicine, Changwon, South Korea

D. You (✉)
Department of Urology, Asan Medical Center, University of Ulsan College of Medicine, Seoul, South Korea
e-mail: dalsanyou@amc.seoul.kr

C. S. Kim (ed.), *Management of Advanced Prostate Cancer*, https://doi.org/10.1007/978-981-10-6943-7_5

The practical role of extended pelvic lymphadenectomy is debatable. In fact, there is controversy between the several guideline committees on the indications and appropriate extent of pelvic lymphadenectomy at the time of radical prostatectomy.

The current European Association of Urology (EAU) guidelines for prostate cancer recommend performing extended pelvic lymphadenectomy in high-risk patients, as the estimated risk for lymph node metastases is 15–40% [5]. And the estimated risk of lymph node metastases over 5% (Briganti nomogram) is an indication to perform an extended pelvic lymphadenectomy [14]. National Comprehensive Cancer Network (NCCN) guideline recommends that performing an extended pelvic lymphadenectomy provides more accurate staging and may cure some patients with microscopic metastases; therefore, the surgeon considers extended pelvic lymphadenectomy in patients with 2% or more estimated risk of lymph node metastases by nomograms [15]. The American Urological Association (AUA) guideline comments that pelvic lymphadenectomy can be considered for localized prostate cancer patients during surgery and is recommended for patients with unfavorable intermediate-risk or high-risk prostate cancer (expert opinion) [16]. However, the AUA guideline does not explain about indication and extent of pelvic lymphadenectomy.

Several nomograms were developed to predict lymph node metastasis. It is decided whether or not to PLND through nomogram. Briganti et al. studied nomograms that predicted non-obturator lymph node metastases in patients with localized prostate cancer [17]. They reported that 11.1% had lymph node metastases. Of those, 3.7% had exclusive non-obturator lymph node metastases. Briganti nomogram uses preoperative factor such as PSA, clinical stage, and Gleason sum. This nomogram suggests that extended pelvic lymphadenectomy should be performed if the lymph node metastasis is greater than 5%. NCCN guideline recommends the nomogram developed at Memorial Sloan Kettering Cancer Center that uses preoperative factor such as PSA, clinical stage, and Gleason score to predict the risk of lymph node metastases at the time of surgery [4]. These nomograms may be used to avoid unnecessary extended pelvic lymphadenectomy which can increase postoperative morbidity and treatment cost in patient with high-risk prostate cancer.

5.2 Extent of Pelvic Lymphadenectomy (Limited Vs. Extended)

The more lymph nodes removed, the more accurate staging could be determined. Pelvic lymphadenectomy has become the standard for assessing lymph node metastasis. However, the optimal extent of pelvic lymphadenectomy (limited vs. extended) and candidates to select for this procedure are still points of discussion. Abdollah et al. determined that an extended pelvic lymphadenectomy should remove at least 20 lymph nodes to provide accurate lymph node staging in 90% of cases, regardless of tumor characteristics [18]. Information on the spreading sites of lymph node metastases will help to guide the management of patients with high-risk prostate cancer. However, there is insufficient evidence as to whether or not the removal of lymph nodes has therapeutic benefit in patients with high-risk prostate cancer (Table 5.1).

Much of the controversy surrounding the extent and proper candidates of pelvic lymphadenectomy is due to disagreement over the exact lymphatic drainage pattern of the prostate. About one-third of the primary lymph nodes are contained within a limited pelvic lymphadenectomy template; two-thirds of the primary nodes are contained within an extended pelvic lymphadenectomy template that includes not only the regions of external iliac vessels and obturator fossa as well as the medial and lateral region of internal iliac vessels but also the nodes overlying the common iliac vessels up to the ureteric crossing [19]. Recently, single-photon emission CT/MRI and indocyanine green injection have been used in a fashion to show that lymph node spread

Table 5.1 Summary of studies determining oncologic outcomes after pelvic lymphadenectomy in patients with high-risk prostate cancer

	Data source	Time period	Retro/pros	Study design	n	Outcome	f/u
Berglund et al. [8]	CAPSURE database	1995–2005	Retro	LPLND vs. no PLND and all risk categories	4693	No difference in 5-y bRFS in high-risk PCa (*P* = 0.45)	LPLND: 49.5 m No PLND: 31.9 M
Schiavina et al. [9]	University of Bologna, Italy	1995–2009	Retro	Effect of number of LNs removed on BFS	872	More extensive PLND positively affects the BCR-free survival in patients with PCa at intermediate and high-risk of LN metastasis (≤2)	Mean f/u: 55.8 m
Lestingi et al. [10]		2012–2016	RCT	– Intermediate- and high-risk PCa – LPLND vs. EPLND	216	No difference in biochemical recurrence (*P* = 0.39)	
Schwerfeld et al. [11]		2011–2013	RCT	– Intermediate- and high-risk PCa – LPLND vs. EPLND	244	Complication EPLND prolongs time for surgery for about 30 min more often after the extended procedure is a lymphocele	
Ku et al. [12]	Seoul National University	1997–2009	Retro	– High-risk PCa – No PLND vs. PLND	199	No significant difference in BCR-free survival rates was observed between PLND vs. no PLND (P=0.355)	37.0 months (range: 1.0–143.0)
Abdollah et al. [2]	Milan, Italy	2000–2012	Retro	– pN1 patients and EPLND – The relationship between the number of removed lymph nodes (RLNs) and cancer-specific mortality (CSM)	124	Higher number of removed LNs during RP was associated with improvement in cancer-specific survival rate ($p = 0.02$)	Mean f/u: 63 m, median f/u: 54 m
Moschini et al. [13]		1987–2012	Retro	– pT3-4p PCa patients treated with RP + EPLND – Relationship between the number of removed lymph nodes (RLNs) and cancer-specific mortality (CSM)	1586	Higher number of removed LNs during RP was associated with higher cancer-specific survival rates	Mean f/u: 80 m Median f/u: 72 m

Table 5.2 Currently available guidelines regarding the need for and the extent of pelvic lymphadenectomy in prostate cancer

Guidelines	Indication	Extent
EAU (2017)	The estimated risk of nodal metastases over 5% (Briganti nomogram)	Extended
AUA (2017)	Unfavorable intermediate-risk or high-risk prostate cancer (expert opinion)	Not indicated
NCCN (2017)	Include in patients with ≥2% predicated probability of nodal metastases by nomograms	Extended

included obturator and external/internal iliac chains [20] (Tables 5.2 and 5.3).

The extent to a pelvic lymphadenectomy during radical prostatectomy varies among centers, and the terminologies and definitions of limited and extended pelvic lymphadenectomy have not been standardized. The limited pelvic lymphadenectomy generally includes the obturator fossa and external iliac regions. The definition of an extended pelvic lymphadenectomy is not yet determined, and the exact extent of the lymphadenectomy varies for each study. Most authors agree at a minimum that an extended pelvic lymphadenectomy should include the limited template (obturator fossa and region of external iliac vessel) and lymph nodes of the common iliac artery, in addition to the hypogastric nodes [22]. Extended pelvic lymphadenectomy in EAU guideline includes removal of the nodes overlying the external iliac vessels, the nodes within the obturator fossa located around the obturator nerve, the nodes surrounding the internal iliac artery, and the nodes overlying the common iliac vessels up to the ureteral crossing. It is recommended that the removed nodes should be sent separately for pathologic analysis in each region [14]. NCCN guideline recommends that extended pelvic lymphadenectomy includes removal of all node-bearing tissue from an area bound by the anterior external iliac vein, the lateral sidewall of pelvic cavity, the medical bladder wall, the posterior pelvic floor, distal Cooper's ligament, and the proximal internal iliac artery [15] (Fig. 5.1).

5.3 Robotic Surgery and Pelvic Lymphadenectomy

Robot-assisted radical prostatectomy is a commonly performed method of operation for prostate cancer patients in recent years. Several studies reported that robot-assisted radical prostatectomy has been proven safe and oncologically effective treatment even in the high-risk prostate cancer [24–26]. However, the role of extended pelvic lymphadenectomy in robot-assisted radical prostatectomy has not been well investigated. The current EAU prostate cancer guidelines recommend performing extended pelvic lymphadenectomy in all high-risk patients, but the value of the robotic pelvic lymphadenectomy is still controversial.

Table 5.4 shows several studies of robot-assisted radical prostatectomy, pelvic lymphadenectomy and complication in patients with high-risk prostate cancer. Ham et al. reported that extended pelvic lymphadenectomy at the time of robot-assisted radical prostatectomy may be performed safely on patients with locally advanced prostate cancer without serious side effects, and there were no significant differences in estimated blood loss, operation time, initiation of a normal postoperative diet, duration of bladder catheterization, and hospital stay in locally advanced prostate cancer [27]. Sagalovich et al. suggested that patients with high-risk prostate cancer should undergo an extended pelvic lymphadenectomy with at least 13 lymph nodes removed for accurate staging. Extended pelvic lymphadenectomy with lymph node yields of 20 or more is associated with deteriorated sexual function [28]. Yuh et al. reported that robotic extended pelvic lymphadenectomy at the time of surgery can be performed safely and increases nodal yield and number of positive node [29]. Jung et al. also reported that complications associated with pelvic lymphadenectomy were not significantly different between standard pelvic lymphadenectomy and extended pelvic lymphadenectomy. Extended pelvic lymphadenectomy (including the internal iliac region) provides an accurate pathologic staging and may have oncological benefits in patients with high-risk prostate cancer [30].

Table 5.3 Studies using lymphography to define prostate lymphatic drainage

		n	Median LNs (range)	External iliac LN (%)	Obturator LN (%)	Internal iliac LN (%)	Common iliac LN (%)	Para-aortic/caval (%)	Presacral + pararectal LN (%)
Mattei et al. [19]	SPECT/CT or SPECT/MRI	34 (EPLND)	10 (3–19)	38		25	16	12	8
Inoue et al. [20]	Fluorescence navigation approach with intraoperatively injected indocyanine green	14 (LPLND)	11 (4–24)	32	43	24			
Joniau et al. [21]	SPECT/CT	74 (EPLND)		16	17	23	19	10	7

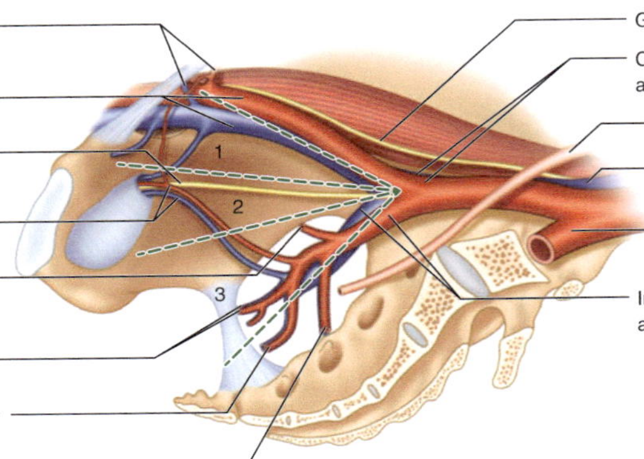

Fig. 5.1 Anatomical extent of pelvic lymphadenectomy during the radical prostatectomy. (1) External iliac, (2) obturator, and (3) internal iliac [23]

Finally, the review of Yuh et al. reported that robot-assisted radical prostatectomy appears to be a safe and effective option for selected patients with high-risk prostate cancer, particularly extended pelvic lymphadenectomy improves staging, increases detection of positive lymph nodes, and can be done safely and thoroughly robotically [26].

5.4 Clinical Outcome of Pelvic Lymphadenectomy

Several retrospective studies resulted that higher number of removed lymph nodes during radical prostatectomy was associated with higher positive lymph nodes and higher cancer-specific survival rates or BCR-free survival rates in high-risk prostate cancer [2, 9, 13]. Other studies comparing no pelvic lymphadenectomy with any type of pelvic lymphadenectomy reported that there was no difference in a 5-year bRFS or BCR-free survival rate [8, 12]. The usefulness of pelvic lymphadenectomy in high-risk prostate cancer is debatable. There was no randomized controlled trial to identify for this controversy. Recently, two randomized controlled trials that were not published reported in AUA annual meeting and annual EAU congress that they did not conclude the oncologic benefic due to short-term follow-up after surgery [10, 11] (Table 5.1).

5.5 Complication of Pelvic Lymphadenectomy

Although there is no doubt that the extended pelvic lymphadenectomy increases the detection rate of pN+ prostate cancer, there is a difficulty with applying these principles to all patients. Several studies reported that extended pelvic lymphadenectomy prolonged surgical time intraoperative complications, bleeding, and hospital stay compared to limited pelvic lymphadenectomy. In addition, complications of pelvic lymphadenectomy for prostate cancer include thromboembolic events (deep venous thrombosis), neurologic injury, ureteral injury, vascular injury, and lower extremity edema. In some study, lymphocele development was the most common complication after extended pelvic lymphadenectomy. Clinically significant lymphocele development after pelvic lymphadenectomy is the most common complication, with an estimated incidence between 0.8% and 9.0% in limited pelvic lymphadenectomy and between 2.4% and 10.3% in extended pelvic lymphadenectomy [32]. Keegan et al. reported that extent of lymphadenectomy, prior radiation, excessive use of cautery, use of heparin, infection, and surgical technique have been implicated as risk factors of lymphocele [32]. Heidenreich et al. suggest several principles to decrease postoperative complications after pelvic lymphadenectomy: (i) all lateral lymphatic vessels in the

Table 5.4 Summary of high-risk robot-assisted radical prostatectomy series: pelvic lymphadenectomy and complications

	Cases, *n*	LN dissection template, %	% of patients with LN dissection (%)	Median or mean LN yield	LN positive rate, %	pT2, *n* (%)	Positive margins, %	Lymphocele, %	Operative time, min
Ham et al. [27]	121	Extended	100	18.6	24.0	21 (17.4)	48.8	2.5	214
Jayram et al. [31]	148	Standard	100	15	12.3	67 (46.0)	20.5	1.4	–
Sagalovich et al. [28]	82	Extended	100	13	13.4	–	12.0	2.4	111
Yuh et al. [29]	30	Extended	100	22	33.3	9 (30.0)	26.7	6.6	186
Jung et al. [30]	200	Standard: 78/ Extended: 23	100	Standard: 15/ Extended: 24	Overall: 9/ Extended: 22	96 (48.0)	41.5	3.0	190

external artery are reserved, (ii) the distal end of the lymphatic vessels is either clipped or ligated with small clips applying a higher pressure to the lymphatic vessels than large clips, (iii) two drains are located in each side of the pelvic cavity, (iv) the drains are removed when the drainage amount is <50 mL/d, and (v) low-molecular-weight heparin is injected into the upper arm [33]. Lebeis et al. also suggested the peritoneal flap interposition as the novel technique to prevent lymphocele after transperitoneal robotic pelvic lymphadenectomy that was the peritoneal interposition flap formed by advancing and rotating of a peritoneum around the both sides of the bladder [34].

5.6 Summary

- Extended pelvic lymphadenectomy is the most accurate way for assessing lymph node metastasis when compared to limited pelvic lymphadenectomy, but the benefit of extended pelvic lymphadenectomy remains controversial.
- The increased risk of nodal metastases by nomogram considers extended pelvic lymphadenectomy.
- Robotic extended or limited pelvic lymphadenectomy can be performed safely.
- Lymphocele development is the most common complication after extended or limited pelvic lymphadenectomy.

References

1. Gerber GS, Thisted RA, Chodak GW, Schroder FH, Frohmuller HG, Scardino PT, et al. Results of radical prostatectomy in men with locally advanced prostate cancer: multi-institutional pooled analysis. Eur Urol. 1997;32(4):385–90.
2. Abdollah F, Gandaglia G, Suardi N, Capitanio U, Salonia A, Nini A, et al. More extensive pelvic lymph node dissection improves survival in patients with node-positive prostate cancer. Eur Urol. 2015;67(2):212–9.
3. Makarov DV, Trock BJ, Humphreys EB, Mangold LA, Walsh PC, Epstein JI, et al. Updated nomogram to predict pathologic stage of prostate cancer given prostate-specific antigen level, clinical stage, and biopsy Gleason score (Partin tables) based on cases from 2000 to 2005. Urology. 2007;69(6):1095–101.
4. Cagiannos I, Karakiewicz P, Eastham JA, Ohori M, Rabbani F, Gerigk C, et al. A preoperative nomogram identifying decreased risk of positive pelvic lymph nodes in patients with prostate cancer. J Urol. 2003;170(5):1798–803.
5. Briganti A, Larcher A, Abdollah F, Capitanio U, Gallina A, Suardi N, et al. Updated nomogram predicting lymph node invasion in patients with prostate cancer undergoing extended pelvic lymph node dissection: the essential importance of percentage of positive cores. Eur Urol. 2012;61(3):480–7.
6. Joslyn SA, Konety BR. Impact of extent of lymphadenectomy on survival after radical prostatectomy for prostate cancer. Urology. 2006;68(1):121–5.
7. von Bodman C, Godoy G, Chade DC, Cronin A, Tafe LJ, Fine SW, et al. Predicting biochemical recurrence-free survival for patients with positive pelvic lymph nodes at radical prostatectomy. J Urol. 2010;184(1):143–8.
8. Berglund RK, Sadetsky N, DuChane J, Carroll PR, Klein EA. Limited pelvic lymph node dissection at the time of radical prostatectomy does not affect 5-year failure rates for low, intermediate and high risk prostate cancer: results from CaPSURE. J Urol. 2007;177(2):526–9; discussion 9–30.
9. Schiavina R, Manferrari F, Garofalo M, Bertaccini A, Vagnoni V, Guidi M, et al. The extent of pelvic lymph node dissection correlates with the biochemical recurrence rate in patients with intermediate- and high-risk prostate cancer. BJU Int. 2011;108(8):1262–8.
10. Lestingi JFP, Pontes Jr J, Borges LL, Ravanini J, Guglielmetti GB, Cordeiro MD, et al. Pd43-06 extended vs limited pelvic lymphadenectomy during radical prostatectomy for intermediate- and high-risk prostate cancer: a prospective randomized trial. J Urol. 2015;193(4):e893-e4.
11. Schwerfeld-Bohr J, Kaemper M, Krege S, Heidenreich A. 270 Prospective randomized multicenter study comparing limited vs extended pelvic lymphadenectomy in intermediate and high risk prostate cancer: comparison of complications (SEAL, AUO AP 55/09). Eur Urol Suppl. 2014;13(1):e270.
12. Ku JH, Jeong CW, Park YH, Cho MC, Kwak C, Kim HH. Biochemical recurrence after radical prostatectomy with or without pelvic lymphadenectomy in Korean men with high-risk prostate cancer. Jpn J Clin Oncol. 2011;41(5):656–62.
13. Moschini M, Fossati N, Abdollah F, Gandaglia G, Cucchiara V, Dell'Oglio P, et al. Determinants of long-term survival of patients with locally advanced prostate cancer: the role of extensive pelvic lymph node dissection. Prostate Cancer Prostatic Dis. 2016;19(1):63–7.
14. Mottet N, Bellmunt J, Bolla M, Briers E, Cumberbatch MG, De Santis M, et al. EAU-ESTRO-SIOG guidelines on prostate cancer. Part 1: screening, diagnosis, and local treatment with curative intent. Eur Urol. 2017;71(4):618–29.

15. Mohler JL, Antonarakis ES, Armstrong AJ, Bahnson RR, Clark C, D'Amico AV, et al. Prostate cancer, version 2.2017. J Natl Compr Canc Netw. 2017;11:1471–9.
16. Sanda MG, Chen RC, Crispino T, Freedland S, Greene K, Klotz LH, et al. Clinically localized prostate cancer: AUA/ASTRO/SUO guideline. Part I: risk stratification, shared decision making, and care options. J Urol. 2017. pii: S0022-5347(17)78003-2. https://doi.org/10.1016/j.juro.2017.11.095. [Epub ahead of print].
17. Briganti A, Chun FK, Salonia A, Zanni G, Gallina A, Deho F, et al. A nomogram for staging of exclusive nonobturator lymph node metastases in men with localized prostate cancer. Eur Urol. 2007;51(1):112–9; discussion 9–20.
18. Abdollah F, Sun M, Thuret R, Jeldres C, Tian Z, Briganti A, et al. Lymph node count threshold for optimal pelvic lymph node staging in prostate cancer. Int J Urol. 2012;19(7):645–51.
19. Mattei A, Fuechsel FG, Bhatta Dhar N, Warncke SH, Thalmann GN, Krause T, et al. The template of the primary lymphatic landing sites of the prostate should be revisited: results of a multimodality mapping study. Eur Urol. 2008;53(1):118–25.
20. Inoue S, Shiina H, Arichi N, Mitsui Y, Hiraoka T, Wake K, et al. Identification of lymphatic pathway involved in the spreading of prostate cancer by fluorescence navigation approach with intraoperatively injected indocyanine green. Can Urol Assoc J. 2011;5(4):254–9.
21. Joniau S, Van den Bergh L, Lerut E, Deroose CM, Haustermans K, Oyen R, et al. Mapping of pelvic lymph node metastases in prostate cancer. Eur Urol. 2013;63(3):450–8.
22. Bader P, Burkhard FC, Markwalder R, Studer UE. Is a limited lymph node dissection an adequate staging procedure for prostate cancer? J Urol. 2002;168(2):514–8.
23. Burkhard FC, Bader P, Schneider E, Markwalder R, Studer UE. Reliability of preoperative values to determine the need for lymphadenectomy in patients with prostate cancer and meticulous lymph node dissection. Eur Urol. 2002;42(2):84–90; discussion 2.
24. Suardi N, Dell'Oglio P, Gallina A, Gandaglia G, Buffi N, Moschini M, et al. Evaluation of positive surgical margins in patients undergoing robot-assisted and open radical prostatectomy according to preoperative risk groups. Urol Oncol. 2016;34(2):57.e1–7.
25. Abdollah F, Sood A, Sammon JD, Hsu L, Beyer B, Moschini M, et al. Long-term cancer control outcomes in patients with clinically high-risk prostate cancer treated with robot-assisted radical prostatectomy: results from a multi-institutional study of 1100 patients. Eur Urol. 2015;68(3):497–505.
26. Yuh B, Artibani W, Heidenreich A, Kimm S, Menon M, Novara G, et al. The role of robot-assisted radical prostatectomy and pelvic lymph node dissection in the management of high-risk prostate cancer: a systematic review. Eur Urol. 2014;65(5):918–27.
27. Ham WS, Park SY, Rha KH, Kim WT, Choi YD. Robotic radical prostatectomy for patients with locally advanced prostate cancer is feasible: results of a single-institution study. J Laparoendosc Adv Surg Tech A. 2009;19(3):329–32.
28. Sagalovich D, Calaway A, Srivastava A, Sooriakumaran P, Tewari AK. Assessment of required nodal yield in a high risk cohort undergoing extended pelvic lymphadenectomy in robotic-assisted radical prostatectomy and its impact on functional outcomes. BJU Int. 2013;111(1):85–94.
29. Yuh BE, Ruel NH, Mejia R, Wilson CM, Wilson TG. Robotic extended pelvic lymphadenectomy for intermediate- and high-risk prostate cancer. Eur Urol. 2012;61(5):1004–10.
30. Jung JH, Seo JW, Lim MS, Lee JW, Chung BH, Hong SJ, et al. Extended pelvic lymph node dissection including internal iliac packet should be performed during robot-assisted laparoscopic radical prostatectomy for high-risk prostate cancer. Journal of Laparoendosc Adv Surg Tech A. 2012;22(8):785–90.
31. Jayram G, Decastro GJ, Large MC, Razmaria A, Zagaja GP, Shalhav AL, et al. Robotic radical prostatectomy in patients with high-risk disease: a review of short-term outcomes from a high-volume center. J Endourol. 2011;25(3):455–7.
32. Keegan KA, Cookson MS. Complications of pelvic lymph node dissection for prostate cancer. Curr Urol Rep. 2011;12(3):203–8.
33. Heidenreich A, Ohlmann CH, Polyakov S. Anatomical Extent of Pelvic Lymphadenectomy in Patients Undergoing Radical Prostatectomy. Eur Urol. 2007;52(1):29–37.
34. Lebeis C, Canes D, Sorcini A, Moinzadeh A. Novel technique prevents lymphoceles after transperitoneal robotic-assisted pelvic lymph node dissection: peritoneal flap interposition. Urology. 2015;85(6):1505–9.

6 Adjuvant Therapy in Locally Advanced Prostate Cancer

Jae Heon Kim

6.1 Introduction

Historically, RP has been considered the gold standard for treatment of localized PCa (even in cases of low- or intermediate-risk PCa). However, RP still retains a somewhat controversial role when considered as a potential therapeutic option to treat locally advanced PCa. RT and HT are usually used as primary and adjuvant therapies, respectively. Unlike the standard role of RP and RT (as generally accepted and established standardized treatment for localized PCa), treatment plans for locally advanced PCa still reside in a gray zone and without any definite treatment protocols or strategies awaiting implementation.

Nowadays, the expanded role of RP has widened to include locally advanced PCa or high-risk PCa patients [1–6]. To date, there are only three treatment modalities as an adjuvant treatment method including early adjuvant or late salvage RT or HT. As basic treatment options currently available to address locally advanced PCa, RT, RP, and HT could be prescribed and administered to patients according to need and by clinicians according to preference based in experience in outcome [7, 8]. However, regarding adjuvant treatment modalities, limited academic evidence existed before now, and accordingly, current guidelines do not provide clear direction with regard to available and potentially effective treatment modalities for locally advanced PCa [9].

6.2 Definition

The definition of "locally advanced PCa" is "invasion of localized cancer into the prostatic capsule, with invasion of per-capsular tissue, bladder neck or seminal vesicle (SV)." However, in locally advanced PCa, there is no lymph node invasion or metastasis to more distant body parts. Clinical staging for locally advanced PCa could be T3-T4 N0 M0 PCa. Indeed, the current definition of locally advanced PCa has a tendency to include any patient with positive lymph nodes (LNs), regardless of the actual presence or absence of evidence of invasion of the prostate capsule (which is sometimes confused by high-risk or high-grade PCa). However, it is clear that "locally advanced PCa" has a different definition in the context of cases of high-risk or high-grade PCa. Recently, high PSA was detected and identified as an independent predictor for LN metastasis in high-grade PCa [10]. High-grade PCa is called "poorly differentiated PCa with Gleason scores from 8 to 10." In this chapter, suggested treatment options would be described by locally advanced PCa itself and additional information

J. H. Kim
Department of Urology, Soonchunhyang University Hospital, Soonchunhyang University College of Medicine, Seoul, South Korea

C. S. Kim (ed.), *Management of Advanced Prostate Cancer*,
https://doi.org/10.1007/978-981-10-6943-7_6

about suggested treatment options according to risk degree of PCa; National Comprehensive Cancer Network (NCCN) guidelines could provide helpful information.

6.3 General Guidelines by NCCN

In NCCN guidelines, locally advanced PCa could be divided into four subgroups for adjuvant treatment: "low risk," "intermediate risk," "high risk," and "very high risk." Regardless of low-risk or high-risk PCa, in accordance with various test results, namely, no high-risk features or cancer in lymph node, high-risk features but no cancer in lymph nodes, and cancer in lymph nodes, appropriate treatment options could be suggested which are observation HT or RT, to include external beam radiation therapy (EBRT). Table 6.1 summarizes the treatment options according to various clinical conditions in from low-risk PCa to very high-risk PCa.

6.4 RP for Locally Advanced PCa

Traditionally, the classic role of RP in locally advanced PCa was limited because of its inability to achieve complete surgical resection of tumor and of expected higher rate of positive surgical margin or LN metastasis [7, 8]. Although some nomograms have been developed to predict the pathologic stage of PCa and SV invasion at RP [11, 12], to date, the application of those nomograms is not realistic due to common pitfalls including over-staging of T2, over-grading, and under-staging of T4.

RP in locally advanced T3 PCa involves a radical prostate extirpation, including an extended lymph node dissection (LND), clean apical dissection, neurovascular bundle resection at the tumor involving side, complete resection of the SV, and wide resection of the bladder neck (BN) [13, 14]. Due to skill development and also emergence of robotic RP, positive surgical margin (PSM) has been improved by 75% in 1987–1994,

Table 6.1 Adjuvant treatment options according to risk grade of PCa and test results after RP or RT

Risk grade of PCa	Primary treatment	Test results	Adjuvant treatment options #1	Adjuvant treatment options #2
Low risk	After RP	No high-risk features or cancer in lymph node	Observation	
		High-risk features but no cancer in lymph node	EBRT	Observation
		Cancer in lymph node	ADT with or without EBRT	Observation
Intermediate risk	After RP	No high-risk features or cancer in lymph node	Observation	
		High-risk features but no cancer in lymph node	EBRT	Observation
		Cancer in lymph node	ADT with or without EBRT	Observation
High risk	After RP	No high-risk features or cancer in lymph node	Observation	
		High-risk features but no cancer in lymph node	EBRT	Observation
		Cancer in lymph node	ADT with or without EBRT	Observation
	After RT		ADT, continue to complete 2–3 years of ADT	
Very high risk	After RP	No high-risk features or cancer in lymph node	Observation	
		High-risk features but no cancer in lymph node	EBRT	Observation
		Cancer in lymph node	ADT with or without EBRT	Observation
	After RT		ADT, continue to complete 2–3 years of ADT	

42% in 1995–1999, and 10.4% in 2000–2004) [14]. Extended LND is mainly indicated in locally advanced PCa and high-grade PCa, due to the heightened possibility of LN involvement by cancer. In cT3 PCa, the expected node positive rate is between 27% and 41% [15]. Nowadays, RP has more extended role in the treatment of locally advanced PCa in US [1–6]. Johnstone et al. reported that those PCa patients with cT4 who underwent RP ($n = 72$) had a better survival rate than those who underwent HT alone or RT alone, which was similar to the survival of those patients who received RT plus HT [16].

6.5 RT in Locally Advanced PCa

In contrast to recent reporting to the effect that RP could provide superior long-term survival to RT in localized PCa [17], RT still represents the treatment of choice in diagnosed cases of locally advanced PCa [18]. However, a recent study supports a superior role as a significant part of the framework of a multimodality therapeutic setting for treating locally advanced PCa [19]. Basically, there are three basic treatment options for framework including RP, RT, and HT in locally advanced PCa [9]. Although RP has a superior clinical outcome on posttreatment incontinence to RT, there are no superior clinical outcomes on other side effects (which include erectile dysfunction, acute and late genitourinary, or gastrointestinal toxicity) [9, 20]. Moreover, to date, there are no existing studies which served to compare the health-related QoL in RP and RT.

6.6 Multimodality Treatment in Locally Advanced PCa

To date there have been no randomized trials to compare the clinical outcomes serving to measure the relative efficacy of RT when compared to RP as an initial treatment option for locally advanced PCa. In a study by Ward et al. [15] (a 15-year arc observational study), it was reported that eventually, 78% of patients required adjuvant or salvage RT or HT after RP as a basic framework treatment option in cT3 patients. Whereas Hsu et al. reported that eventually, 56% of patients of unilateral cT3a disease who underwent RP needed adjuvant or salvage treatment [13]. These studies revealed excellent 5–15-year overall survival (OS) rates and cancer-specific survival (CSS) rates, which are closely comparable to the OS and CSS of cT2 patients. In addition, the Ward and Hsu studies reported similar survival rates: 95% and 98.7% for 5-year CSS, respectively, and 90% and 91.6% for 10-year CSS, respectively, after adjuvant or salvage treatment [13, 15]. As well, Ward et al. [15] reported that 15-year CSS rate mark to be about 79%.

There are two randomized clinical trials to compare the clinical outcome between solitary RP and RP plus adjuvant radiotherapy in the treatment of locally advanced PCa. Bolla et al. [21] reported that patients with adjuvant RT group yielded superior clinical outcomes, which included biochemical progression-free survival to solitary RP group (BPFS) (74% and 52.6%, respectively, $p < 0.0001$). However, there was no significant difference in CSS at the time of their extended follow-ups. The other randomized trial, by Thompson et al. [22], reported that adjuvant RT after RP showed evidence of superior clinical outcomes, when compared to RP alone relative to PSA relapse rates (median PSA relapse-free survival was 10.3 years for adjuvant RT group and 3.1 years for solitary RP group, $p < 0.001$) and disease recurrence (median recurrence-free survival was 13.3 years for adjuvant RT group and 9.9 years for solitary RT group, respectively, $p < 0.001$).

Recently, Fahmy et al. reported in their meta-analysis that there is a superiority of both RP and RT over HT as the base framework treatment options for locally advanced PCa [23]. Moreover, RP could significantly improve survival outcomes when compared to any other base framework treatment options including RT and HT. To date, adjuvant RT could significantly improve the outcome of base framework treatment of RP, but, yet adjuvant HT after RP still requires validation by documented long-term survival numbers. EAU guidelines also recommend not to offer adjuvant HT after RP for no LN-positive patients

[9]. Moreover, recently, there have been various reports that HT, itself, has a close association with OS through its direct or indirect effect on cardiovascular disease, diabetes, osteoporosis, dementia, and so on [6, 24–26]. However, there is a significant beneficial clinical outcome through adjuvant HT after RT in high-risk or high-grade localized PCa [27].

6.7 Adjuvant Postoperative RT

There are two generally accepted, established modalities for postoperative radiotherapy including adjuvant RT and salvage RT. There are three randomized clinical trials which reported the efficacy of adjuvant RT after RP for high-risk PCa patients [21, 28, 29]. Among these high-risk PCa patients, quite a few of them could be defined as "locally advanced PCa patients." In the USA, there is a published guideline designed and developed by urology/oncology teams which specifies that adjuvant RT after RP should be performed in those patients with prominent locally advanced findings at RP (including seminal vesicle invasion or extracapsular extension or positive surgical margin) to prevent biochemical and clinical recurrence or progression [30]. They also recommended to consider short- and long-term adverse events of RT and to consider adjuvant postoperative RT. However and with regard to the actual timing of adjuvant RT in locally advanced PCa, there remained some residual controversy due to the risk of overtreatment and its related complications.

To date, there has been only one randomized study involving controlled clinical trials with RCT positive clinical outcomes with regard to issues of distant metastasis and long-term survival after adjuvant RT [28]. Other randomized controlled trials [21, 29] (including the EORTC trial) have reported only improved clinical outcome in biochemical failure rate after adjuvant RT. However, in these trials, there exist some limitations with regard to the validity of the biochemical failure-free survival rate as a surrogate endpoint.

Recently, Ku et al. reported in their meta-analysis that the adjuvant RT patient group showed superior clinical outcomes when compared to salvage RT groups, in relation to the specific issue of long-term survival [31]. They reported superiority in terms of the biochemical recurrence-free survival period of 5 years and progression-free survival period of 5 years. However, there was no appreciable benefit in terms of OS at the 5- and 10-year marks. To date, it is recommended that prompt adjuvant RT after RP be performed in diagnosed cases of locally advanced RP because in those cases of biochemical relapse by reason of deferred adjuvant treatment, there might well be a corresponding decrease in survival rate.

6.8 Adjuvant HT

Several randomized, controlled trials have confirmed that the implementation of RP, or RT plus HT, yields superior clinical outcomes when compared to courses of care consisting of RP or RT alone (especially in intermediate- or high-risk PCa) [32–34].

Recently, Zhou et al. [35] reported in their meta-analysis (which included nine randomized controlled trials and a total of 4743 patients) that there exist seven randomized controlled trials to compare the clinical outcomes between courses of RT plus short-term (not more than 6 months) adjuvant HT and RT plus long-term (more than 6 months) adjuvant HT and two randomized clinical trials that RP plus short-term adjuvant HT and RP plus long-term adjuvant HT.

This meta-analysis ultimately served to demonstrate no significant difference in OS and disease-free survival rates, but the long-term HT was superior to short-term HT as an adjuvant treatment in biochemical failure rate, clinical progression rate, and prostate cancer-specific mortality rates. However, adverse events possibly connected to long-term HT were seen less frequently in cases of short-term HT. In this meta-analysis, in the comparison of RP plus short-term HT and RP plus long-term HT, HT was not usually performed as adjuvant but rather as neo-adjuvant treatment [36, 37].

For neo-adjuvant HT issue, Roach et al. have reported (in their RTOG 9413 trial) that there was no significant difference of survival benefit between neo-adjuvant HT and adjuvant HT. This was, historically, the first study to seriously investigate this issue, with head-to-head comparison trials [38]. Based on the long-time follow-up contemporary studies (including RTOG 8513 and RTOG 8610), neo-adjuvant HT and adjuvant HT showed similar OS in relation to diagnosed cases of locally advanced PCa [33, 34].

6.9 Adjuvant Chemotherapy

Adjuvant chemotherapy after RP in high-risk PCa is still a controversial issue. Lin et al. [39] reported that early adjuvant chemotherapy using docetaxel and prednisolone given to those patients with high-risk PCa who undergone RP without HT showed well-tolerated response; however, it did not guarantee the statistical superiority in progression-free survival. Several issues are still being existed to be more clarified about the stratified indication among high-risk PCa.

6.10 Summary

To date, RP plus adjuvant RT and primary RT plus adjuvant HT have been thought to represent the optimal and most appropriate treatment modalities for locally advanced PCa without metastasis and the courses of care thought to best assure the best survival outcome. Further studies are necessary to further explore and evaluate whether, in patients diagnosed with clinically positive LNs (high-risk PCa), head-to-head clinical trials are needed between RP with extended lymphadenectomy for the base framework plus adjuvant RT and RP with extended lymphadenectomy alone or between RP with extended lymphadenectomy for base framework plus adjuvant RT and total pelvic RT plus adjuvant HT. It is thought that long-term HT may be even more beneficial, especially in high-risk PCa, but to date there has been no academic evidence to illuminate the potential benefits of long-term adjuvant HT after RP. During HT, clinicians should probably focus more on the possible adverse events, which could incidentally and inevitably compromise the OS of the PCa patients.

References

1. Berglund RK, Jones JS, Ulchaker JC, Fergany A, Gill I, Kaouk J, et al. Radical prostatectomy as primary treatment modality for locally advanced prostate cancer: a prospective analysis. Urology. 2006;67(6):1253–6.
2. Carver BS, Bianco FJ Jr, Scardino PT, Eastham JA. Long-term outcome following radical prostatectomy in men with clinical stage T3 prostate cancer. J Urol. 2006;176(2):564–8.
3. Freedland SJ, Partin AW, Humphreys EB, Mangold LA, Walsh PC. Radical prostatectomy for clinical stage T3a disease. Cancer. 2007;109(7):1273–8.
4. Loeb S, Smith ND, Roehl KA, Catalona WJ. Intermediate-term potency, continence, and survival outcomes of radical prostatectomy for clinically high-risk or locally advanced prostate cancer. Urology. 2007;69(6):1170–5.
5. Masterson TA, Pettus JA, Middleton RG, Stephenson RA. Isolated seminal vesicle invasion imparts better outcomes after radical retropubic prostatectomy for clinically localized prostate cancer: prognostic stratification of pt3b disease by nodal and margin status. Urology. 2005;66(1):152–5.
6. Secin FP, Bianco FJ Jr, Vickers AJ, Reuter V, Wheeler T, Fearn PA, et al. Cancer-specific survival and predictors of prostate-specific antigen recurrence and survival in patients with seminal vesicle invasion after radical prostatectomy. Cancer. 2006;106(11):2369–75.
7. Boccon-Gibod L, Bertaccini A, Bono AV, Dev Sarmah B, Holtl W, Mottet N, et al. Management of locally advanced prostate cancer: a European consensus. Int J Clin Pract. 2003;57(3):187–94.
8. Hodgson D, Warde P, Gospodarowicz M. The management of locally advanced prostate cancer. Urol Oncol. 1998;4(1):3–12.
9. Heidenreich A, Bastian PJ, Bellmunt J, Bolla M, Joniau S, van der Kwast T, et al. EAU guidelines on prostate cancer. Part 1: screening, diagnosis, and local treatment with curative intent-update 2013. Eur Urol. 2014;65(1):124–37.
10. Porcaro AB, De Luyk N, Corsi P, Sebben M, Tafuri A, Processali T, et al. Clinical factors predicting bilateral lymph node invasion in high-risk prostate cancer. Urol Int. 2017;99:392–9.

11. Gallina A, Chun FK, Briganti A, Shariat SF, Montorsi F, Salonia A, et al. Development and split-sample validation of a nomogram predicting the probability of seminal vesicle invasion at radical prostatectomy. Eur Urol. 2007;52(1):98–105.
12. Joniau S, Hsu CY, Lerut E, Van Baelen A, Haustermans K, Roskams T, et al. A pretreatment table for the prediction of final histopathology after radical prostatectomy in clinical unilateral T3a prostate cancer. Eur Urol. 2007;51(2):388–94. discussion 95-6.
13. Hsu CY, Joniau S, Oyen R, Roskams T, Van Poppel H. Outcome of surgery for clinical unilateral T3a prostate cancer: a single-institution experience. Eur Urol. 2007;51(1):121–8. discussion 8-9
14. Hsu CY, Joniau S, Roskams T, Oyen R, Van Poppel H. Comparing results after surgery in patients with clinical unilateral T3a prostate cancer treated with or without neoadjuvant androgen-deprivation therapy. BJU Int. 2007;99(2):311–4.
15. Ward JF, Slezak JM, Blute ML, Bergstralh EJ, Zincke H. Radical prostatectomy for clinically advanced (cT3) prostate cancer since the advent of prostate-specific antigen testing: 15-year outcome. BJU Int. 2005;95(6):751–6.
16. Johnstone PA, Ward KC, Goodman M, Assikis V, Petros JA. Radical prostatectomy for clinical T4 prostate cancer. Cancer. 2006;106(12):2603–9.
17. Wallis CJD, Saskin R, Choo R, Herschorn S, Kodama RT, Satkunasivam R, et al. Surgery versus radiotherapy for clinically-localized prostate cancer: a systematic review and meta-analysis. Eur Urol. 2016;70(1):21–30.
18. Mason MD, Parulekar WR, Sydes MR, Brundage M, Kirkbride P, Gospodarowicz M, et al. Final report of the intergroup randomized study of combined androgen-deprivation therapy plus radiotherapy versus androgen-deprivation therapy alone in locally advanced prostate cancer. J Clin Oncol. 2015;33(19):2143–50.
19. Yamamoto S, Kawakami S, Yonese J, Fujii Y, Urakami S, Kitsukawa S, et al. Long-term oncological outcome in men with T3 prostate cancer: radical prostatectomy versus external-beam radiation therapy at a single institution. Int J Clin Oncol. 2014;19(6):1085–91.
20. Raina R, Agarwal A, Goyal KK, Jackson C, Ulchaker J, Angermeier K, et al. Long-term potency after iodine-125 radiotherapy for prostate cancer and role of sildenafil citrate. Urology. 2003;62(6):1103–8.
21. Bolla M, van Poppel H, Tombal B, Vekemans K, Da Pozzo L, de Reijke TM, et al. Postoperative radiotherapy after radical prostatectomy for high-risk prostate cancer: long-term results of a randomised controlled trial (EORTC trial 22911). Lancet. 2012;380(9858):2018–27.
22. Thompson IM Jr, Tangen CM, Paradelo J, Lucia MS, Miller G, Troyer D, et al. Adjuvant radiotherapy for pathologically advanced prostate cancer: a randomized clinical trial. JAMA. 2006;296(19):2329–35.
23. Fahmy O, Khairul-Asri MG, Hadi S, Gakis G, Stenzl A. The role of radical prostatectomy and radiotherapy in treatment of locally advanced prostate cancer: a systematic review and meta-analysis. Urol Int. 2017;99:249–56.
24. Crawford ED, Schally AV, Pinthus JH, Block NL, Rick FG, Garnick MB, et al. The potential role of follicle-stimulating hormone in the cardiovascular, metabolic, skeletal, and cognitive effects associated with androgen deprivation therapy. Urol Oncol. 2017;35(5):183–91.
25. Gupta D, Salmane C, Slovin S, Steingart RM. Cardiovascular complications of androgen deprivation therapy for prostate cancer. Curr Treat Options Cardiovasc Med. 2017;19(8):61.
26. Keating NL. Type of androgen deprivation therapy and risk of cardiovascular disease. Eur Urol. 2017;72:929–30.
27. Bolla M, Van Tienhoven G, Warde P, Dubois JB, Mirimanoff RO, Storme G, et al. External irradiation with or without long-term androgen suppression for prostate cancer with high metastatic risk: 10-year results of an EORTC randomised study. Lancet Oncol. 2010;11(11):1066–73.
28. Thompson IM, Tangen CM, Paradelo J, Lucia MS, Miller G, Troyer D, et al. Adjuvant radiotherapy for pathological T3N0M0 prostate cancer significantly reduces risk of metastases and improves survival: long-term followup of a randomized clinical trial. J Urol. 2009;181(3):956–62.
29. Wiegel T, Bartkowiak D, Bottke D, Bronner C, Steiner U, Siegmann A, et al. Adjuvant radiotherapy versus wait-and-see after radical prostatectomy: 10-year follow-up of the ARO 96-02/AUO AP 09/95 trial. Eur Urol. 2014;66(2):243–50.
30. Thompson IM, Valicenti RK, Albertsen P, Davis BJ, Goldenberg SL, Hahn C, et al. Adjuvant and salvage radiotherapy after prostatectomy: AUA/ASTRO guideline. J Urol. 2013;190(2):441–9.
31. Ku JY, Lee CH, Ha HK. Long-term oncologic outcomes of postoperative adjuvant versus salvage radiotherapy in prostate cancer: systemic review and meta-analysis of 5-year and 10-year follow-up data. Korean J Urol. 2015;56(11):735–41.
32. Denham JW, Wilcox C, Joseph D, Spry NA, Lamb DS, Tai KH, et al. Quality of life in men with locally advanced prostate cancer treated with leuprorelin and radiotherapy with or without zoledronic acid (TROG 03.04 RADAR): secondary endpoints from a randomised phase 3 factorial trial. Lancet Oncol. 2012;13(12):1260–70.
33. Pilepich MV, Winter K, Lawton CA, Krisch RE, Wolkov HB, Movsas B, et al. Androgen suppression adjuvant to definitive radiotherapy in prostate carcinoma: long-term results of phase III RTOG 85-31. Int J Radiat Oncol Biol Phys. 2005;61(5):1285–90.
34. Roach M 3rd, Bae K, Speight J, Wolkov HB, Rubin P, Lee RJ, et al. Short-term neoadjuvant androgen deprivation therapy and external-beam radiotherapy for locally advanced prostate cancer: long-term results of RTOG 8610. J Clin Oncol. 2008;26(4):585–91.
35. Zhou ZR, Zhu XD, Xia J, Zou ZY, Qu S, Zeng XT, et al. Short-term versus long-term hormone therapy

plus radiotherapy or prostatectomy for prostate cancer: a systematic review and meta-analysis. J Cancer Res Clin Oncol. 2013;139(5):783–96.

36. Gleave ME, Goldenberg SL, Chin JL, Warner J, Saad F, Klotz LH, et al. Randomized comparative study of 3 versus 8-month neoadjuvant hormonal therapy before radical prostatectomy: biochemical and pathological effects. J Urol. 2001;166(2):500–6. discussion 6-7.
37. Pu XY, Wang XH, Wu YL, Wang HP. Comparative study of the impact of 3- versus 8-month neoadjuvant hormonal therapy on outcome of laparoscopic radical prostatectomy. J Cancer Res Clin Oncol. 2007;133(8):555–62.
38. Roach M 3rd, DeSilvio M, Lawton C, Uhl V, Machtay M, Seider MJ, et al. Phase III trial comparing whole-pelvic versus prostate-only radiotherapy and neoadjuvant versus adjuvant combined androgen suppression: Radiation Therapy Oncology Group 9413. J Clin Oncol. 2003;21(10):1904–11.
39. Montgomery B, Lavori P, Garzotto M, Lee K, Brophy M, Thaneemit-Chen S, et al. Veterans Affairs Cooperative Studies Program study 553: chemotherapy after prostatectomy, a phase III randomized study of prostatectomy versus prostatectomy with adjuvant docetaxel for patients with high-risk, localized prostate cancer. Urology. 2008;72(3):474–80.

7 Role of Radical Prostatectomy in the Management of Metastatic Prostate Cancer

Hyeong Dong Yuk and Cheol Kwak

Most of prostate cancers diagnosed at localized disease were regarded as less aggressive malignancy because of their indolent course; nonetheless, metastatic prostate cancer is still lethal. The 5-year survival rate approaches 100% for patients within localized disease, but it declined to 28% for metastatic disease [1]. About 4% of prostate cancer present metastasis on initial diagnosis, and about one-third of localized prostate cancer patients experience disease progression [2, 3].

The standard treatment for patients with metastatic prostate cancer is systemic therapy based on androgen axis control [1, 4, 5]. Conventionally, local therapy such as radical prostatectomy (RP) or radiation therapy (RT) places only for palliative arm in metastatic prostate cancer management. Unlike other malignancies, cytoreductive RP dose is not recommended because of lack of evidences on benefit and potential harm. However, recent advance in surgical procedure and clinical evidence suggests potential role of RP in advanced disease even for the metastatic prostate cancer [6–9]. There are still none of level 1 evidence supporting oncological benefit of cytoreductive RP in metastatic disease; careful selection of eligible patients should be important.

H. D. Yuk · C. Kwak (✉)
Department of Urology, Seoul National University Hospital, Seoul, South Korea
e-mail: mdrafael@snu.ac.kr

7.1 Classic Role of Radical Prostatectomy for Palliative Local Symptom Control

Management of locoregional symptoms in metastatic prostate cancer is a very important issue, because of high incidence within their life expectancy. Over half of metastatic prostate cancer patients without local control develop lower urinary tract complication, and about 25% of patient needs definitive treatment. Patients with previous local therapy either RT or RP present lower incidence of local complications. However, RP was more effective to prevent and lower urinary tract impairment in castration-resistant prostate cancer (CRPC) [1, 10].

Transurethral resection of prostate (TURP) and radical prostatectomy (RP) place palliative role to relieve or lower urinary tract complications in metastatic prostate cancer. Palliative TURP is regarded as surgical treatment of choice in sub-vesical level obstruction; however, about 10% who experience recurrence needed surgical intervention. Palliative RP and palliative cystoprostatectomy are considered as definitive treatments used to reduce pain, bleeding, and obstruction of voiding. Both RT and RP reduce 20–50% of symptoms caused by local progression in castration-resistant prostate cancer (CRPC) patients [1].

However, palliative RP for symptom control in these patients with metastatic prostate cancer is

C. S. Kim (ed.), *Management of Advanced Prostate Cancer*,
https://doi.org/10.1007/978-981-10-6943-7_7

associated with various complications and needs for additional treatment. Particularly, palliative RP performed for end-stage prostate cancer patients who have a severe local symptom may involve more extensive surgery and lead to several complications. A study investigating the role of palliative RP and cystoprostatectomy with urinary diversion in patients with symptomatic metastatic prostate cancer found that 13% of patients showed rectal injuries and 24% required additional surgical procedures. Another study reported that 10% of patients evaluated required massive intraoperative transfusion [1, 4]. Initiation of early local therapy instead of palliative management for metastatic prostate cancer reduces complications and morbidity and improves functional outcomes.

7.2 Feasibility of Radical Prostatectomy in Metastatic Prostate Cancer

There were several retrospective studies that have discussed the safety and feasibility of cytoreductive RP [1]. A case control study has compared RP and pelvic lymph node dissection (PLND) with M1b (23 patients) and androgen deprivation therapy (ADT) alone without local therapy (38 patients). Complications observed in the RP and PLND group were similar to those previously reported in a high-risk localized RP series [1]. Clavien-Dindo classification showed no grade 4.5, grade 3 was 13%, grade 2 was 8%, and grade 1 was 17%. Among patients belonging to the ADT group, approximately 30% patients showed local progression and required additional surgical treatment or intervention, while those belonging to the cytoreductive RP group did not show late genitourinary complications due to local progression. A multicenter study evaluating cases of distant metastatic prostate cancer found that complications occurred in 21% of patients and intervention was required in 8%. Functional outcomes were not significantly different from RP in high-risk prostate cancer. At 1 year postoperatively, less than one pad was 82%, and no pad was 64%. Another retrospective study investigating oligometastatic prostate cancer reported that Clavien grade 3 complications were observed in only 18% of patients after 5 years of follow-up following RP [1]. And cancer-specific survival was 45% (95% CI, 30–85%), and overall survival was 82% (95% CI, 62–99%) [1].

Limited to prostate sites, the biological characteristics of metastatic prostate cancer are similar with locally advanced prostate cancer except for distant metastasis. Thus, cytoreductive radical prostatectomy is feasible and is not significantly different from high-risk prostate cancer surgery in terms of safety and functional outcomes.

7.3 Possible Rationale for Cytoreductive Radical Prostatectomy in Metastatic Prostate Cancer

The underlying mechanism of cytoreductive surgery in metastatic disease is still unclear; however, there are some hypotheses to explain this phenomenon to gain positive oncological outcome.

Kaplan et al. presented the concept of a "premetastatic niche" to indicate that metastasis occurs through circulation and thereby dissemination of tumor cells from the primary tumor. Tumor-specific chemokines activate progenitor cell proliferation and act on niche-dependent compartments in the bone marrow, leading to migration of progenitor cells into the circulation. The migrated progenitor cells form clusters and cause microenvironmental changes necessary/conducive to metastasis [11].

A similar "tumor self-seeding theory" explains that self-seeding of solid tumors such as breast and colon cancers and melanoma is mediated by circulating tumor cells. Circulating tumor cells are intermediaries between primary tumor and metastatic sites, mediating metastasis from the origin and accelerating tumor growth by promoting angiogenesis and stromal recruitment through seed-derived factors. It also returns to the primary tumor at the derived metastatic site and grows [1].

Another concept popularly discussed in this context is "tumor microenvironment." The microenvironment of the tumor affects maintenance of androgens that affect tumor growth.

When the activity of androgens is inhibited, the microenvironment of the tumor changes in a manner that increases the sensitivity of androgens. This change in microenvironment allows the tumor to survive even in low androgenic environments. Based on this concept, removal or reduction in the size of the primary tumor may result in therapeutic benefits and affect survival. The presence and extent of residual tumor noted after local treatment of metastatic cancer may affect tumor progression and survival [12].

7.4 Indirect Evidence Supporting the Effectiveness of Cytoreductive Radical Prostatectomy

Reduction of primary tumor burden has shown survival benefit in many malignancies. Cytoreductive surgery has shown increasing survival on colon, breast, and ovarian cancer. Radical surgery on primary site in metastatic disease proves beneficial effect on ovarian cancer and renal cell carcinoma. Although the underlying mechanism of cytoreductive surgery of metastatic disease is unclear, cytoreductive RP expected to increase survival and the response to systemic therapy [12].

There is level 1 evidence of effectiveness; additional locoregional therapy provides better survival benefit than systemic therapy alone in high-risk prostate cancer. Malcom et al. compared 1205 locally advanced prostate cancer patients, he randomly divided the patients into two groups, androgen deprivation therapy (ADT) alone group with RT and ADT combination group. Patients receiving a combination of RT and ADT for locally advanced prostate cancer demonstrate significantly improved overall survival and decreased cancer-specific morality compared to patients who receive only ADT. Another multicenter randomized trial (SPCG-7/SFUO-3) also reports that additional local radiation therapy has beneficial effect in a 10-year cancer-specific mortality and biochemical recurrence relapse-free survival than ADT alone [10].

Such studies provide a solid body of evidence to support the addition of local therapy to systemic therapy in patients with advanced prostate cancer to achieve positive clinical outcomes such as survival.

In the case of regional nodal metastasis, radical prostatectomy with extended pelvic lymph node dissection (PLND) has accepted for one of the standard treatment options [1, 2]. It has been demonstrated that in cases with node-positive prostate cancer, combined treatment using radical prostatectomy and adjuvant hormone therapy resulted in 80% cancer-specific survival for >10 years [13]. A prospective randomized study showed that 14% of patients with node-positive disease who underwent only radical prostatectomy (RP) with pelvic lymph node dissection (PLND) without adjuvant hormone therapy showed a disease-free survival period of 12 years. Recent studies have shown survival results after RP in node-positive prostate cancer with 5, 10, and 15 years of cancer-specific survival reaching 84–95%, 51–86%, and 45% postoperatively. Overall survival rates at 5, 10, and 15 years were 79–85%, 36–69%, and 42%, respectively [1, 10].

Though not a cytoreductive RP, there was randomized controlled study compare potential benefit of surgery in metastatic disease. SWOG (Southwest Oncology Group) randomized control study, patients with metastatic disease initially diagnosed or who had progressed after surgical castration. Patients who underwent RP showed a better response to androgen ablation and a better survival rate than untreated patients [1], suggesting that even in patients diagnosed with progressive prostate cancer, RP itself is worthy of survival, and even in node-positive patients, RP abandonment may not be justified.

7.5 Direct Evidence Supporting the Effectiveness of Cytoreductive Radical Prostatectomy in Metastatic Prostate Cancer

The oncological benefit of cytoreductive RP in metastatic disease is actively collected by in vitro studies and animal model. Several preclinical trials have evaluated the role of cytoreductive surgery in the treatment of metastatic prostate cancer. The R3327/MAT-Lu tumor and a prostate cancer cell line were implanted subcutaneously into the flank of rats, and the lungs were subjected to 100% metastasis. These rats were treated using surgery, chemotherapy, and a combination of surgery for primary tumor and chemotherapy, and the clinical prognosis was compared between the groups. A positive survival benefit was noted in the group that received a combination of surgery and chemotherapy compared to the group that did not undergo surgery. In other animal studies, metastasis after resection of prostate was smaller and had longer-lasting effect than the control group [1].

There is some ongoing prospective randomized trial to analyze the risk and benefit of cytoreductive RP by the University of Texas MD Anderson Cancer Center (NCT01751438), Martini-Klinik am UKE GmbH (NCT02454543), and Oxford University (ISRCTN15704862). The result from these well-designed studies should provide more powerful evidence of the oncological role of cytoreductive RP. There are none of level 1 evidence supporting oncological benefit of cytoreductive RP in metastatic disease right now; we gathered evidences from large retrospective databases.

A recent Surveillance, Epidemiology, and End Results (SEER) database study comprising patients with metastatic prostate cancer compared patients who received local therapy with those who did not. The local therapy group that received RP or brachytherapy showed a significantly higher survival rate and lower mortality. In another population-based study, all-cause mortality and cancer-specific mortality were reduced by approximately 70% in patients who underwent RP after a diagnosis of metastatic prostate cancer [1].

A study based on the Munich Cancer Registry showed that patients with metastatic prostate cancer who underwent RP were more likely to demonstrate a significantly higher 5-year overall survival rate than those who did not receive RP (55% vs. 22%, respectively) [1].

Löppenberg et al. showed benefit of local treatment in metastatic prostate cancer using the data of 15,501 patients from the National Cancer Database (NCDB). 20% patients of local treatment group underwent cytoreductive RP. In the propensity-matched analysis, the 3-year overall mortality-free survival was higher in local treatment group than nonlocal treatment group (69% vs. 54%; $p < 0.001$) [14]. In the 3-year survival stratified by treatment type, RP shows almost similar survival benefit with brachytherapy (78% vs. 80%; $p < 0.001$). Another NCDB studies have compared ADT with RT, ADT with RP, and use of ADT alone in patients with metastatic prostate cancer. Overall survival was found to be improved in those who received ADT with RT and ADT with RP compared to those who received only ADT [1].

7.6 Limitations of Radical Prostatectomy in Metastatic Prostate Cancer

Cytoreductive RP is an important first step in the treatment of de novo metastatic disease in cases diagnosed with metastatic prostate cancer. However, there is no prospective evidence that local therapy has a better survival benefit in patients with metastatic prostate cancer.

Most previous studies that have evaluated the role of cytoreductive RP for treatment of metastatic prostate cancer primarily included patients without visceral metastasis and oligometastatic disease, patients with low volume, and those with a low prostate-specific antigen (PSA) nadir using systemic therapy. Additionally, most studies were population based and retrospective case control studies.

Currently ongoing prospective and randomized control studies, in addition to non-biased studies evaluating the role of cytoreductive RP, are needed to assess patients with the most benefit from local control of primary tumors.

7.7 Summary

- Cytoreductive radical prostatectomy is feasible: similar with locally advanced prostate cancer except for distant metastasis.
- Possible rationale for cytoreductive radical prostatectomy gains positive oncological outcome: pre-metastatic niche, tumor self-seeding theory, and tumor microenvironment.

- There is still none of level 1 evidence supporting oncological benefit of cytoreductive RP in metastatic disease; careful selection of eligible patients should be important.

References

1. Metcalfe MJ, Smaldone MC, Lin DW, Aparicio AM, Chapin BF. Role of radical prostatectomy in metastatic prostate cancer: a review. Urol Oncol. 2017;35(4):125–34.
2. David N, Spears MR, Clarke NW, et al. Survival with newly diagnosed metastatic prostate cancer in the "Docetaxel Era": data from 917 patients in the control arm of the STAMPEDE trial (MRC PR08, CRUK/06/019). Eur Urol. 2015;67(6):1028–38.
3. Norum J, Nieder C. Treatments for metastatic prostate cancer (mPC): a review of costing evidence. Pharmacoeconomics. 2017;35:1–14.
4. Faiena I, Singer EA, Pumill C, Kim IY. Cytoreductive prostatectomy: evidence in support of a new surgical paradigm (review). Int J Oncol. 2014;45(6):2193–8.
5. Cornford P, Bellmunt J, Bolla M, et al. EAU-ESTRO-SIOG guidelines on prostate cancer. Part II: treatment of relapsing, metastatic, and castration-resistant prostate cancer. Eur Urol. 2017;71(4):630–42.
6. Eddy C, Guillaume P, Mohamed MD, Vaudoyer D. Management of peritoneal carcinomatosis from colorectal cancer. Cancer J. 2009;15(3):243–8.
7. Mitchell CR, Boorjian SA, Umbreit EC, Rangel LJ, Carlson RE, Karnes RJ. 20-year survival after radical prostatectomy as initial treatment for cT3 prostate cancer. BJU Int. 2012;110(11):1709–13.
8. Loeb S, Schaeffer EM, Trock BJ, Epstein JI, Elizabeth B, Walsh PC. What are the outcomes of radical prostatectomy for high-risk prostate cancer? Urology. 2011;76(3):710–4.
9. Kane CJ. Palliative transurethral prostate resection for bladder outlet obstruction in patients with locally advanced prostate cancer. J Urol. 2004;171:668–71.
10. Ristau BT, Cahn D, Uzzo RG, Chapin BF, Smaldone MC. The role of radical prostatectomy in high-risk localized, node-positive and metastatic prostate cancer. Future Oncol. 2016;12(5):687–99.
11. Kaplan RN, Rafii S, Lyden D. Preparing the "Soil": the premetastatic niche rosandra. Cancer Res. 2010;66(23):1 089–93.
12. Cole BF, Gelber RD, Gelber S, Coates AS, Goldhirsch A. Polychemotherapy for early breast cancer: an overview of the randomised clinical trials with quality-adjusted survival analysis. Lancet. 2001;358(7):277–86.
13. Joniau S, Spahn M, Briganti A, et al. Pretreatment tables predicting pathologic stage of locally advanced prostate cancer. Eur Urol. 2014;67(2):319–25.
14. Löppenberg B, Dalela D, Karabon P, et al. The impact of local treatment on overall survival in patients with metastatic prostate cancer on diagnosis: a national cancer data base analysis. Eur Urol. 2017;72(1):14–9.

Part II

Radiotherapy for Advanced Prostate Cancer

Young Seok Kim

The Roles of Radiotherapy, Androgen Deprivation Therapy, and Their Combination for Locally Advanced Prostate Cancer

8

Sung Uk Lee and Kwan Ho Cho

8.1 Introduction

Men with locally advanced or high-risk prostate cancer have a substantial risk of dying and developing distant metastases. Historically, androgen deprivation therapy (ADT) by bilateral orchiectomy was frequently used as an effective systemic treatment for advanced prostate cancer. In the 1980s, luteinizing hormone-releasing hormone (LHRH) analogs and antiandrogens emerged and have been used as a medical castration alternative to bilateral orchiectomy. After its success as a palliative treatment for metastatic prostate cancer, a number of trials were initiated to investigate the role of radiotherapy (RT), ADT, and their combination in multimodal treatment for locally advanced or high-risk prostate cancer. In this chapter, we highlighted important randomized trials of combined therapy for locally advanced or high-risk prostate cancer and tried to define the individual roles of RT, ADT, and their combination. A comprehensive review of this topic has been published elsewhere [1], and a large part of the content has been duplicated.

S. U. Lee, M.D. · K. H. Cho, M.D. (✉)
The Proton Therapy Center, Research Institute and Hospital, National Cancer Center, Ilsandong-gu, South Korea
e-mail: kwancho@ncc.re.kr

8.2 Radiotherapy Alone Versus Radiotherapy Plus Androgen Deprivation Therapy

Several multicenter randomized controlled trials designed to demonstrate the effectiveness of ADT in locally advanced or high-risk prostate cancer treated with definitive RT were executed in the late 1980s and early 1990s; these were Radiation Therapy Oncology Group (RTOG) 8531 [2], RTOG 8610 [3], and European Organisation for Research and Treatment of Cancer (EORTC) 22863 [4] (Table 8.1). When combined with RT, ADT schedules were varied from short-term (ST-ADT) to long-term (LT-ADT). Arbitrarily, duration of ST-ADT and LT-ADT were 4–6 months and over 2 years, respectively. During this period, conventional RT was standard of care which delivered with 45 Gy to whole pelvis followed by 20–25 Gy to prostate boost (total dose 65–70 Gy).

RTOG 8531 [2] was designed to compare between RT alone and RT plus lifelong ADT using goserelin (LT-ADT). Eligible criteria for RTOG 8531 were prostate adenocarcinoma extending beyond the prostate (cT3) or those with regional lymph node metastasis (N1). Nine hundred and seventy-seven patients were randomly allocated to RT alone ($n = 488$) and RT combined with LT-ADT ($n = 489$). In RT-alone group, goserelin was applied at the time of disease relapse. In addition patients who had

C. S. Kim (ed.), *Management of Advanced Prostate Cancer*,
https://doi.org/10.1007/978-981-10-6943-7_8

Table 8.1 The results of randomized controlled trials for radiotherapy plus ADT versus radiotherapy alone for locally advanced or high-risk prostate cancer

			Patient characteristics					Treatments			Clinical outcomes at 10 years (%)				
Study	Treatment arms	*n*	Age (med)	T3–4 (%)	(+)*N* (%)	GS ≥ 8	iPSA≥20	RT (Gy)	ADT duration	Med F/U (yr)	BCF	LP	DM	OS	DSM
RTOG 8531 [2]	RT + LT-ADT	489		>70	29	32		65–70	Lifelong	7.6	69[a]	23[a]	24[a]	49[a]	16[a]
	RT	488		>70	26	32		65–70			91	38	39	39	22
RTOG 8610 [3]	RT + ST-ADT	224	70	70	7	26		65–70	4 months	11.9	65[a]	NS	35[a]	43	23[a]
	RT	232	71	70	9	30		65–70		13.2	80		47	34	36
EORTC 22863 [4]	RT + LT-ADT	207	71	91	4		72	70	36 months	9.1		6[a]	49[a]	58[a]	10[a]
	RT	208	70	89	3		73	70				24	70	40	30
TROG 9601 [5]	RT + ST-ADT (6 months)	267	68	39	0	16	33	66	6 months	10.6	53[a]	13[a]	10	71[a]	11[a]
	RT + ST-ADT (3 months)	265	68	42	0	20	37	66	3 months		60[a]	16[a]	15	63	19
	RT	270	67	39	0	15	43	66			74	28	14	57	22

Abbreviations: *ADT* androgen deprivation therapy, *RT* radiation treatment, *BCF* biochemical failure, *LP* local progression, *DM* distant metastasis, *OS* overall survival, *DSM* disease-specific mortality, *NS* no significant difference, *LT* long term, *ST* short term

[a]Statistically significant difference compared to RT alone

received radical prostatectomy were included if pathologic specimen showed extracapsular extension to the resection margin and/or with seminal vesicle involvement (15%). At a median follow-up of 7.6 years, adjuvant lifelong LT-ADT was significantly related to reductions in local progression (23 vs. 38%, $p < 0.001$) and distant metastasis (24 vs. 39%, $p < 0.001$) at 10 years. LT-ADT also showed survival benefits with an increase in 10-year overall survival (49 vs. 39%, $p = 0.002$) and a reduction in disease-specific mortality (16 vs. 22%, $p = 0.005$) compared to RT alone. The improvements in survival were shown preferentially in patients who had Gleason score of 7–10.

RTOG 8610 [3] evaluated whether RT plus 4-month ST-ADT improves locoregional control and consequently survival when compared with RT alone. Eligibility was prostate cancer patients with cT2–T4 bulky tumors with or without regional lymph node metastasis and no evidence of distant metastasis. Four hundred and fifty-six patients (median age, 70 years) were randomly assigned to receive RT alone ($n = 232$) or RT plus ST-ADT ($n = 224$). ST-ADT composed of goserelin (3.6 mg every month) and flutamide (250 mg of three times a day for 2 months) before and during RT. Estimated 10-year biochemical failure (BCF) (65 vs. 80%, $p < 0.001$) and distant metastasis (35 vs. 47%, $p = 0.006$) favored RT plus ST-ADT, respectively. A local effect of ST-ADT was shown until the 8-year estimates [6] but disappeared in the 10-year estimates [3]. The 4-month ADT showed a significant reduction in 10-year disease-specific mortality (23 vs. 36%, $p = 0.02$) but no significant improvement in overall survival (43 vs. 34%, $p = 0.12$).

EORTC 22863 [4] conducted a randomized controlled trial to evaluate the benefits of LT-ADT for 36 months with LHRH analogs compared with RT alone in prostate cancer with a high risk of metastases. Inclusion criteria were younger than 80 years old and had cT1–2 prostate cancer with World Health Organization histological grade 3 (10%) or cT3–4 prostate cancer of any histological grade (90%). A total of 415 patients were randomly allocated to two groups, 208 in radiotherapy alone and 207 in radiotherapy plus LT-ADT. At a median 9.1 years of follow-up, RT combined with LT-ADT significantly improved 10-year local progression (6 vs. 24%, $p < 0.001$) and distant metastasis (49 vs. 70%, $p < 0.001$) compared to RT alone. Long-term survival benefits were also associated with combined treatment by an improvement in 10-year overall survival (58 vs. 40%, $p < 0.001$) and a reduction in 10-year disease-specific mortality (10 vs. 30%, $p < 0.001$). There was no significant difference in cardiovascular toxicity between two groups regardless of the presence of underlying heart diseases at study entry.

In the late 1990s, Trans-Tasman Radiation Oncology Group (TROG 9601) trial was conducted to compare neoadjuvant 3- and 6-month ST-ADT when combined with radiotherapy for advanced prostate cancer [5]. A total of 802 men with cT2b-T4 N0M0 prostate adenocarcinoma were randomized to receive RT alone ($n = 270$), 3-month ST-ADT plus RT ($n = 265$), or 6-month ST-ADT plus RT ($n = 267$). All patients received 66 Gy of RT to the prostate target (without pelvic RT). Long-term outcomes were reported at a median follow-up of 10.6 years after the randomization. Compared with RT alone, 3-month ST-ADT decreased the 10-year BCF ($p = 0.003$) and local progression ($p < 0.001$) significantly, but had no improvement in distant metastasis, overall survival, and disease-specific mortality. In contrast, 6-month ADT offers further reductions in BCF ($p < 0.001$) and local progression ($p < 0.001$) as well as decreased distant metastasis ($p = 0.001$) and disease-specific mortality ($p < 0.001$) and improved overall survival ($p < 0.001$) compared to RT alone. Treatment-related toxicity rate was not affected by ST-ADT in the first 5 years.

8.3 Androgen Deprivation Therapy Alone Versus Radiotherapy Plus Androgen Deprivation Therapy

The major benefit of ADT in advanced prostate cancer may be associated with the control of occult micro-metastases, with delayed progression at the prostate by some local effect [7]. For ADT alone as a treatment for locally advanced prostate cancer, lifelong ADT with either surgical castration or LHRH analogs is maintained until disease recurrence or death. In a randomized study for patients with cT2-T4 prostate cancer, in the 1980s, a total of 277 patients were allocated to undergo orchiectomy alone (n = 90), to receive RT alone (n = 88), and to undergo combined therapy (n = 99) [8]. Orchiectomy either alone or combined with RT produced a significant delay in distant metastasis when compared with RT alone [8]. There were no differences in survival between those three groups; however, the number of participants was not sufficient to show statistically significant survival differences due to poor accrual [9]. In the early 1990s, after a data has emerged which suggested that ADT combined with RT improves clinical outcomes when compared to RT alone, several randomized controlled trials were commenced to assess the benefit of addition of RT to ADT in locally advanced or high-risk prostate cancer. The long-term results comparing ADT alone and RT plus LT-ADT were available in two multicenter prospective studies (Table 8.2).

National Cancer Institute of Canada Clinical Trial Group and Medical Research Council (NCIC CTG/MRC) trial [10] randomized a total of 1205 patients to ADT-alone group (n = 602) and RT plus LT-ADT group (n = 603). Patients with cT3–4 prostate adenocarcinoma (n = 1057) or organ-confined disease (cT2) with either an initial serum prostate-specific antigen (PSA) value higher than 40 ng/mL (n = 119) or a PSA value higher than 20 ng/mL and a Gleason score 8–10 (n = 25) were included. Node-positive disease was excluded. RT dose was delivered to 45 Gy for the regional lymphatic chain and total 65–69 Gy to the prostate and seminal vesicles. All patients received lifelong ADT either LHRH analogs (93%) or bilateral orchiectomy (7%). The median age of all patients was 70 years old. At a median 8-year follow-up, the addition of RT led to a 30% reduction of the overall mortality (hazard ratio 0.70, 95% CI 0.57–0.85, P < 0.001) and significantly reduced deaths from prostate cancer (hazard ratio 0.46, 95% CI 0.34–0.61, P < 0.001). The 10-year BCF was 73% with ADT alone and 37% with RT plus LT-ADT, respectively, with no reports on local progression or distant metastasis. Patients in RT plus LT-ADT group reported more frequent bowel toxicity, but most were grades 1–2. Regarding the ADT-related toxicity, the three most common grade 3 or higher toxicities were impotence (29–33%), hot flush (5–8%), and urinary frequency (4–7%), and there were no significant differences. The difference in reported cardiac events between two groups was also nonsignificant.

In the Scandinavian Prostate Cancer Group Study No. 7/the Swedish Association for Urological Oncology-3 (SPCG-7/SFUO-3) trial [11], a total of 875 men with advanced prostate cancer (T3; 78%; N0; M0; PSA <70) were randomly allocated to ADT alone (n = 439) or to RT plus LT-ADT (n = 436). Notably, SPCG-7/SFUO3 enrolled younger patients (median 66 years) than other randomized trials (median 70–71 years). ADT consisted of total androgen blockade for 3 months followed by antiandrogen treatment using flutamide. Total RT dose of minimum 70 Gy was prescribed to prostate target with or without pelvic RT. After a median 7.6 years of follow-up, the addition of RT halved the rate of disease-specific mortality at 10 years compared to ADT alone (12 vs. 24%, p < 0.001) and substantially increased overall survival at 10 years (70 vs. 60%, p = 0.004). Incidence of BCF at 10 years was significantly higher in the ADT-alone group (26 vs. 75%, p < 0.001). Slightly more frequent urinary, bowel, and sexual problems were shown after addition of RT to ADT, but it was fully acceptable compared to ADT alone.

In 2000s, Mottet et al. [12] conducted a multicenter prospective trial to evaluate the addition of RT in patients who received temporary LT-ADT (3 years) for cT3–4 or pT3N0 M0 (4%) prostate adenocarcinoma. After randomization, ADT alone was given to 130 patients and combined treatment to 133 patients. In LT-ADT plus RT arm, a total of 68–70 Gy was prescribed to prostate target. After a median follow-up of 5.6 years, additional local RT improved 5-year clinical outcomes significantly with decreased BCF (35 vs.

Table 8.2 The results of randomized controlled trials for radiotherapy plus ADT versus ADT alone for locally advanced or high-risk prostate cancer

Study	Treatment arms	Patient characteristics						Treatment		Clinical outcomes at 5–10 years[b] (%)					
		n	Age (med)	T3–4 (%)	(+)*N* (%)	GS ≥ 8	iPSA≥20	RT (Gy)	ADT duration	Med F/U (yr)	BCF	LP	DM	OS	DSM
NCIC CTG/ MRC [10]	ADT + RT	603	70	88		36	64	65–69	Lifelong	8	37[a]			55[a]	15[a]
	ADT	602	70	87		36	63		Lifelong		73			49	25
SPCG-7/SFUO3 [11]	ADT + RT	436	66	77			40	70	Lifelong	7.6	26[a]			70[a]	12[a]
	ADT	439	66	79			40		Lifelong		75			60	24
Mottet et al. [12]	ADT + RT	133	72	100	1	24	65	68–70	36 months	5.6	35[a]	10[a]	3[a]	71	7
	ADT	130	71	100	1	17	62		36 months		85	29	11	72	14

Abbreviations: *ADT* androgen deprivation therapy, *RT* radiation treatment, *BCF* biochemical failure, *LP* local progression, *DM* distant metastasis, *OS* overall survival, *DSM* disease-specific mortality, *LT* long term, *ST* short term

[a]Statistically significant difference compared to ADT alone

[b]10-year outcomes in NCIC CTG/MRC and SPCG-7/SFUO3; 5-year outcomes in Mottet et al.

85%, $p < 0.001$), local progression (10 vs. 29%, $p < 0.001$), and distant metastasis (3 vs. 11%, $p = 0.018$). A difference in 5-year overall survival was not significant, but a difference in 5-year disease-specific mortality was shown borderline significance (7 vs. 14%, $p = 0.0586$) between two groups. This trial has limitations such as a small cohort with a short follow-up period to show the survival benefit. Genitourinary and gastrointestinal toxicities were more common in LT-ADT plus RT than with ADT alone. At 6 months, grades 2–4 toxicity were reported in bladder/urethra (18% ADT alone vs. 29% in LT-ADT plus RT), rectum (2 vs. 14%), and small intestine/colon (3 vs. 13%), respectively, but decreased gradually with time. Cardiovascular problems were observed at a similar rate between the two arms.

8.4 Short-Term Versus Long-Term Androgen Deprivation Therapy When Combined with Radiotherapy

The randomized controlled trials comparing RT alone and the combined treatment in 1980s reported superior outcomes of combined treatment either ST-ADT or LT-ADT with RT in their initial analysis. Subsequently, the optimal ADT duration when combined with RT has been questioned continuously. Prolonged ADT can deteriorate the quality of life and heighten the risk of long-term morbidities including cardiovascular events, sarcopenia, osteopenia, and fractures [13]. Short-term use of ADT may effectively reduce these risks if it can achieve comparable clinical outcome to LT-ADT. Several multicenter randomized trials were performed to determine whether ST-ADT would achieve disease control and survival rate obtained by LT-ADT and preserve the quality of life (Table 8.3).

RTOG 9202 [14] was performed to compare 4-month ST-ADT and 28-month LT-ADT when combined with RT in patients with cT2c-4 prostate cancer and a serum PSA value below 150 ng/mL. After all patients received a combined treatment with 4-month ST-ADT and RT, a total of 1554 patients were randomized to receive no more treatment ($n = 763$) or additional 24-month ADT ($n = 758$). Approximately 55% of the patients were clinically T3-T4, and 30% had positive pelvic nodal spread. Median follow-up period was over 11 years. The LT-ADT plus RT group showed significantly better outcomes for most of end points than ST-ADT plus RT group, but not for overall survival. Improvements in 10-year BCF (52 vs. 68%, $p < 0.001$), local progression (12 vs. 22%, $p < 0.001$), and distant metastasis (15 vs. 23%, $p < 0.001$) were observed in LT-ADT when compared with ST-ADT, respectively. Although 10-year disease-specific mortality was significantly reduced by LT-ADT (11 vs. 16%, $p = 0.004$), 10-year overall survival was not (54 vs. 52%, $p = 0.36$). An increase in overall survival was restricted to a subgroup of patients with a Gleason score 8 or higher (45 vs. 32%, $p = 0.006$). One patient in RT plus LT-ADT died of chemical hepatitis caused by ADT during the hormone treatment. LT-ADT exhibits slightly more severe late RT-related toxicity with grade 3 (ST-ADT 6% vs. LT-ADT 7%) and grade 4 (ST-ADT 1% vs. LT-ADT 3%). No significant difference in cardiovascular toxicity was seen between two groups.

EORTC 22961 [15] reported the comparison between 6-month ST-ADT and 36-month LT-ADT when combined with RT for cT1c-T2b with N1-2 prostate cancer or cT2c-T4 with N0-N2 prostate cancer. A total of 970 patients were randomly allocated, 483 to ST-ADT and 487 to LT-ADT. Approximately 95% were at cT2c-T4 stage, and 9% were node positive. Total of 70 Gy RT (pelvic RT 50 Gy + prostate boost 20 Gy) was delivered to all patients. A hazard ratio 1.35 or less was adapted to establish the noninferiority of ST-ADT to LT-ADT for overall survival. After a median 6.4 years of follow-up, ST-ADT combined with RT provides inferior survival compared with LT-ADT combined with RT. The 5-year overall mortality in ST-ADT arm and LT-ADT arm was 19.0 and 15.2%, respectively, corresponding to a hazard ratio of 1.42 (upper 95.71% confidence limit, 1.79; $p = 0.65$ for noninferiority), and higher 5-year disease-specific mortality (5 vs. 3%, $p = 0.002$ by the

Table 8.3 The results of randomized controlled trials for the optimal durations of ADT when combined with RT for locally advanced or high-risk prostate cancer

Study	Treatment arms	Patient characteristics						Treatment		Clinical outcomes at 5–10 years[b] (%)					
		n	Age (med)	T3–4 (%)	(+)*N* (%)	GS ≥ 8	iPSA≥20	RT (Gy)	ADT duration	Med F/U (yr)	BCF	LP	DM	OS	DSM
RTOG 9202 [14]	RT + LT-ADT	758	70	55	3	46	>33	65–70	28 months	11.3	52[a]	12[a]	15[a]	54	11[a]
	RT + ST-ADT	763	70	55	4	49	>33	65–70	4 months		68	22	23	52	16
EORTC 22961 [15]	RT + LT-ADT	487	69	76	9	19		70	36 months	6.4				85	3[a]
	RT + ST-ADT	483	70	79	9	19		70	6 months					81	5

Abbreviations: *ADT* androgen deprivation therapy, *RT* radiation treatment, *BCF* biochemical failure, *LP* local progression, *DM* distant metastasis, *OS* overall survival, *DSM* disease-specific mortality, *LT* long term, *ST* short term

[a]Statistically significant difference

[b]10-year outcomes in RTOG 9202; 5-year outcomes in EORTC 22961

log-rank test) was observed in ST-ADT arm. In terms of adverse events, LT-ADT arm was associated with higher scores of hot flushes and reduced sexual interest and sexual activity than ST-ADT arm. Fatal cardiovascular toxicity at 5 years was not significantly different between two groups.

8.5 Other Issues

The role of radiation dose intensification in multimodal therapy has been studied as well. ASCENDE-RT phase III trial investigated the efficacy of brachytherapy as a boost to external beam RT (EBRT) in intermediate- and high-risk prostate cancer [16–18]. A total of 398 patients received 12-month ADT and pelvic irradiation to 46 Gy and then were randomly assigned to EBRT boost arm (total dose up to 78 Gy) or low-dose-rate prostate brachytherapy boost (LDR-PB) arm. After a median 6.5 years of follow-up, LDR-PB halved the risk of BCF compared to EBRT boost; however, no significant improvement in OS was observed. Urinary function impairment was significantly more in LDR-PB arm than EBRT boost arm [16–18]. However, no trial has been conducted to define the role of radiation dose intensification using EBRT (conventional or hypo-fractionation) or brachytherapy boost solely for locally advanced or high-risk prostate cancer; hence, the role has not been well established yet. In patients with locally advanced or high-risk prostate cancer, it should be noted that the risk of distant metastases was higher than those of local progression after the current standard treatment of RT plus LT-ADT [1]. Thus, the intensification of systemic treatment may have more potential to improve the clinical outcome than those of local treatment. A couple of studies demonstrated that the addition of docetaxel to ADT led to an improvement in overall survival in locally advanced or high-risk patients in their interim analyses [19, 20]. Similarly, ADT plus abiraterone showed significantly improved overall survival in patients with newly diagnosed, metastatic, castration-sensitive prostate cancer [21]. It is worthy to evaluate the role of the intensification of systemic treatment by addition of these new agents for locally advanced or high-risk prostate cancer in the future trials.

8.6 Conclusions

To determine the contributions of each treatment (RT, ST-ADT and LT-ADT) and their combinations on clinical outcome after multimodal treatment for locally advanced prostate cancer, the 10-year clinical outcomes were extracted from published articles, and then their average rates were calculated by weighting the cohort number to depict a roughly estimated trend (Fig. 8.1) [1] (adapted from a previous publication by the same authors). Although ADT alone tends to show higher estimated 10-year overall survival than RT alone, the 10-year disease-specific mortality rate was almost similar between two groups. When combined with RT, ADT either ST- or LT-ADT provides notable local and systemic effect. Compared to RT alone, the 10-year local progression was profoundly decreased by addition of ST-ADT and further by those of LT-ADT. Likewise, the 10-year distant metastasis and disease-specific mortality also had a similar trend, as well as the most favorable 10-year overall survival was seen in RT plus LT-ADT. In summary, the best long-term clinical outcomes were resulted by the combined treatment with RT and LT-ADT, indicating that both RT and ADT are crucial parts of multimodal treatment and should be considered as the current standard of care for locally advanced or high-risk prostate cancers. Further refinement of combined treatment is warranted.

8.7 Summary

Locally advanced prostate cancer has a substantial risk of occurrence of distant metastasis. Androgen deprivation therapy by either surgical or medical castrations is considered as the most effective systemic therapy for advanced prostate cancer. Numerous trials have been executed to investigate the role of radiotherapy, androgen deprivation therapy, and their combination in multimodal

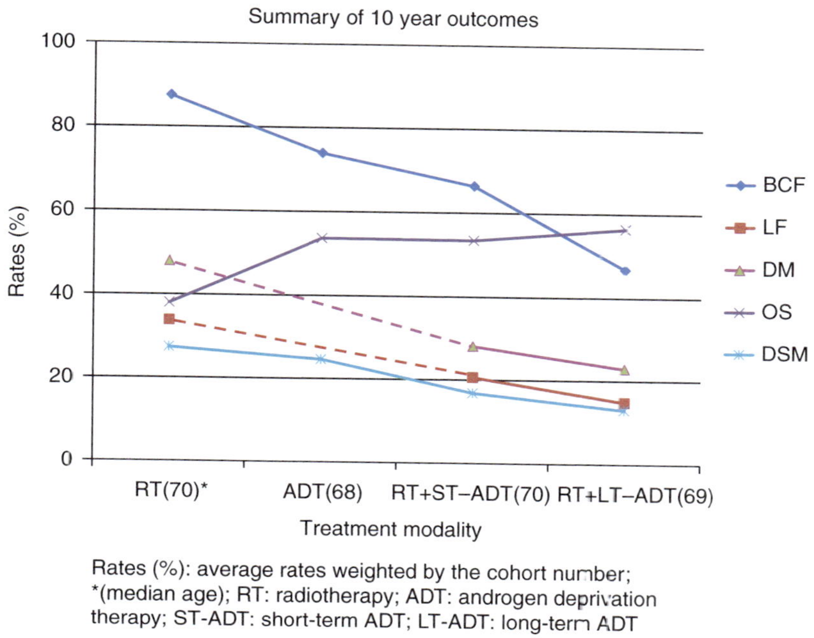

Fig. 8.1 The relative contributions of individual treatment in multimodal therapy for locally advanced prostate cancer [1]

treatment for locally advanced or high-risk prostate cancer. The best long-term clinical outcomes resulted from the combined treatment with radiotherapy and long-term androgen deprivation therapy, indicating that both RT and ADT are crucial parts of multimodal treatment and should be considered as the current standard of care.

References

1. Lee SU, Cho KH. Multimodal therapy for locally advanced prostate cancer: the roles of radiotherapy, androgen deprivation therapy, and their combination. J Radiat Oncol. 2017;35(3):189–97.
2. Pilepich MV, Winter K, Lawton CA, Krisch RE, Wolkov HB, Movsas B, et al. Androgen suppression adjuvant to definitive radiotherapy in prostate carcinoma--long-term results of phase III RTOG 85-31. Int J Radiat Oncol Biol Phys. 2005;61(5):1285–90.
3. Roach M 3rd, Bae K, Speight J, Wolkov HB, Rubin P, Lee RJ, et al. Short-term neoadjuvant androgen deprivation therapy and external-beam radiotherapy for locally advanced prostate cancer: long-term results of RTOG 8610. J Clin Oncol. 2008;26(4):585–91.
4. Bolla M, Van Tienhoven G, Warde P, Dubois JB, Mirimanoff R-O, Storme G, et al. External irradiation with or without long-term androgen suppression for prostate cancer with high metastatic risk: 10-year results of an EORTC randomised study. Lancet Oncol. 2010;11(11) 1066–73.
5. Denham JW, Steigler A, Lamb DS, Joseph D, Turner S, Matthews J, et al. Short-term neoadjuvant androgen deprivation and radiotherapy for locally advanced prostate cancer: 10-year data from the TROG 96.01 randomised trial. Lancet Oncol. 2011;12(5):451–9.
6. Pilepich MV, Winter K, John MJ, Mesic JB, Sause W, Rubin P, et al. Phase III radiation therapy oncology group (RTOG) trial 86-10 of androgen deprivation adjuvant to definitive radiotherapy in locally advanced carcinoma of the prostate. Int J Radiat Oncol Biol Phys. 2001;50(5):1243–52.
7. McLaughlin PW, Liss AL, Nguyen PL, Assimos DG, D'Amico AV, Gottschalk AR, et al. ACR appropriateness criteria(R) locally advanced, high-risk prostate cancer. Am J Clin Oncol. 2017;40(1):1–10.
8. Fellows GJ, Clark PB, Beynon LL, Boreham J, Keen C, Parkinson MC, et al. Treatment of advanced localised prostatic cancer by orchiectomy, radiotherapy, or combined treatment. A Medical Research Council Study. Urological Cancer Working Party--Subgroup on Prostatic Cancer. Br J Urol. 1992;70(3):304–9.
9. Warde P, Mason M, Ding K, Kirkbride P, Brundage M, Cowan R, et al. Combined androgen deprivation therapy and radiation therapy for locally advanced prostate cancer: a randomised, phase 3 trial. Lancet. 2011;378(9809):2104–11.

10. Mason MD, Parulekar WR, Sydes MR, Brundage M, Kirkbride P, Gospodarowicz M, et al. Final report of the intergroup randomized study of combined androgen-deprivation therapy plus radiotherapy versus androgen-deprivation therapy alone in locally advanced prostate cancer. J Clin Oncol. 2015;33(19):2143–50.
11. Widmark A, Klepp O, Solberg A, Damber JE, Angelsen A, Fransson P, et al. Endocrine treatment, with or without radiotherapy, in locally advanced prostate cancer (SPCG-7/SFUO-3): an open randomised phase III trial. Lancet. 2009;373(9660):301–8.
12. Mottet N, Peneau M, Mazeron JJ, Molinie V, Richaud P. Addition of radiotherapy to long-term androgen deprivation in locally advanced prostate cancer: an open randomised phase 3 trial. Eur Urol. 2012;62(2):213–9.
13. Freedland SJ, Eastham J, Shore N. Androgen deprivation therapy and estrogen deficiency induced adverse effects in the treatment of prostate cancer. Prostate Cancer Prostatic Dis. 2009;12(4):333–8.
14. Horwitz EM, Bae K, Hanks GE, Porter A, Grignon DJ, Brereton HD, et al. Ten-year follow-up of radiation therapy oncology group protocol 92-02: a phase III trial of the duration of elective androgen deprivation in locally advanced prostate cancer. J Clin Oncol. 2008;26(15):2497–504.
15. Bolla M, de Reijke TM, Van Tienhoven G, Van den Bergh AC, Oddens J, Poortmans PM, et al. Duration of androgen suppression in the treatment of prostate cancer. N Engl J Med. 2009;360(24):2516–27.
16. Morris WJ, Tyldesley S, Rodda S, Halperin R, Pai H, McKenzie M, et al. Androgen suppression combined with elective nodal and dose escalated radiation therapy (the ASCENDE-RT trial): an analysis of survival endpoints for a randomized trial comparing a low-dose-rate brachytherapy boost to a dose-escalated external beam boost for high- and intermediate-risk prostate cancer. Int J Radiat Oncol Biol Phys. 2017;98(2):275–85.
17. Rodda S, Tyldesley S, Morris WJ, Keyes M, Halperin R, Pai H, et al. ASCENDE-RT: an analysis of treatment-related morbidity for a randomized trial comparing a low-dose-rate brachytherapy boost with a dose-escalated external beam boost for high- and intermediate-risk prostate cancer. Int J Radiat Oncol Biol Phys. 2017;98(2):286–95.
18. Rodda S, Morris WJ, Hamm J, Duncan G. ASCENDE-RT: an analysis of health-related quality of life for a randomized trial comparing low-dose-rate brachytherapy boost with dose-escalated external beam boost for high- and intermediate-risk prostate cancer. Int J Radiat Oncol Biol Phys. 2017;98(3):581–9.
19. James N, Mason M. Docetaxel and/or zoledronic acid for hormone-naïve prostate cancer: first survival results from STAMPEDE. J Clin Oncol. 2015;33(suppl):5001.
20. Sandler HM, Hu C, Rosenthal SA, et al. A phase III protocol of androgen suppression (AS) and 3DCRT/IMRT versus AS and 3DCRT/IMRT followed by chemotherapy (CT) with docetaxel and prednisone for localized, high-risk prostate cancer (RTOG 0521). J Clin Oncol. 2015;33(suppl):5002.
21. Fizazi K, Tran N, Fein L, Matsubara N, Rodriguez-Antolin A, Alekseev BY, et al. Abiraterone plus prednisone in metastatic, castration-sensitive prostate cancer. N Engl J Med. 2017;377:352–60.

External Beam Radiotherapy for Advanced Prostate Cancer: Dose, Technique, and Fractionation

9

Yeon Joo Kim and Young Seok Kim

9.1 Introduction

Prostate cancer is generally considered to have a low α/β ratio. With this biological rationale and the development of radiation techniques, hypofractionation is now rapidly performed in radiation oncology field. Several prospective trials have been conducted to evaluate the moderate hypofractionation and demonstrated that moderate hypofractionation is not superior but equivalent to conventional fractionation regimen in terms of biochemical control. The data on extreme hypofractionation is still immature, but promising. Also, combined treatment with external beam radiotherapy and brachytherapy has demonstrated better biochemical control than that of external beam radiotherapy alone. In this chapter, we review the dose, technique, and fractionation scheme for the prostate cancer.

9.2 Dose Escalation and Rationale for Hypofractionation

Several randomized clinical trials have reported long-term outcomes that high-dose external beam radiotherapy (EBRT) is more effective in treating localized prostate cancer including low-, intermediate-, and high-risk disease in the aspect of biochemical failure (BCF) [1–3]. As a result, the prescription dose for EBRT has increased from the ranges of 68–70 Gy to 76–80 Gy, especially for intermediate- and high-risk patients. However, increased adverse events were the results of dose escalation. In a meta-analysis with seven randomized trials, there were more incidences of late grade >2 gastrointestinal (GI) toxicity after high-dose RT with an odds ratio (OR) of 1.58 [4]. However, highly conformal irradiation techniques such as intensity-modulated radiotherapy (IMRT) and image-guided radiotherapy (IGRT) have been proven to reduce the risks of toxicities and now widely used in clinics [5, 6].

In addition, hypofractionation has been proposed to improve therapeutic ratio. Hypofractionation scheme is based on an assumption that prostate cancer has a low α/β ratio compare to healthy normal tissues. Many studies have evaluated the α/β ratio for prostate cancer about 1.5 Gy [7, 8] while that for the late-responding normal organs nearby (rectum, bladder, and urethra) has been estimated to be ≥3 Gy. This low α/β ratio indicates greater sensitivity to higher doses per fraction, which could yield improved local tumor control without increased toxicity. Moreover, shorten RT course could save the health care costs and provide convenience for the patients.

Y. J. Kim, M.D. · Y. S. Kim, M.D. (✉)
Depatment of Radiation Oncology, Asan Medical Center, Seoul, South Korea
e-mail: ysk@amc.seoul.kr

C. S. Kim (ed.), *Management of Advanced Prostate Cancer*,
https://doi.org/10.1007/978-981-10-6943-7_9

Although there is no clear consensus on definition for fractionation schemes, conventional fractionation is commonly defined as a fraction size of 1.8–2.0 Gy (7–9 weeks). Following the general concept, we defined the moderate hypofractionation with doses per fraction between 2.5 and 4.0 Gy (4–6 weeks) and severe/extreme hypofractionation with a single dose ≥5 Gy (4–5 fractions) for the organization of the present review.

9.3 Moderate Hypofractionation

The trials on moderate hypofractionation (MH) could be divided into superiority and non-inferiority studies. Superiority trials are listed in Table 9.1. Except for the abstract from the University of Texas MD Anderson Cancer Center [11], most studies reported negative results for superiority of MH. The largest superiority study was HYPRO study which enrolled a total of 804 patients [12]. The subjects were randomized to conventional arm (78 Gy in 39 fractions, every weekday) and MH arm (64.6 Gy in 19 fractions, three fractions in a week). The majority of patients (73–74%) were high-risk group. With median follow-up time of 60 months, 5-year BCFFS was 80.5% in MH arm and 77.1% in conventional arm ($p = 0.36$). HYPRO study also evaluated late toxicity in non-inferiority setting with an endpoint of the event of grade 2 or worse acute and late genitourinary (GU) and GI toxicity. HYPRO study could not demonstrate that MH was not inferior for cumulative late GU and GI toxicity compared with the conventional fractionation since estimated hazard ratio (HR) was not met to reject inferiority. Late grade ≥3 genitourinary (GU) toxicities were significantly worse in hypofractionation arm (19 vs. 12.9%, $p = 0.021$) [13]. The other studies in superiority settings reported that biochemical control and toxicities were not significantly different between conventional and MH arm [9, 10]. HYPRO study used higher biologically effective dose of 137.8 Gy with α/β ratio of 3 Gy for the bladder and rectum in MH arm than those of the other studies (126.1–133.4 Gy_3), and this could be the reason for the higher late toxicity. Although superiority trials failed to demonstrate the superiority of MH in either reducing late toxicity or increasing efficacy, the results were comparable to the conventional fractionations.

Long-waited results of three non-inferiority trials with over 5000 patients were published recently and summarized in Table 9.2. There was no difference in BCFFS in all studies [14–16]. In the aspect of late toxicities, the results were slightly different. RTOG 0415 reported increased late grade ≥2 GI and GU toxicities in MH arm, while PROFIT and CHHiP reported no significant difference in late toxicities between two fractionation regimens.

The largest non-inferiority study was CHHiP study which enrolled 3216 patients. Patients were randomly allocated to conventional regimen of 74 Gy in 37 fractions or either 60 Gy in

Table 9.1 Superiority trials for moderate hypofractionation

Trial	N	Median FU (Y)	Risk group/ GS	Dose (TD/SD)	ADT	BCFFS	Late toxicity
Rome [9]	85 83	9	High	80/2 62/3.1	100%	NS	NS
FCCC [10]	152 151	5.5	Low Intermediate High	76/2 70.2/2.7	~45% (high risk)	NS	NS
MDACC [11] abs	206	8.4	GS 6–7	75.6/1.8 72/2.4	24%	SS	NS
HYPRO [12, 13]	397 407	5	Intermediate High	78/2 64.6/3.4	67%	NS	SS (↑G3+ GU in hypofractionation)

ADT androgen deprivation therapy, *abs* data derived from abstract, *BCFFS* biochemical failure-free survival, *FU* follow-up, *GI* gastrointestinal, *G* grade, *GS* Gleason score, *GU* genitourinary, *NS* not significant, *SS* statistically significant, *SD* single dose, *TD* total dose, *Y* years

Table 9.2 Non-inferiority trials for moderate hypofractionation

Trial	N	Median FU (Y)	Risk group/GS	Dose (TD/SD)	ADT	BCFFS	Late toxicity
PROFIT [14]	598 608	6	Intermediate	78/2 60/3	0%	NS	NS
RTOG 0415 [16]	542 550	5.8	Low	73.8/1.8 70/2.5	0%	NS	SS (↑G2+ GI/GU in hypofractionation)
CHHiP [15]	1065 1074 1077	5.2	Low Intermediate High	74/2 60/3 57/3	97%	NS	NS

ADT androgen deprivation therapy, *abs* data derived from abstract, *BCFFS* biochemical failure-free survival, *FU* follow-up, *GI* gastrointestinal, *G* grade, *GS* Gleason score, *GU* genitourinary, *NS* not significant, *SS* statistically significant, *SD* single dose, *TD* total dose, *Y* years

20 fractions or 57 Gy in 19 fractions. With a median follow-up of 62.4 months, 5-year biochemical or clinical failure-free survival rate was 88.3% in the 74 Gy arm, 90.6% in the 60 Gy arm, and 85.9% in the 57 Gy arm. Sixty Gy was non-inferior to 74 Gy, but 57 Gy failed to show non-inferiority compared with 74 Gy. Late complications were similar in the hypofractionated regimens compared to those of the conventional group. Five-year cumulative incidences of grade ≥ 2 GI toxicity were 13.7% for 74 Gy group, 11.9% for 60 Gy group, and 11.3% for 57 Gy group with no statistical significance. Five-year cumulative incidences of grade ≥ 2 GU toxicity were 9.1% for 74 Gy group, 11.7% for 60 Gy group (HR 1.34, $p = 0.07$), and 6.6% for 57 Gy group (HR 0.85, $p = 0.37$).

The RTOG 0415 study randomized 1092 patients with low-risk disease to conventional arm (73.8 Gy in 41 fractions) or MH arm (70 Gy in 28 fractions). With a median follow-up time of 5.8 years, there was no significant difference in 5-year BCFFS and acute complications. However, the late grades 2–3 GI toxicities were about 60% more likely in MH group. The majority of the late toxicities were grade 2 (11.4% vs. MF 18.3%, relative risk (RR) 1.59), and grade 3 were 2.4% in conventional arm and 4.1% in MF arm (RR, 1.55). Likewise, grade 2 late GU complications were 20.5% in conventional and 26.2% in MR arm (RR, 1.31), and grade 3 events were 2.1% and 3.5% (RR, 1.56), respectively.

The first possible reason for the worse toxicity outcomes in MH of RTOG 0415 seemed the prescription doses in both control and MH arms. BED of conventional arm was 118.1 Gy_3 in RTOG 0415 which is lower than those of the CHHiP (123.3 Gy_3) and PROFIT (130 Gy_3). On the other hand, BED of MH arm was higher in RTOG 0415 (128.3 Gy_3) than the other studies (120 Gy_3). BED difference control and MF arm were most prominent in RTOG trial. Second, RTOG 0415 had more generous organs at risk (OAR) dose constraint protocol. These factors might affect significant differences in late toxicities.

Overall, superiority and non-inferiority studies have consistently demonstrated that hypofractionation is not inferior to conventional fractionation. Although there is a little worrisome on potential higher late toxicities, the absolute difference was only about 6% and mostly confined to grade 2 adverse effects [13, 16]. Routine use of IMRT and IGRT could further decrease the toxicity rate. Also, baseline check on preexisting inflammatory bowel disease or urinary dysfunction must be preceded.

MH regimen of 60 Gy with 3 Gy per fraction demonstrated its efficacy and safety in PROFIT and CHHiP trials. There might be a question on further dose escalation in MH. A phase II study assessing further dose-escalated hypofractionation regimen (66 Gy in 22 fractions) enrolled patients from 2001 to 2005, and its long-term outcomes were reported [17]. Median follow-up was 128 months for 60 Gy and 108 months for 66 Gy. Enrollment of 66 Gy arm closed early due to excessive grades 3–4 late toxicity; 66 Gy was related to significantly higher late toxicity. From the non-inferiority trials and this phase II study,

BED of 60 Gy with fraction size of 3 Gy (120 Gy_3) would be appropriate for MH and also comparable to conventional fractionation in terms of safety and efficacy.

9.4 Extreme Hypofractionation

Extreme hypofractionation (EH) was defined as a ≥5 Gy per fraction, and usually 6.25–8 Gy per fraction with a total dose of 35–40 Gy. EH is possible owing to the development of techniques for inter- and intra-fractional movement control such as fiducial markers insertion and image-guided radiotherapy. Both robotic non-coplanar (Cyberknife™) and gantry-based techniques can be used for EH.

Several phase I–II studies on EH reported comparable efficacy and toxicity outcomes to those of conventional RT [18–21] (Table 9.3). The 5-year BCFFS was 95–97% in low-risk disease, 83–97% in intermediate-risk group, and 69–78% in high-risk group. Higher EH dose of 40 Gy demonstrated higher 4-year cumulative incidence of grade ≥2 GI/GU toxicities than those of 35 Gy [21], the difference was observed in grade 2 toxicities, and rate of grade ≥3 late toxicities were below 2%.

The phase III data is awaited and there are three phase III studies comparing EH with conventional regimens. The Scandinavian trial "HYPO-RT-PC" (ISRCTN45905321) enrolled 1200 intermediate-risk prostate cancer patients and randomized them to either conventional (78 Gy in 39 fractions) or EH (42.7 Gy in 7 fractions, every other weekday). They reported early toxicity result with the 866 patients who reached 2-year follow-up, and there was no difference [22]. The tumor control outcomes would take more time.

Another ongoing trial is PACE B (NCT01584258) comparing EH (36.25 Gy/five fractions), MH (62 Gy/20 fractions), and conventional regimen (78 Gy/39 fractions). The last one is HEAT trial (NCT01794403) which compare MH (70.2 Gy/26 fractions) with EH (36.25 Gy/5 fractions).

The PATRIOT study (NCT01423474) is a randomized phase II study comparing two EH schedules delivered every other day over 11 days and once per week over 29-day schedule with prescription dose of 40 Gy in 5 fractions. The study reported early results with median follow-up time of 13.1 months; 29-day group was associated with superior bowel and urinary quality of life than those of 11-day arm [23].

Table 9.3 Phase I–II trials for extreme hypofractionation

Trial	N	Median FU (Y)	Risk group/GS	Technique	Dose (TD/SD)	ADT	5-year BCFFS	Late toxicity
Meier [18] abs	309	5.1	Low Intermediate	Robotic	40/8	No report	97.3% 97.1%	G3 ~1.5% No G4+
King [19]	1100	3	Low Intermediate High	Robotic	35–40/7–8	14%	95% 83% 78%	No report
Katz [20]	515	6	Low Intermediate High	Robotic	35–36.25/7–7.25	14%	96% (7Y) 89% 69%	G2 GI 4%, GU 9.1% G3 GU 1.7%
Musunuru [21]	114	6.2 3	Low Intermediate	Gantry	35–40/7–8	<1%	98.7% (4Y) 100%	G4 GI <1% More G2+ toxicities in 40 Gy (5–7.6% vs. 24.2–26.2%)

ADT androgen deprivation therapy, *abs* data derived from abstract, *BCFFS* biochemical failure-free survival, *FU* follow-up, *GI* gastrointestinal, *G* grade, *GS* Gleason score, *GU* genitourinary, *NS* not significant, *SS* statistically significant, *SD* single dose, *TD* total dose, *Y* years

9.5 Boost Modalities: External Beam Radiotherapy Versus Brachytherapy

In a comparative analysis, brachytherapy demonstrates its value in all risk groups [24]. In terms of biochemical control, brachytherapy provides superior results in patients with low-risk group. For intermediate-risk group, the combination of EBRT and brachytherapy appears comparable to brachytherapy alone. For high-risk diseases, combination therapies including EBRT, brachytherapy, and androgen deprivation therapy (ADT) appear superior to localized treatment alone.

There was an attempt to compare the EBRT alone and combined treatment consisting of low-dose rate (LDR) brachytherapy and EBRT. A total of 870 patients with intermediate-risk prostate cancer treated with either 86.4 Gy of EBRT alone ($n = 470$) or combined treatment with 50.4 Gy of EBRT ($n = 400$). The 7-year BCFFS was 81.4 in EBRT vs. 92.0% in combined treatment ($p < 0.001$), and distant metastasis-free survival (DMFS) rates were 93.0 vs. 97.2% ($p = 0.04$), respectively [25]. Although a higher incidence of acute GU toxicities observed in combined treatment arm, late toxicity outcomes were similar between the two groups.

Recently, the results of a randomized phase III study (ASCEND-RT trial) were published. The ASCEND-RT trial enrolled 398 patients with intermediate or high-risk disease. After pelvic irradiation to 46 Gy, patients were randomized to an EBRT boost to 78 Gy ($n = 200$) or LDR boost ($n = 198$). Patients randomized to EBRT boost arm were twice as likely to experience biochemical failure (multivariable analysis HR 2.04; $p = 0.004$) with the 9-year BCFFS of 83% (EBRT) and 62% (LDR) [26]. Toxicity data were also reported, and 5-year cumulative incidence of grade 3 GU toxicities was 18.4% for LDR and 5.2% for EBRT boost ($p < 0.001$) [27].

Previous trials suggested that combined therapy with EBRT and brachytherapy would be better than EBRT alone. To escalate the efficacy of EBRT alone, there is attempt to introduce EH as a boost therapy. There have been several reports that EH could achieve a comparable dose distribution to that of brachytherapy [28, 29]. ADEBAR trial (NCT03322020) is conducted in Asan Medical Center, which evaluated the feasibility of CyberKnife boost with two EH regimens (18 Gy/3 fractions and 21 Gy/3 fractions). The participant accrual is over and the study is waiting for data maturation.

9.6 Summary

Moderate hypofractionation is effective and safe for prostate cancer. Moderate hypofractionation regimen of 60 Gy in 20 fractions could be considered as another standard care for prostate cancer. Next question for radiation oncologists is the feasibility of extreme hypofractionation. The results of ongoing randomized trials are now awaited. Brachytherapy seems superior modality for boost treatment to external beam radiotherapy, and boost using extreme hypofractionation is under evaluation.

References

1. Zietman AL, Bae K, Slater JD, Shipley WU, Efstathiou JA, Coen JJ, et al. Randomized trial comparing conventional-dose with high-dose conformal radiation therapy in early-stage adenocarcinoma of the prostate: long-term results from proton radiation oncology group/american college of radiology 95-09. J Clin Oncol. 2010;28(7):1106–11. https://doi.org/10.1200/jco.2009.25.8475.
2. Dearnaley DP, Jovic G, Syndikus I, Khoo V, Cowan RA, Graham JD, et al. Escalated-dose versus control-dose conformal radiotherapy for prostate cancer: long-term results from the MRC RT01 randomised controlled trial. Lancet Oncol. 2014;15(4):464–73.
3. Heemsbergen WD, Al-Mamgani A, Slot A, Dielwart MFH, Lebesque JV. Long-term results of the Dutch randomized prostate cancer trial: Impact of dose-escalation on local, biochemical, clinical failure, and survival. Radiother Oncol. 2014;110(1):104–9. https://doi.org/10.1016/j.radonc.2013.09.026.
4. Viani GA, Stefano EJ, Afonso SL. Higher-than-conventional radiation doses in localized prostate cancer treatment: a meta-analysis of randomized, controlled trials. Int J Radiat Oncol Biol Phys. 2009;74(5):1405–18. https://doi.org/10.1016/j.ijrobp.2008.10.091.

5. Al-Mamgani A, Heemsbergen WD, Peeters STH, Lebesque JV. Role of intensity-modulated radiotherapy in reducing toxicity in dose escalation for localized prostate cancer. Int J Radiat Oncol Biol Phys. 2009;73(3):685–91. https://doi.org/10.1016/j.ijrobp.2008.04.063.
6. Zelefsky MJ, Kollmeier M, Cox B, Fidaleo A, Sperling D, Pei X, et al. Improved clinical outcomes with high-dose image guided radiotherapy compared with non-IGRT for the treatment of clinically localized prostate cancer. Int J Radiat Oncol Biol Phys. 2012;84(1):125–9. https://doi.org/10.1016/j.ijrobp.2011.11.047.
7. Miralbell R, Roberts SA, Zubizarreta E, Hendry JH. Dose-fractionation sensitivity of prostate cancer deduced from radiotherapy outcomes of 5,969 patients in seven international institutional datasets: α/β= 1.4 (0.9–2.2) Gy. Int J Radiat Oncol Biol Phys. 2012;82(1):e17–24.
8. Dasu A, Toma-Dasu I. Prostate alpha/beta revisited–an analysis of clinical results from 14 168 patients. Acta Oncol. 2012;51(8):963–74.
9. Arcangeli G, Saracino B, Arcangeli S, Gomellini S, Petrongari MG, Sanguineti G, et al. Moderate hypofractionation in high-risk, organ-confined prostate cancer: final results of a phase III randomized trial. J Clin Oncol. 2017;35:1891–7.
10. Pollack A, Walker G, Horwitz EM, Price R, Feigenberg S, Konski AA, et al. Randomized trial of hypofractionated external-beam radiotherapy for prostate cancer. J Clin Oncol. 2013;31(31):3860–8. https://doi.org/10.1200/jco.2013.51.1972.
11. Hoffman KE, Voong KR, Levy LB, Pugh TJ, Choi S, Du W, et al. Randomized trial of hypofractionated dose-escalated intensity modulated radiation therapy versus conventionally fractionated intensity modulated radiation therapy for localized prostate cancer. Int J Radiat Oncol Biol Phys. 2016;96(2):S32. https://doi.org/10.1016/j.ijrobp.2016.06.091.
12. Incrocci L, Wortel RC, Alemayehu WG, Aluwini S, Schimmel E, Krol S, et al. Hypofractionated versus conventionally fractionated radiotherapy for patients with localised prostate cancer (HYPRO): final efficacy results from a randomised, multicentre, open-label, phase 3 trial. Lancet Oncol. 2016;17(8):1061–9. https://doi.org/10.1016/S1470-2045(16)30070-5.
13. Aluwini S, Pos F, Schimmel E, Krol S, van der Toorn PP, de Jager H, et al. Hypofractionated versus conventionally fractionated radiotherapy for patients with prostate cancer (HYPRO): late toxicity results from a randomised, non-inferiority, phase 3 trial. Lancet Oncol. 2016;17(4):464–74. https://doi.org/10.1016/S1470-2045(15)00567-7.
14. Catton CN, Lukka H, Gu C-S, Martin JM, Supiot S, Chung PWM, et al. Randomized trial of a hypofractionated radiation regimen for the treatment of localized prostate cancer. J Clin Oncol. 2017;35(17):1884–90. https://doi.org/10.1200/jco.2016.71.7397.
15. Dearnaley D, Syndikus I, Mossop H, Khoo V, Birtle A, Bloomfield D, et al. Conventional versus hypofractionated high-dose intensity-modulated radiotherapy for prostate cancer: 5-year outcomes of the randomised, non-inferiority, phase 3 CHHiP trial. Lancet Oncol. 2016;17(8):1047–60.
16. Lee WR, Dignam JJ, Amin MB, Bruner DW, Low D, Swanson GP, et al. Randomized phase III noninferiority study comparing two radiotherapy fractionation schedules in patients with low-risk prostate cancer. J Clin Oncol. 2016;34(20):2325–32. https://doi.org/10.1200/JCO.2016.67.0448.
17. Lieng H, Pintilie M, Bayley A, Berlin A, Bristow R, Chung P, et al. Long-term outcomes of a phase II trial of moderate hypofractionated image-guided intensity modulated radiotherapy (IG-IMRT) for localized prostate cancer. Radiother Oncol. 2017;122(1):93–8. https://doi.org/10.1016/j.radonc.2016.10.017.
18. Meier R, Beckman A, Henning G, Mohideen N, Woodhouse S, Cotrutz C et al. Five-year outcomes from a multi-center trial of stereotactic body radiotherapy for low-and intermediate-risk prostate cancer. 2016.
19. King CR, Freeman D, Kaplan I, Fuller D, Bolzicco G, Collins S, et al. Stereotactic body radiotherapy for localized prostate cancer: pooled analysis from a multi-institutional consortium of prospective phase II trials. Radiother Oncol. 2013;109(2):217–21.
20. Katz AJ, Kang J. Stereotactic body radiotherapy as treatment for organ confined low-and intermediate-risk prostate carcinoma, a 7-year study. Front Oncol. 2014;4:240.
21. Musunuru HB, Quon H, Davidson M, Cheung P, Zhang L, D'Alimonte L, et al. Dose-escalation of five-fraction SABR in prostate cancer: toxicity comparison of two prospective trials. Radiother Oncol. 2016;118(1):112–7. https://doi.org/10.1016/j.radonc.2015.12.020.
22. Widmark A, Gunnlaugsson A, Beckman L, Thellenberg-Karlsson C, Hoyer M, Lagerlund M, et al. Extreme hypofractionation versus conventionally fractionated radiotherapy for intermediate risk prostate cancer: early toxicity results from the scandinavian randomized phase III trial "HYPO-RT-PC". Int J Radiat Oncol Biol Phys. 2016;96(5):938–9. https://doi.org/10.1016/j.ijrobp.2016.09.049.
23. Quon HC, Ong A, Cheung P, Chu W, Chung HT, Vesprini D, et al. PATRIOT trial: randomized phase II study of prostate stereotactic body radiotherapy comparing 11 versus 29 days overall treatment time. J Clin Oncol. 2015;33(7_suppl):6. https://doi.org/10.1200/jco.2015.33.7_suppl.6.
24. Grimm P, Billiet I, Bostwick D, Dicker AP, Frank S, Immerzeel J, et al. Comparative analysis of prostate-specific antigen free survival outcomes for patients with low, intermediate and high risk prostate cancer treatment by radical therapy. Results from the Prostate Cancer Results Study Group. BJU Int. 2012;109(Suppl 1):22–9. https://doi.org/10.1111/j.1464-410X.2011.10827.x.
25. Spratt DE, Zumsteg ZS, Ghadjar P, Kollmeier MA, Pei X, Cohen G, et al. Comparison of high-dose (86.4 Gy) IMRT vs combined brachytherapy plus

IMRT for intermediate-risk prostate cancer. BJU Int. 2014;114(3):360–7. https://doi.org/10.1111/bju.12514.

26. Morris WJ, Tyldesley S, Rodda S, Halperin R, Pai H, McKenzie M, et al. Androgen suppression combined with elective nodal and dose escalated radiation therapy (the ASCENDE-RT Trial): an analysis of survival endpoints for a randomized trial comparing a low-dose-rate brachytherapy boost to a dose-escalated external beam boost for high- and intermediate-risk prostate cancer. Int J Radiat Oncol Biol Phys. 2017;98(2):275–85. https://doi.org/10.1016/j.ijrobp.2016.11.026.
27. Rodda S, Tyldesley S, Morris WJ, Keyes M, Halperin R, Pai H, et al. ASCENDE-RT: an analysis of treatment-related morbidity for a randomized trial comparing a low-dose-rate brachytherapy boost with a dose-escalated external beam boost for high- and intermediate-risk prostate cancer. Int J Radiat Oncol Biol Phys. 2017;98(2):286–95. https://doi.org/10.1016/j.ijrobp.2017.01.008.
28. Fuller DB, Naitoh J, Lee C, Hardy S, Jin H. Virtual HDRSM CyberKnife treatment for localized prostatic carcinoma: dosimetry comparison with HDR brachytherapy and preliminary clinical observations. Int J Radiat Oncol Biol Phys. 2008;70(5):1588–97. https://doi.org/10.1016/j.ijrobp.2007.11.067.
29. Spratt DE, Scala LM, Folkert M, Voros L, Cohen GN, Happersett L, et al. A comparative dosimetric analysis of virtual stereotactic body radiotherapy to high-dose-rate monotherapy for intermediate-risk prostate cancer. Brachytherapy. 2013;12(5):428–33. https://doi.org/10.1016/j.brachy.2013.03.003.

Radiotherapy for Prostate Cancer Patients with Pelvic Lymph Node Metastasis

10

Seung Gyu Park and Won Park

10.1 Introduction

The prostate cancer (PCA) disseminates by the lymphatics, the perineural spaces, and the venous routes through the Santorini's venous plexus. The lymphatic dissemination includes external iliac nodes, hypogastric nodes, and lateral and subaortic sacral nodes [1].

In the United States, among 230,000 patients diagnosed with PCA, 12% have regional lymph node involvements (LNI) [2]. In the absence of exact statistical data about LNI in South Korea, it is expected more than 12% of patients would have LNI, based on the study that showed South Korean patients had more aggressive clinical features than Caucasian an African American [3].

Imaging techniques are useful but show poor sensitivity for staging and detecting metastases and tumor recurrences. The guidelines recommend computed tomography (CT) or magnetic resonance imaging (MRI) for staging workup in patients with longer life expectancies, T3 or T4 disease, or probability of lymph node involvement >10% [4]. However, diagnostic accuracy of CT and MRI in nodal staging was poor. A meta-analysis for nodal staging showed pooled sensitivity of 0.42 (95% CI 0.26–0.56) and pooled specificity of 0.82 (95% CI 0.80–0.83) in CT and pooled sensitivity of 0.39 (95% CI 0.22–0.56) and pooled specificity of 0.82 (95% CI 0.79–0.83) in MRI [5]. In prospective comparison studies of CT, diffusion-weighted MRI and ^{11}C–choline positron emission tomography (PET)/CT; sensitivity, specificity and accuracy were 57, 68, and 64% for CT; 57, 79, and 70% for MRI; and 57, 90, and 88% for ^{11}C–choline PET/CT, respectively [6]. All imaging techniques showed low diagnostic efficacy, but ^{11}C–choline PET/CT were better in specificity. Thus, in detecting clinically node-positive patients, not only imaging studies but also patients' clinical information should be considered carefully and staging pelvic lymphadenectomy could be considered, if needed.

Several prognostic factors and models to predict LNI are demonstrated for years [7]. At present, the Partin tables, Memorial Sloan Kettering Cancer Center (MSKCC), and Briganti nomograms are widely used to predict LNI in PCA patients. The Partin tables included preoperative prostate-specific antigen (PSA) level, clinical stage, and biopsy Gleason score to predict trends in clinical features and pathologic stage for patients with localized PCA [8]. The MSKCC nomograms also used three clinical variables (pretreatment PSA, clinical stage, and Gleason score) to predict pathological LNI [9]. The Briganti nomograms are most recent and widely used nomograms for patients undergoing extended

S. G. Park · W. Park (✉)
Department of Radiation Oncology, Samsung Medical Center, Sungkyunkwan University School of Medicine, Seoul, South Korea
e-mail: wonro.park@samsung.com

C. S. Kim (ed.), *Management of Advanced Prostate Cancer*,
https://doi.org/10.1007/978-981-10-6943-7_10

pelvic lymphadenectomy [10]. They included same variables with other nomograms and added the percentage of positive biopsy cores.

Once regional LNI are found, PCA is categorized as stage IV. Although stage IV PCA also includes distant metastatic disease, management of node-positive patients needs to be in contrast with distant metastatic disease, and some of node-positive patients can be cured by multimodality therapy [11]. However, few studies have focused on node-positive patients; thus majority of evidences are derived from the studies for locally advanced PCA or metastatic diseases.

We will review the current evidences in two different clinical situations. First, studies for the patients who are diagnosed with LNI via imaging studies or pathologic nodal staging (definitive radiotherapy). Second, for situation that LNI are identified during radical prostatectomy (adjuvant radiotherapy).

10.2 The Role of Definitive Radiotherapy for Node-Positive Prostate Cancer

In European Organization for Research and Treatment of Cancer (EORTC) 30846 study, from 1986 to 1998, 234 patients with LNI confirmed after lymphadenectomy without prostatectomy or other local treatment were randomized to immediate androgen deprivation therapy (ADT) or ADT given at time of clinical progression. ADT consisted of luteinizing hormone-releasing hormone (LHRH) agonist and 1 month of antiandrogen treatment or surgical castration [12]. After 13 years of follow-up time, the median overall survival (OS) was 7.6 years (95% CI 6.3–8.3) for immediate ADT arm and 6.1 years (95% CI 5.7–7.3) for delayed ADT arm. The intention to treat analysis showed a 22% relative increase in the risk of death. PCA-specific mortality at 10 years was 52.1 and 55.6% for immediate and delayed ADT arm, respectively. None of the results showed statistical significances [13]. There is still no clear evidence whether immediate ADT is better than delayed ADT or not for node-positive patients.

The concept of definitive radiotherapy in node-positive PCA was largely derived from randomized studies for locally advanced or high-risk patients. Recently, two large randomized trials showed effectiveness of radiotherapy combined with ADT. Radiotherapy improved absolute survival by 8–10% and cancer-specific survival (CSS) by approximately 50% [14–16]. However, the trials didn't fully examined nodal status and excluded node-positive patients if there was an evidence of LNI. To date, there is no randomized trial directly compared efficacy of definitive radiotherapy in node-positive patients. However, several studies supported the efficacy of radiotherapy.

In a retrospective analysis of 225 patients with lymphadenectomy-proven LNI between 1984 and 1998, it compared ADT alone and ADT plus radiotherapy [17]. None of the patients received prostatectomy. ADT consisted of either orchiectomy or medical castration. Total radiation dose ranged from 60 to 78 Gy (median 68 Gy). With a median follow-up of 9.4 years, a 10-year OS was 46% for ADT alone and 67% for ADT plus radiotherapy. The 10-year freedom from relapse or rising PSA rate and freedom from distant metastasis 25 and 56%, respectively, for ADT alone, and 80 and 85% for ADT and radiotherapy, respectively. ADT plus radiotherapy showed statistically significant outcomes in both univariate and multivariate analyses.

Studies analyzing Surveillance, Epidemiology and End Results (SEER) data also showed a survival benefit from radiotherapy [18, 19]. Tward et al. analyzed 1100 clinically node-positive patients diagnosed between 1988 and 2006. Most patients had clinically palpable PCA and high-grade tumors with Gleason scores of eight or higher. It compared radiotherapy (external beam radiotherapy with or without brachytherapy) and no radiotherapy of any kind. After median follow-up of 7.5 years, radiotherapy showed improved 5-year cancer-specific survival (CSS, 78.1% for radiotherapy and 71.1% for no radiotherapy, HR 0.66, 95% CI 0.54–0.82) and 5-year OS (67.8% for radiotherapy and 56.2% for no radiotherapy, HR 0.70, 95% CI 0.59–0.81) in both univariate and multivariate analysis [19].

Rusthoven et al. analyzed 3787 patients with LNI diagnosed between 1995 and 2005. The study included both clinically and pathologically confirmed node-positive patients. Outcomes for clinically node-positive patients (796 patients) showed radiotherapy significantly improved 10-year OS (45% for radiotherapy and 29% for no radiotherapy, $p < 0.001$) and 10-year CSS (67% for radiotherapy and 53% for no radiotherapy, $p < 0.001$). Similar improvement for survival was also noted in pathologically node-positive patients (2991 patients) [18]. However, both reported SEER data analyses had some weaknesses for that no information on ADT was available.

Lin et al. analyzed 3540 clinically node-positive patients diagnosed between 2004 and 2011 from National Cancer Database (NCDB) of the United States [20]. Most patients had at least one high-risk feature, high Gleason scores [8–10], high PSA level (≥20 ng/mL), or clinical stage T3 or T4. Among the patients, 32.2% of patients received ADT alone and 51.4% received ADT plus radiotherapy. Survival analyses were performed in 983 patients diagnosed between 2004 and 2006 to obtain sufficient follow-up time. Five-year OS was 49.4% for patients received ADT alone and 72.4% for patients received ADT plus radiotherapy (HR 0.51, 95% CI 0.40–0.65, $p < 0.001$). A decreased risk in ADT plus radiotherapy was also reproduced in propensity-matched cohort (HR 0.50, 95% CI 0.37–0.67, $p < 0.001$).

Cohort study from control arms of the STAMPEDE trial described the impact of radiotherapy on survival by nodal involvement. The STAMPEDE trial is a multi-arm, multi-stage randomized clinical trial to test the addition of further treatment to ADT-based therapy. While control arm of the trial received various additional therapies, the control arm has consistently been use of long-term hormonal therapy with or without radiotherapy. Radiotherapy was delivered using intensity modulated radiotherapy or conformal radiotherapy technique. Recommended dose was 74 Gy in 37 fractions or the equivalent dose using hypofractionated dose to prostate and seminal vesicles, with pelvic node dose of 46–50 Gy in 2-Gy fractions or equivalent. In 177 node-positive patients, 2-year failure-free survival was better with radiotherapy (81 vs. 53%, adjusted HR 0.48, 95% CI 0.29–0.79). Using the control arms of large prospective trial, the data were collected in a consistent, prospective fashion. However, there are still limitations, because radiotherapy was not randomized and the median follow-up time was too short; thus survival data are still immature [21].

Like addition of radiotherapy to ADT above, the addition of ADT to definitive radiotherapy is also based on the randomized studies for locally advanced or high-risk patients. Multiple randomized trials showed improved survival from addition of ADT to radiotherapy. Some of these trials didn't include node-positive patients [22]. But other trials included some node-positive patients [23–25].

The Radiation Therapy Oncology Group (RTOG) 85-31 study was designed to evaluate the efficacy of ADT to definitive radiotherapy. The trial randomized 977 patients with clinical stage T3 patients or those with LNI [25]. In a subgroup analysis of RTOG 85-31, authors evaluated efficacy of radiotherapy plus ADT for 173 patients with clinically or pathologically proven node-positive PCA [26]. Among them, 21 patients in each arm received prostatectomy; thus 77 patients in immediate ADT arm and 54 patients in radiotherapy alone arm received definitive radiotherapy. For radiotherapy, the initial target volume including pelvic lymph nodes was to receive a total of 44–46 Gy with boost volume encompassing prostate with enough margins to receive up to 65–70 Gy. In median follow-up of 6.5 years, univariate analysis showed better biochemical control and distant control in immediate ADT plus radiotherapy arm for regardless of prostatectomy status. Although CSS and OS didn't show statistical significance on univariate analysis, multivariate analysis after adjusting variables showed statistically significant benefit in all end points analyzed including OS (RR 1.62, $p = 0.03$) and CSS (RR 0.014, $p = 0.014$). Gleason score 8–10 was another factor that negatively impact on end points.

Another randomized trial of Granfors et al. compared combination of radiotherapy and ADT to radiotherapy alone [27]. Authors randomized 91 patients who underwent surgical node staging without prostatectomy, and 43% of patients had LNI. ADT was achieved by orchiectomy in all patients. After relatively long-term follow-up times (mean 9.7 years in all patients, 16.5 years in survivors), radiotherapy plus ADT showed statistically significant improvement on OS ($p = 0.03$). Especially, this result was mainly due to lymph node-positive patients, because in subgroup analysis of node-positive patients had statistically better OS ($p = 0.005$), while subgroup of node-negative patients didn't show any statistical differences.

Although there is no randomized trial for definitive radiotherapy in node-positive patients, several studies consistently showed improved OS and CSS improvement compared to ADT only or conservative management only (Table 10.1). Based on many studies demonstrating a survival benefit of both adding radiotherapy to ADT and adding ADT to radiotherapy, implementation of radiotherapy as a part of locoregional treatment seemed to be reasonable to consider. Unlike distant metastatic disease, long-term survival can be achieved by using multimodality treatment. However, it should be noted that evidences are limited by their retrospective study. Current guidelines recommend either long-term ADT alone or long-term ADT plus definitive radiotherapy as treatment option in clinically or pathologically proven node-positive patients who didn't receive prostatectomy [4].

10.3 The Role of Adjuvant Radiotherapy for Pathologically Node-Positive Patients After Prostatectomy

The Eastern Cooperative Oncology Group (ECOG) 3886 trial randomized 98 patients who were proven LNI after prostatectomy and pelvic lymphadenectomy to immediate ADT or delayed ADT [28]. At median follow-up of 11.9 years, unlike the results of EORTC 30846 for node-positive patients who confirmed after lymphadenectomy without prostatectomy, the trial showed that immediate ADT resulted in statistically better OS (HR 1.84, 95% CI 1.01–3.35, $p = 0.04$), CSS (HR 4.09, 95% CI 1.76–9.49, $p = 0.0004$), and progression-free survival (HR 3.42, 95% CI 1.96–5.98, $p < 0.0001$). According to the authors' opinion, ADT is most effective in prostatectomy patients, but not in patients without prostatectomy due to larger quantities of tumor burden. To date, ECOG 3886 trial provides the only level 1 evidence for adjuvant treatment for pathologically positive lymph node patients after prostatectomy and lymphadenectomy [11].

Several randomized studies demonstrated survival benefit of adjuvant radiotherapy after radical prostatectomy for patients with locally advanced PCA such as pT3 disease or positive resection margins [29–31]. Although the studies showed that maximizing local control resulted better outcomes, the studies didn't include node-positive patients. RTOG 96–08 study was the only randomized trial to attempt to demonstrate the advantage of radiotherapy for node-positive patients, but the study was closed prematurely because of poor accrual. No randomized or prospective results for node-positive patients are published, but several retrospective studies tried to demonstrate the efficacy of adjuvant radiotherapy.

Briganti et al. reported the impact of adjuvant radiotherapy and ADT for pathologically node-positive patients [32]. They analyzed 364 patients who undergone radical prostatectomy and pelvic lymphadenectomy between 1988 and 2003. All patients received ADT via orchiectomy, or LHRH agonist and radiotherapy were treated in 117 patients. In most cases (85%), radiotherapy consisted of a four-field whole pelvis irradiation to a median dose of 50.4 Gy (range 45–50.4), followed by boost to prostatic bed up to a median dose of 68.4 Gy (range 55.8–72). After a median follow-up of 95.1 months, patients treated with adjuvant radiotherapy showed significantly higher CSS (at 8-year 91 vs. 78%, $p = 0.004$) and OS (at 8-year 84 vs. 65%, $p < 0.001$) compared with patients treated with ADT alone. Subgroup

Table 10.1 Studies of definitive treatment for node positive prostate cancer

Author/study name	Study type	Inclusion criteria	Arms	N	Median follow-up (year)	Outcomes			
						OS	Statistic	CSS	Statistic
EORTC 30846 [13]	Randomized trial	cT2-3, pN+	Immediate ADT	119	13	Median 7.6 years	NS	(10-year) 47.9%	NS
			Delayed ADT	115		Median 6.1 years		(10-year) 44.4%	
Zagars et al. [17]	Retrospective	cT1-3, pN+	ADT plus radiotherapy	72	9.4	(10-year) 67%	0.008		
			ADT alone	183		(10-year) 44%			
Tward et al. [19]	Retrospective (SEER data)	any T, cN+	ADT plus radiotherapy	397	5.3	(5-year) 67.8%	<0.01	(5-year) 78.1%	<0.01
			ADT alone	703		(5-year) 56.2%		(5-year) 71.1%	
Rusthoven et al. [18]	Retrospective (SEER data)	Any T, cN+	ADT plus radiotherapy	340	6.8	(10-year) 45%	<0.01	(10-year) 67%	<0.01
			ADT alone	456		(10-year) 29%		(10-year) 53%	
Lin et al. [20]	Retrospective (from NCDB)	Any T, cN+	ADT plus radiotherapy	595	5.2	(5-year) 72.4%	<0.01		
			ADT alone	388		(5-year) 49.4%			
James et al. [21]	Cohort study		ADT plus radiotherapy	97	1.4			(2-year) 81%	SS
			ADT alone	80				(2-year) 53%	
RTOG 85–31 [26]	Subgroup analysis of randomized trial	T1-3, cN+/pN+	Radiotherapy plus ADT	98	6.5	(Multivariate analysis)	0.03	(Multivariate analysis)	0.014
			Radiotherapy alone	75		Favor radiotherapy plus ADT		Favor radiotherapy plus ADT	
Granfors et al. [27]	Subgroup analysis of randomized trial		Radiotherapy plus ADT	20	Mean 9.7	Favor radiotherapy plus ADT	0.005		
			Radiotherapy alone	19					

N number; *OS* overall survival; *CSS* cancer-specific survival; *EORTC* European Organization for Research and Treatment of Cancer; *RTOG* Radiation Therapy Oncology Group; *SEER* Surveillance, Epidemiology, and End Results; *NCDB* National Cancer Database; *ADT* androgen deprivation therapy; *NS* not significant; *SS* statistically significant analysis showed comparably improved survival for patients with two or fewer positive pelvic nodes as well as patient with more than two positive nodes.

Similar study by Abdollah et al. was published in 2014 [33]. The study included 1107 patients between 1988 and 2010 with pathologically LNI who are treated with prostatectomy and extended pelvic lymphadenectomy followed by ADT. Among them, 386 patients received adjuvant radiotherapy. Authors identified four variables (number of positive nodes, pathologic Gleason score, tumor stage, and surgical margin status) to stratify patients according to their CSS risk. On the basis of these variables, the patients were stratified into five risk groups: very low risk (≤2 positive nodes and Gleason score 2–6), low risk (≤2 positive nodes, Gleason score 7–10, pT2/pT3a stage, and negative surgical margins), intermediate risk (≤2 positive nodes, Gleason score 7–10, and pT3b/pT4 stage or positive surgical margins), high risk (3–4 positive nodes), and very high risk (>4 positive nodes).

After a median follow-up of 7.1 years, adjuvant radiotherapy was associated with improved CSS in intermediate risk (at 8-year, 93.1 vs. 84.2%, p = 0.03) and high risk (at 8-year, 96.5 vs. 78.8%, p = 0.02) groups. This result was also confirmed at multivariate analysis. In all other risk groups (very low, low, and very high risk), adjuvant radiotherapy didn't improve survival significantly. Similar findings were observed for OS. Authors also confirmed their findings via external validation using 3158 patients of SEER data. The study demonstrated that pathologically node-positive patients should not be considered as a single risk category. And clinicians always consider other characteristics of node-positive patients and decided who may benefit from radiotherapy.

Patients' data from the NCDB had recently been published [34]. Inclusion criteria were adenocarcinoma histology, pathologically LNI, and receipt of radical prostatectomy plus subsequent adjuvant ADT. 2569 patients with node-positive patients between 2003 and 2011 were identified, and 906 of them (35.3%) received adjuvant radiotherapy. Radiotherapy showed improved 5-year OS (87 vs. 82%, p = 0.007). After propensity matching, adjuvant radiotherapy still showed improved 5-year OS (88 vs. 81%, p = 0.004), with an HR of 1.43 (95% CI 1.10–1.86). Adjuvant radiotherapy showed improved OS across all strata in tested variables (PSA, Gleason score, surgical margin status, lymph node ratio, and number of lymph node examined and involved).

In contrast to aforementioned studies, SEER data analysis by Kaplan et al. didn't show a benefit from adjuvant radiotherapy [35]. Authors included 577 pathologically node-positive patients between 1995 and 2007. Adjuvant radiotherapy is defined as receipt of radiotherapy within 1 year of surgery. After propensity matching by age, comorbidities, Gleason score, pathologic T stage, PSA level, and number of positive nodes, adjuvant radiotherapy was not associated with OS (5.09 vs. 3.77 events per 100 person-years, p = 0.153) or CSS (2.89 vs. 1.31, p = 0.090). Another SEER data analysis by Rusthoven et al. also showed no statistically significant OS at both univariate and multivariate analysis [36]. But on analyses by identical risk stratification of Abdollah et al., adjuvant radiotherapy showed improved OS for intermediate-risk patients (≤2 positive nodes, Gleason score 7–10, and pT3b/pT4 stage or positive surgical margins). However, unlike the results of Abdollah et al., adjuvant radiotherapy didn't show benefit for high-risk patients.

Up to date, several confounding retrospective results show survival benefit of adjuvant radiotherapy, but negative results also exist (Table 10.2). Although ADT is the only level 1 treatment guideline for adjuvant therapy in pathologically node-positive patients, further extensive locoregional therapy is needed to overcome aggressive tumor burden in selected patients. Clinical trials are needed to verify the efficacy of adjuvant radiotherapy and to find proper indication for adjuvant radiotherapy.

Table 10.2 Studies of adjuvant treatment after prostatectomy for node-positive prostate cancer

Author/study name	Study type	Inclusion criteria	Arms	N	Median follow-up (year)	Outcomes			
						OS	Statistic	CSS	Statistic
ECOG 3886 [28]	Randomized trial	pT1b or 2 N+	Immediate ADT	47	11.9	Median 13.9 years	0.04	Not reached	0.0004
			Delayed ADT	51		median 11.3 years		median 12.3 years	
Briganti et al. [32]	Retrospective	pT2-4 N+	ADT plus radiotherapy	117	8	(8-year) 84%	<0.001	(8-year) 91%	0.004
			ADT alone	247		(8-year) 65%		(8-year) 78%	
Abdollah et al. [33]	Retrospective	pT2-4 N+	ADT plus radiotherapy	386	7.1	(8-year) 87.6%	<0.001	(8-year) 92.4%	0.080
			ADT alone	721		(8-year) 75.1%		(8-year) 86.2%	
Jegadeesh et al. [34]	Retrospective (from NCDB)	pT2-4 N+	ADT plus radiotherapy	906	4.4	(5-year) 87%	0.007		
			ADT alone	1663		(5-year) 82%			
Kaplan et al. [35]	Retrospective (from SEER data)	pT2-4 N+	ADT plus radiotherapy	177		5.09 events per 100 person-years	0.153	2.89 events per 100 person-years	0.090
			ADT alone	400		3.77 events per 100 person-years		1.31 events per 100 person-years	

N number; *OS* overall survival; *CSS* cancer-specific survival; *ECOG* Eastern Cooperative Oncology Group; *NCDB* National Cancer Database; *SEER* Surveillance, Epidemiology, and End Results; *ADT* androgen deprivation therapy

10.4 Summary

In PCA patients, once regional LNI are found, PCA is categorized as stage IV. However, unlike distant metastatic disease, patients with regional LNI can be curable with multimodality therapy [11]. For definitive treatment, several retrospective studies, population-based analyses, and subgroup analyses of randomized trials showed that radiotherapy plus ADT improved survival outcomes compared with ADT alone or radiotherapy alone. Although no clinical trials have directly studied efficacy of radiotherapy for node-positive patients, current guidelines recommend either 2–3 years of ADT with radiotherapy or long-term ADT alone [4]. For adjuvant treatment after prostatectomy, the only level 1 evidence for adjuvant therapy is from ECOG 3886 study supporting immediate adjuvant ADT. Although several retrospective studies showed survival benefit adding radiotherapy to ADT, population-based study showed confounding outcomes. Current guidelines recommend either adjuvant ADT with/without adjuvant radiotherapy or observation [4].

References

1. Porcaro AB, De Luyk N, Corsi P, Sebben M, Tafuri A, Processali T, et al. Clinical factors predicting bilateral lymph node invasion in high-risk prostate cancer. Urol Int. 2017;99(4):392–9.
2. Fast Stats: an interactive tool for access to SEER cancer statistics. www.seer.cancer.gov/faststats.
3. Jeong IG, Dajani D, Verghese M, Hwang J, Cho YM, Hong JH, et al. Differences in the aggressiveness of prostate cancer among Korean, Caucasian, and African American men: A retrospective cohort study of radical prostatectomy. Urol Oncol. 2016;34(1):3 e9–14.
4. James L, Mohler M, Armstrong AJ, Bahnson RR, D'Amico AV, Davis BJ. Prostate cancer, version 1.2016. J Natl Compr Cancer Netw. 2016;14(1):19–30.
5. Hovels AM, Heesakkers RA, Adang EM, Jager GJ, Strum S, Hoogeveen YL, et al. The diagnostic accuracy of CT and MRI in the staging of pelvic lymph nodes in patients with prostate cancer: a meta-analysis. Clin Radiol. 2008;63(4):387–95.
6. Heck MM, Souvatzoglou M, Retz M, Nawroth R, Kubler H, Maurer T, et al. Prospective comparison of computed tomography, diffusion-weighted magnetic resonance imaging and [11C]choline positron emission tomography/computed tomography for preoperative lymph node staging in prostate cancer patients. Eur J Nucl Med Mol Imaging. 2014;41(4):694–701.
7. Cimino S, Reale G, Castelli T, Favilla V, Giardina R, Russo GI, et al. Comparison between Briganti, Partin and MSKCC tools in predicting positive lymph nodes in prostate cancer: a systematic review and meta-analysis. Scand J Urol. 2017;51(5):345–50.
8. Makarov DV, Trock BJ, Humphreys EB, Mangold LA, Walsh PC, Epstein JI, et al. Updated nomogram to predict pathologic stage of prostate cancer given prostate-specific antigen level, clinical stage, and biopsy Gleason score (Partin tables) based on cases from 2000 to 2005. Urology. 2007;69(6):1095–101.
9. Cagiannos I, Karakiewicz P, Eastham JA, Ohori M, Rabbani F, Gerigk C, et al. A preoperative nomogram identifying decreased risk of positive pelvic lymph nodes in patients with prostate cancer. J Urol. 2003;170(5):1798–803.
10. Briganti A, Larcher A, Abdollah F, Capitanio U, Gallina A, Suardi N, et al. Updated nomogram predicting lymph node invasion in patients with prostate cancer undergoing extended pelvic lymph node dissection: the essential importance of percentage of positive cores. Eur Urol. 2012;61(3):480–7.
11. Baker BR, Mohiuddin JJ, Chen RC. The role of radiotherapy in node-positive prostate cancer. Oncology. 2015;29(2):108–14, 16.
12. Schroder FH, Kurth KH, Fossa SD, Hoekstra W, Karthaus PP, Debois M, et al. Early versus delayed endocrine treatment of pN1-3 M0 prostate cancer without local treatment of the primary tumor: results of European Organisation for the Research and Treatment of Cancer 30846--a phase III study. J Urol. 2004;172(3):923–7.
13. Schroder FH, Kurth KH, Fossa SD, Hoekstra W, Karthaus PP, De Prijck L, et al. Early versus delayed endocrine treatment of T2-T3 pN1-3 M0 prostate cancer without local treatment of the primary tumour: final results of European Organisation for the Research and Treatment of Cancer protocol 30846 after 13 years of follow-up (a randomised controlled trial). Eur Urol. 2009;55(1):14–22.
14. Mason MD, Parulekar WR, Sydes MR, Brundage M, Kirkbride P, Gospodarowicz M, et al. Final report of the intergroup randomized study of combined androgen-deprivation therapy plus radiotherapy versus androgen-deprivation therapy alone in locally advanced prostate cancer. J Clin Oncol. 2015;33(19):2143–50.
15. Warde P, Mason M, Ding K, Kirkbride P, Brundage M, Cowan R, et al. Combined androgen deprivation therapy and radiation therapy for locally advanced prostate cancer: a randomised, phase 3 trial. Lancet. 2011;378(9809):2104–11.
16. Widmark A, Klepp O, Solberg A, Damber J-E, Angelsen A, Fransson P, et al. Endocrine treatment, with or without radiotherapy, in locally advanced prostate cancer (SPCG-7/SFUO-3): an open randomised phase III trial. Lancet. 2009;373(9660):301–8.

17. Zagars GK, Pollack A, von Eschenbach AC. Addition of radiation therapy to androgen ablation improves outcome for subclinically node-positive prostate cancer. Urology. 2001;58(2):233–9.
18. Rusthoven CG, Carlson JA, Waxweiler TV, Raben D, Dewitt PE, Crawford ED, et al. The impact of definitive local therapy for lymph node-positive prostate cancer: a population-based study. Int J Radiat Oncol Biol Phys. 2014;88(5):1064–73.
19. Tward JD, Kokeny KE, Shrieve DC. Radiation therapy for clinically node-positive prostate adenocarcinoma is correlated with improved overall and prostate cancer-specific survival. Pract Radiat Oncol. 2013;3(3):234–40.
20. Lin CC, Gray PJ, Jemal A, Efstathiou JA. Androgen deprivation with or without radiation therapy for clinically node-positive prostate cancer. J Natl Cancer Inst. 2015;107(7).
21. James ND, Spears MR, Clarke NW, Dearnaley DP, Mason MD, Parker CC, et al. Failure-free survival and radiotherapy in patients with newly diagnosed non-metastatic prostate cancer: data from patients in the control arm of the STAMPEDE trial. JAMA Oncol. 2016;2(3):348–57.
22. Denham JW, Steigler A, Lamb DS, Joseph D, Mameghan H, Turner S, et al. Short-term androgen deprivation and radiotherapy for locally advanced prostate cancer: results from the Trans-Tasman Radiation Oncology Group 96.01 randomised controlled trial. Lancet Oncol. 2005;6(11):841–50.
23. Bolla M, Collette L, Blank L, Warde P, Dubois JB, Mirimanoff R-O, et al. Long-term results with immediate androgen suppression and external irradiation in patients with locally advanced prostate cancer (an EORTC study): a phase III randomised trial. Lancet. 2002;360(9327):103–8.
24. Roach M 3rd, Bae K, Speight J, Wolkov HB, Rubin P, Lee RJ, et al. Short-term neoadjuvant androgen deprivation therapy and external-beam radiotherapy for locally advanced prostate cancer: long-term results of RTOG 8610. J Clin Oncol. 2008;26(4):585–91.
25. Pilepich MV, Winter K, Lawton CA, Krisch RE, Wolkov HB, Movsas B, et al. Androgen suppression adjuvant to definitive radiotherapy in prostate carcinoma--long-term results of phase III RTOG 85-31. Int J Radiat Oncol Biol Phys. 2005;61(5):1285–90.
26. Lawton CA, Winter K, Grignon D, Pilepich MV. Androgen suppression plus radiation versus radiation alone for patients with stage D1/pathologic node-positive adenocarcinoma of the prostate: updated results based on national prospective randomized trial Radiation Therapy Oncology Group 85-31. J Clin Oncol. 2005;23(4):800–7.
27. Granfors T, Modig H, Damber JE, Tomic R. Long-term followup of a randomized study of locally advanced prostate cancer treated with combined orchiectomy and external radiotherapy versus radiotherapy alone. J Urol. 2006;176(2):544–7.
28. Messing EM, Manola J, Yao J, Kiernan M, Crawford D, Wilding G, et al. Immediate versus deferred androgen deprivation treatment in patients with node-positive prostate cancer after radical prostatectomy and pelvic lymphadenectomy. Lancet Oncol. 2006;7(6):472–9.
29. Thompson IM, Tangen CM, Paradelo J, et al. Adjuvant radiotherapy for pathologically advanced prostate cancer: a randomized clinical trial. JAMA. 2006;296(19):2329–35.
30. Thompson IM, Tangen CM, Paradelo J, Lucia MS, Miller G, Troyer D, et al. Adjuvant radiotherapy for pathological T3N0M0 prostate cancer significantly reduces risk of metastases and improves survival: long-term followup of a randomized clinical trial. J Urol. 2009;181(3):956–62.
31. Wiegel T, Bottke D, Steiner U, Siegmann A, Golz R, Storkel S, et al. Phase III postoperative adjuvant radiotherapy after radical prostatectomy compared with radical prostatectomy alone in pT3 prostate cancer with postoperative undetectable prostate-specific antigen: ARO 96-02/AUO AP 09/95. J Clin Oncol. 2009;27(18):2924–30.
32. Briganti A, Karnes RJ, Da Pozzo LF, Cozzarini C, Capitanio U, Gallina A, et al. Combination of adjuvant hormonal and radiation therapy significantly prolongs survival of patients with pT2-4 pN+ prostate cancer: results of a matched analysis. Eur Urol. 2011;59(5):832–40.
33. Abdollah F, Karnes RJ, Suardi N, Cozzarini C, Gandaglia G, Fossati N, et al. Impact of adjuvant radiotherapy on survival of patients with node-positive prostate cancer. J Clin Oncol. 2014;32(35):3939–47.
34. Jegadeesh N, Liu Y, Zhang C, Zhong J, Cassidy RJ, Gillespie T, et al. The role of adjuvant radiotherapy in pathologically lymph node-positive prostate cancer. Cancer. 2017;123(3):512–20.
35. Kaplan JR, Kowalczyk KJ, Borza T, Gu X, Lipsitz SR, Nguyen PL, et al. Patterns of care and outcomes of radiotherapy for lymph node positivity after radical prostatectomy. BJU Int. 2013;111(8):1208–14.
36. Rusthoven CG, Carlson JA, Kavanagh BD. External validation of the benefit of adjuvant radiotherapy for pathologic N1M0 prostate cancer. J Clin Oncol. 2015;33(17):1987–8.

Emerging Role of Radiotherapy in Stage IV Prostate Cancer

11

Changhoon Song and Jae-Sung Kim

11.1 Introduction

It has been considered that metastatic prostate cancer is incurable and is solely managed by systemic therapy like androgen deprivation therapy (ADT). Like in other cancers, evidences prevailed that prostate cancer patients with "oligometastases," which refer to small number of metastases, have a better outcome than those with extensive metastases [1–3]. Oligometastatic prostate cancer has a favorable prognosis with a median survival over 6 years [2, 3]. Oligometastasis refers to a state where metastases are limited in number and destination organ site. According to the recent expert panel consensus conference which was held in St Gallen, 85% of the panel agreed that the presence of three or fewer synchronous metastases is the most meaningful definition of oligometastatic prostate cancer [4]. Hopefully, a genomic definition of oligometastatic prostate cancer will prevail, but until that time, these radiographic definitions are reasonable. Patients with oligometastatic prostate cancer are an ideal target for local therapy such as stereotactic body radiotherapy (SBRT). Moreover, SBRT can defer ADT, which is the current backbone of treatment but can be harmful on patient's quality of life.

Imaging studies are critical in assessing the presence of metastatic tumor before treatment. Although significant development has been made in imaging techniques, its diagnostic capability for detecting metastasis is limited. It has been recognized that conventional imaging tools like computed tomography (CT) and/or bone scintigraphy have low sensitivity and accuracy to detect limited metastases. New imaging tools also have poor sensitivities for detecting metastases in prostate cancer, even with the multiparametric magnetic resonance imaging and/or positron emission tomography (PET)/CT with 11C- or 18F-labelled choline derivatives [5–7]. Recently, a meta-analysis indicates favorable sensitivity and specificity profiles with PET of 68Ga-labelled prostate-specific membrane antigen compared to choline-based PET [8].

11.2 Metastasis-Directed Radiation Therapy

A systematic review of the literature by Ost et al. [1] evaluated the impact of metastasis-directed local therapy (either radiation therapy or lymph node dissection) in the event of regional or distant recurrences following curative therapy. This review included retrospective studies reporting on a total of 450 patients with oligometastatic pros-

C. Song · J.-S. Kim (✉)
Department of Radiation Oncology, Seoul National University College of Medicine, Seoul National University Bundang Hospital, Gyeonggi-do, South Korea
e-mail: jskim@snubh.org

C. S. Kim (ed.), *Management of Advanced Prostate Cancer*,
https://doi.org/10.1007/978-981-10-6943-7_11

tate cancer. Fifty-one percent of patients were progression-free 1–3 years after metastasis-directed local therapy, with most of them receiving adjuvant ADT. A summary of the selected retrospective studies using radiation therapy as a type of metastasis-directed radiation therapy is shown in Table 11.1 [9–19]. Radiation doses as well as fractionation schedules used were heterogeneous between and within the studies. The series by Schick et al. [13] analyzed 50 patients affected by oligometastatic prostate cancer. Subset of 26 patients received whole-pelvis radiotherapy (50.4 Gy) with a boost (total median dose 65 Gy) to the choline-PET-positive nodes, in addition to limited ADT (median 12 months). After a median follow-up of 31 months, the 3-year clinical failure-free survival and overall survival (OS) rates were 59 and 92%, respectively. A normalized total dose higher than 64 Gy was the only significant factor for better prognosis.

SBRT is emerging as an appropriate treatment option in patients with oligometastatic prostate cancer. Figure 11.1 illustrates a case of oligometastases who underwent SBRT. In a retrospective study by Muldermans et al., 66 patients with 81 metastatic lesions (74 bone, 6 lymph nodes, and 1 liver) underwent SBRT [16]. At the time of the treatment, 62% of patients were castrate resistant. Most common regimen of SBRT was one fraction of a median dose of 16 Gy (range, 16–24 Gy) to 71 lesions (88%). The regimen of 30 Gy in three fractions ($n = 6$) or 50 Gy in five fractions ($n = 4$) was also used. Follow-up duration was 16 months (range, 3–49 months). Two-year local control of metastatic lesion was 82%. OS and distant progression-free survival were 83 and 45%, respectively. The dose of SBRT was the only significant factor for local control by multivariate analysis. Recently, Ponti et al. [20] performed a systematic review to assess outcomes and toxicity of SBRT for patients affected by oligorecurrent prostate cancer limited to lymph nodes. A total of 363 patients from nine studies were collected. Median follow-up was 19.2 months. Local control rate was 98%. Median progression-free survival was 22.5 months (range, 11–30 months). Acute and/or late grade two or higher toxicity was reported in only 5.6% of patients, and no patient developed grade four toxicity.

As reviewed, only small retrospective studies suggest that metastasis-directed radiation therapy provides excellent local control and carries a low risk of adverse events. There are several ongoing clinical trials assessing the role of metastasis-directed radiation therapy in oligometastatic prostate cancer. Results from these ongoing prospective trials will help elucidate the role of radiation therapy in this setting [21–23]. The OLIGOPELVIS–GETUG P07 (NCT02274779) is a multicenter phase II trial to assess the 2-year relapse-free survival in patients with oligometastases treated concurrently with high-dose IMRT (66 Gy to the lymph nodes and 54 Gy to whole pelvis) and ADT for 6 months [21]. The STOMP study (NCT01558427) assesses the impact of metastasis-directed therapy (surgery or SBRT) on the initiation of palliative treatment with ADT compared to patients undergoing active surveillance [22]. ADT will be started in both arms at time of local progression, higher than three metastatic lesions, or developed symptoms. The primary endpoint of the study is ADT-free survival. The conventional care or radioablation in the treatment of extracranial metastases trial (NCT02759783) is examining whether the addition of SBRT to oligometastases can improve progression-free survival compared to current standard of care [23].

11.3 Prostate-Directed Radiation Therapy

Because advances in systemic therapy have improved the control of distant metastases and prolonged survival, local treatment for the primary tumor becomes more important, especially in cancers with relatively long natural histories.

Table 11.1 Studies of metastasis-directed radiation therapy in patients with oligometastatic prostate cancer

Study	No. of patients	Metastatic sites treated: nodes/bone/visceral	Median PSA at time of metastasis (ng/mL)	Staging method	Details of radiation therapy	No. of patients in ADT	Median follow-up (month)	Outcomes	No. of patients with toxicity (grade ≥2)
Casamassima et al. (2011) [9]	25	25/0/0	5.7	Choline PET/CT	SBRT (3 × 10 Gy)	None	29	Median PFS: 24 month; 3-year OS: 92%; 3-year LC: 90%	0
Muacevic et al. (2011) [10]	40	0/40/0	5.4	Choline PET/CT	SBRT (1 × 16.5–22 Gy)	27	10	2-year LC: 96%	0
Jereczek-Fossa et al. (2012) [11]	19	16/1/2	1.8 (nodes) 10.7 (visceral)	Choline PET/CT	SBRT (3 × 11–12 Gy)	19	17	Median PFS not reached; 30-month PFS: 64%	1 (acute); 2 (late)
Ahmed et al. (2012) [12]	17	1/15/1	2.1	Choline PET/CT or MRI	SBRT (1 × 8–24 Gy; 5 × 10 Gy)	15	6	Median PFS: 12 months	2 (acute); 0 (late)
Schick et al. (2013) [13]	50	33/15/2	6.7	Choline or acetate PET/CT or bone scan	3D-CRT (54–74 Gy in conventional fractions); IMRT (28–36 Gy in 5–6 fractions)	49	31	Median PFS not reached; 3-year PFS: 59%; 3-year OS: 92%	0 (grade ≥3)
Decaestecker et al. (2014) [14]	50	27/22/1	3.8	Choline or FDG PET/CT	SBRT (3 × 10 Gy; 5 × 10 Gy)	35	25	Median PFS: 19 months; 2-year LC: 100%, 2-year PFS: 35%	3
Detti et al. (2015) [15]	30	30/0/0	5.0	Choline PET/CT	SBRT (3 × 9–12 Gy; 1 × 24 Gy; 5 × 6 Gy)	14	12	2-year LC: 100%,	1 (acute)

(continued)

Table 11.1 (continued)

Study	No. of patients	Metastatic sites treated: nodes/bone/visceral	Median PSA at time of metastasis (ng/mL)	Staging method	Details of radiation therapy	No. of patients in ADT	Median follow-up (month)	Outcomes	No. of patients with toxicity (grade ≥2)
Muldermans et al. (2016) [16]	66	6/74/1	1.9	Choline PET/CT or MRI	SBRT (1 × 16–24 Gy; 3 × 10 Gy; 5 × 10 Gy)	NR	16	2-year LC: 82%; 2-year PFS: 45%; 2-year OS: 83%	0
Pasqualetti et al. (2016) [17]	29	17/14/0	3.4	Choline PET/CT	SBRT (1 × 24 Gy; 3 × 9 Gy)	0	12	ADT-free survival: 40 months	0
Ingrosso et al. (2017) [18]	40	40/0/0	4.2	Choline PET/CT	SBRT (5 × 6–10 Gy)	19	24	Median PFS: 16 months; ADT-free survival: 26 months; LC 98%	1 (acute); 1 (late)
Ost et al. (2016) [19]	72	72/0/0	3.4	Choline or FDG PET/CT	SBRT (3 × 8–10 Gy; 5 × 6 Gy; 10 × 5 Gy)	31	36	Median PFS: 21 months; 3-year PFS: 34%; ADT-free survival: 44 months; LC 96%	3 (late)

PSA prostate-specific antigen, *ADT* androgen-deprivation therapy, *PET/CT* positron emission tomography with coregistered computed tomography, *SBRT* stereotactic body radiotherapy, *PFS* progression-free survival, *OS* overall survival, *LC* local control, *3D-CRT* 3D-conformal radiotherapy, *IMRT* intensity modulated radiotherapy, *FDG* fluorodeoxyglucose, *NR* not reported

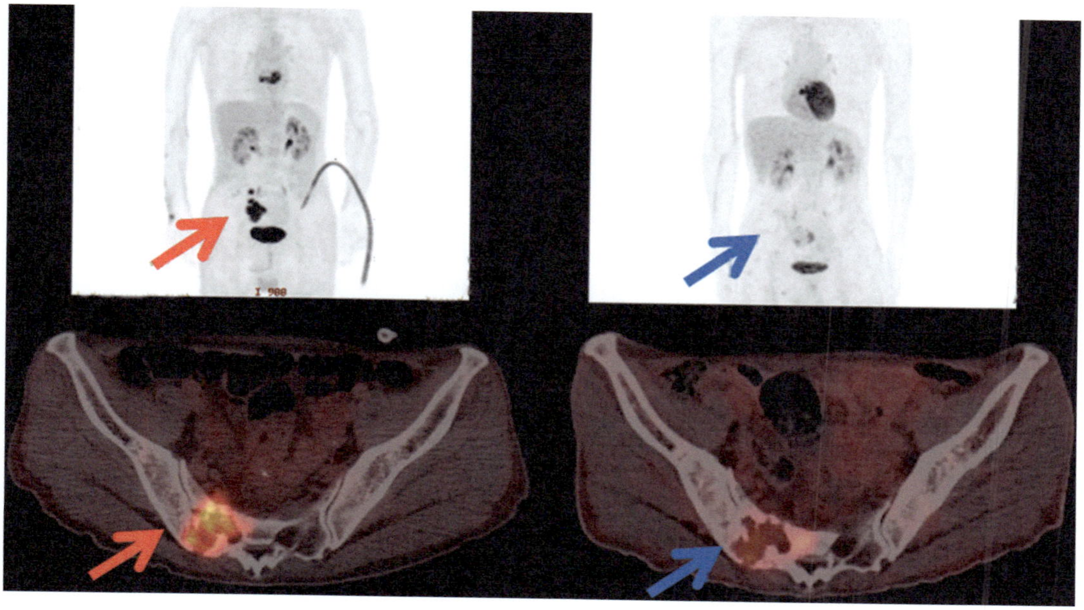

Fig. 11.1 A case of 69-year old man who presented with pelvic pain. Bony oligometastases were detected involving the T-spine and sacrum. Metastatic tumor at sacrum on PET/CT (*red arrow*) received a dose of 30 Gy in 3 fractions with SBRT. Decreased FDG uptake on PET/CT (*blue arrow*) in sacrum is observed at 2 month after SBRT

In metastatic prostate cancer, primary site treatment may not only reduce urologic symptoms but also slow the metastatic progression, as it may reduce the seeding from the primary site or alter the microenvironment and thus minimize the formation of new metastatic sites.

Culp et al. [24] suggested a survival benefit of local treatment of the prostate in patients with metastatic prostate cancer by using the data from public access Surveillance, Epidemiology, and End Results (SEER) registry. Among 8185 patients identified, 245 patients received radical prostatectomy (RP), 129 patients received brachytherapy, and 7811 patients were not treated with local therapy. The 5-year OS rate and cancer-specific survival (CSS) rate were higher in patients treated with RP (67 and 76%, respectively) or brachytherapy (53 and 61%, respectively) than in patients without local therapy (23 and 49%, respectively). Leyh-Bannurah et al. [25] suggested that patients who were treated with RP had better survival than those with radiotherapy using the SEER database from 2004 to 2013. However, this study had no access to radiotherapy doses, and it is likely that a substantial proportion of patients in the radiotherapy group received low-dose palliative radiotherapy. Using the SEER-Medicare linked database from 2004 to 2009, Satkunasivam et al. [26] were able to evaluate CSS rates of 47 patients treated with RP and 88 patients treated with intensity-modulated radiotherapy (IMRT) or 107 three-dimensional conformal radiotherapy (3D-CRT). They found that local therapy with IMRT or RP but not with 3D-CRT was associated with an improved survival. The adjusted cancer-specific mortality rate was 52 and 62% lower [hazard ratio (HR) 0.48 and HR 0.38] in patients treated with RP and IMRT, respectively, compared to no local therapy. Rusthoven et al. [27] have used the National Cancer Database (NCDB) to evaluate the impact of radiotherapy on OS of patients with metastatic prostate cancer. The treatment information of NCDB contains data not available in the SEER database, including detailed information of radiation therapy regarding treatment intent, treatment site, radiation dose, and receipt of ADT. The study included 6382 men treated with ADT, of whom 538 (8.4%) received radiotherapy to prostate. With a median follow-up of 5.1 years, OS was improved in men who received radiotherapy plus ADT versus those who received ADT alone (HR 0.624; 95% CI 0.551–0.706). A propensity analysis that made adjustments for clinically relevant factors such as age, race, comorbidities, prostate-specific antigen level, and Gleason score showed that RT was associated with an 18-month improvement in median OS (55 vs. 37 months) and a 16% improvement in 5-year OS (49 vs. 33%). They also compared the survival outcomes for patients treated with therapeutic dose radiotherapy (≥65 Gy) with ADT versus RP with ADT and demonstrated no significant differences in OS. Outcomes of these population-based studies are summarized in Table 11.2. However, readers should interpret these population-based analyses with caution, these studies all have the same potential inherent biases. There is no available data in these registries describing patient comorbidities, performance status, and extent of metastatic disease. Unbalanced patient and disease characteristics between comparison groups can explain much of the survival differences seen.

Several clinical trials are ongoing to investigate the survival impact of prostate-directed radiotherapy in addition to ADT (NCT00268476; NCT01957436; ISRCTN06890529) or local therapy (radiotherapy or surgery) in addition to best systemic therapy (NCT01751438) for patients with metastatic prostate cancer. Surgical trials in the oligometastatic bone setting are also being conducted (NCT02454543; ISRCTN15704862). Results from these ongoing clinical trials will help elucidate the role for prostate-directed radiation therapy in the setting of oligometastatic prostate cancer. For now, efforts to provide local control should be limited to patients entering a clinical trial or those with local symptoms that warrant additional therapeutic intervention.

11.4 Palliative Radiotherapy

Radiotherapy is an effective treatment to palliate symptoms caused by prostate cancer. External beam radiotherapy (EBRT) has been recognized as effective palliative tool for metastatic bone lesions. Most commonly used schedules for palliating bone metastases are reported as 30 Gy in ten fractions, 20 Gy in five fractions, and 8 Gy in a single fraction. Chow et al. [28] conducted a meta-analysis of 19 studies which compared conventional multiple fractionated radiotherapy with a single-fraction radiotherapy for initial treatment of bone metastases for various sites of cancers, including prostate cancer. The results showed similar response of relieved symptoms and rates of pathologic fracture and spinal cord compression. When deciding on the appropriate radiation treatment schedule for patients with long life expectancy, the durability of radiation treatment effect is one of the important considerations. If a single radiation dose is used, re-irradiation of the same metastatic lesion is 2.5 more likely. The reason as to what is causing the higher re-irradiation rate is unclear; it may be due to the decreased durability of treatment effect or radiation oncologist's willingness to re-irradiate following a single dose. According to a recent SEER-Medicare analysis of 3050 patients who were treated for bone metastases between 2006 and 2009, only 3% of patients were treated with a single fraction, while 50% received more than ten [29].

For multiple bone metastases, systemic radiopharmaceuticals can reduce pain, and the improved survival benefit of radium-223 was proved in randomized controlled trials [30]. Although bone metastases are the most common cause of morbidity in patients with castration-resistant prostate cancer, pelvic symptoms can also be developed. Hematuria, bladder outlet obstruction, ureteral obstruction, pelvic pain, and rectal obstruction can be improved with palliative EBRT.

Table 11.2 Population-based studies of prostate-directed radiation therapy in patients with oligometastatic prostate cancer

Study	Database, period	No. of identified patients	Type of local treatment (*n*)	Median follow-up (month)	5-year overall survival	5-year cancer-specific survival	Multivariable analysis (HR (95% CI, *p*)) for CSM
Culp et al. (2014) [24]	SEER, 2004–2010	8185	RP (245) Brachytherapy (129) NLT (7811)	16	67% 53% 23%	76% 61% 49%	0.38 (0.27–0.53, $p < 0.001$) 0.68 (0.49–0.93, $p = 0.018$) Reference
Satkunasivam et al. (2015) [26]	SEER-Medicare, 2004–2009	4069	RP (47) IMRT (88) 3D-CRT (107) NLT (3827)	20	73%[a] 72%[a] 37%[a] 34%[a]	79%[a] 82%[a] 49%[a] 46%[a]	0.48 (0.27–0.85, $p = 0.01$) 0.38 (0.24–0.61, $p < 0.001$) 0.85 (0.64–1.14, $p = 0.3$) Reference
Rusthoven et al. (2016) [27]	NCDB, 2004–2012	6382	ADT plus RT (538) ADT alone (5844)	61	49% 33%	NR	0.62 (0.55–0.71, $p < 0.001$)[b] Reference
Leyh-Bannurah et al. (2017) [25]	SEER, 2004–2013	13692	RP (313) RT (161) NLT (13218)	39 56 31	NR	NR	0.35 (0.26–0.46, $p < 0.001$) 0.48 (0.35–0.66, $p < 0.001$) Reference

HR hazard ratio, *CI* confidence interval, *CSM* cancer-specific mortality, *SEER* Surveillance, epidemiology, and end results, *RP* radical prostatectomy, *NLT* no local treatment, *IMRT* intensity modulated radiotherapy, *3D CRT* 3D Conformal radiotherapy, *NCDB* National Cancer Data Base, *ADT* androgen-deprivation therapy, *RT* radiotherapy, *NR* not reported

[a]At 3-year result

[b]For overall survival

11.5 Summary

Based on the small retrospective studies, metastasis-directed radiation therapy, such as SBRT, is associated with minimal toxicity and provides excellent local control for oligometastatic prostate cancer. The survival benefit of prostate-directed radiation therapy was suggested in population-based studies. Clinical trials evaluating the role of radiation therapy in the oligometastatic setting are ongoing. Although radiation therapy for oligometastatic setting is promising, it should be validated in randomized controlled trials.

References

1. Ost P, Bossi A, Decaestecker K, De Meerleer G, Giannarini G, Karnes RJ, et al. Metastasis-directed therapy of regional and distant recurrences after curative treatment of prostate cancer: a systematic review of the literature. Eur Urol. 2015;67(5):852–63.
2. Schweizer MT, Zhou XC, Wang H, Yang T, Shaukat F, Partin AW, et al. Metastasis-free survival is associated with overall survival in men with PSA-recurrent prostate cancer treated with deferred androgen deprivation therapy. Ann Oncol. 2013;24(11):2881–6.
3. Ost P, Decaestecker K, Lambert B, Fonteyne V, Delrue L, Lumen N, et al. Prognostic factors influencing prostate cancer-specific survival in non-castrate patients with metastatic prostate cancer. Prostate. 2014;74(3):297–305.
4. Gillessen S, Omlin A, Attard G, de Bono JS, Efstathiou E, Fizazi K, et al. Management of patients with advanced prostate cancer: recommendations of the St Gallen Advanced Prostate Cancer Consensus Conference (APCCC) 2015. Ann Oncol. 2015;26(8):1589–604.
5. Thoeny HC, Forstner R, De Keyzer F. Genitourinary applications of diffusion-weighted MR imaging in the pelvis. Radiology. 2012;263(2):326–42.
6. Paparo F, Piccardo A, Bacigalupo L, Romagnoli A, Piccazzo R, Monticone M, et al. Value of bimodal (18)F-choline-PET/MRI and trimodal (18)F-choline-PET/MRI/TRUS for the assessment of prostate cancer recurrence after radiation therapy and radical prostatectomy. Abdom Imaging. 2015;40(6):1772–87.
7. Kitajima K, Murphy RC, Nathan MA, Froemming AT, Hagen CE, Takahashi N, et al. Detection of recurrent prostate cancer after radical prostatectomy: comparison of 11C-choline PET/CT with pelvic multiparametric MR imaging with endorectal coil. J Nucl Med. 2014;55(2):223–32.
8. Perera M, Papa N, Christidis D, Wetherell D, Hofman MS, Murphy DG, et al. Sensitivity, specificity, and predictors of positive 68Ga-prostate-specific membrane antigen positron emission tomography in advanced prostate cancer: a systematic review and meta-analysis. Eur Urol. 2016;70(6):926–37.
9. Casamassima F, Masi L, Menichelli C, Bonucci I, Casamassima E, Lazzeri M, et al. Efficacy of eradicative radiotherapy for limited nodal metastases detected with choline PET scan in prostate cancer patients. Tumori. 2011;97(1):49–55.
10. Muacevic A, Kufeld M, Rist C, Wowra B, Stief C, Staehler M. Safety and feasibility of image-guided robotic radiosurgery for patients with limited bone metastases of prostate cancer. Urol Oncol. 2013;31(4):455–60.
11. Jereczek-Fossa BA, Beltramo G, Fariselli L, Fodor C, Santoro L, Vavassori A, et al. Robotic image-guided stereotactic radiotherapy, for isolated recurrent primary, lymph node or metastatic prostate cancer. Int J Radiat Oncol Biol Phys. 2012;82(2):889–97.
12. Ahmed KA, Barney BM, Davis BJ, Park SS, Kwon ED, Olivier KR. Stereotactic body radiation therapy in the treatment of oligometastatic prostate cancer. Front Oncol. 2012;2:215.
13. Schick U, Jorcano S, Nouet P, Rouzaud M, Vees H, Zilli T, et al. Androgen deprivation and high-dose radiotherapy for oligometastatic prostate cancer patients with less than five regional and/or distant metastases. Acta Oncol. 2013;52(8):1622–8.
14. Decaestecker K, De Meerleer G, Lambert B, Delrue L, Fonteyne V, Claeys T, et al. Repeated stereotactic body radiotherapy for oligometastatic prostate cancer recurrence. Radiat Oncol. 2014;9:135.
15. Detti B, Bonomo P, Masi L, Doro R, Cipressi S, Iermano C, et al. Stereotactic radiotherapy for isolated nodal recurrence of prostate cancer. World J Urol. 2015;33(8):1197–203.
16. Muldermans JL, Romak LB, Kwon ED, Park SS, Olivier KR. Stereotactic body radiation therapy for oligometastatic prostate cancer. Int J Radiat Oncol Biol Phys. 2016;95(2):696–702.
17. Pasqualetti F, Panichi M, Sainato A, Matteucci F, Galli L, Cocuzza P, et al. [(18)F]Choline PET/CT and stereotactic body radiotherapy on treatment decision making of oligometastatic prostate cancer patients: preliminary results. Radiat Oncol. 2016;11:9.
18. Ingrosso G, Trippa F, Maranzano E, Carosi A, Ponti E, Arcidiacono F, et al. Stereotactic body radiotherapy in oligometastatic prostate cancer patients with isolated lymph nodes involvement: a two-institution experience. World J Urol. 2017;35(1):45–9.
19. Ost P, Jereczek-Fossa BA, Van As N, Zilli T, Tree A, Henderson D, et al. Pattern of progression after stereotactic body radiotherapy for oligometastatic prostate cancer nodal recurrences. Clin Oncol. 2016;28(9):e115–20.
20. Ponti E, Lancia A, Ost P, Trippa F, Triggiani L, Detti B, et al. Exploring all avenues for radiotherapy in oligo recurrent prostate cancer disease limited to

lymph nodes: a systematic review of the role of stereotactic body radiotherapy. Eur Urol Focus. 2017.
21. Supiot S, Rio E, Pacteau V, Mauboussin MH, Campion L, Pein F. OLIGOPELVIS - GETUG P07: a multicentre phase II trial of combined salvage radiotherapy and hormone therapy in oligometastatic pelvic node relapses of prostate cancer. BMC Cancer. 2015;15:646.
22. Decaestecker K, De Meerleer G, Ameye F, Fonteyne V, Lambert B, Joniau S, et al. Surveillance or metastasis-directed Therapy for OligoMetastatic Prostate cancer recurrence (STOMP): study protocol for a randomized phase II trial. BMC Cancer. 2014;14:671.
23. Conventional care versus radioablation (stereotactic body radiotherapy) for extracranial oligometastases—full text view. Clinicaltrials.gov. https://clinicaltrials.gov/ct2/show/NCT02759783. Accessed 20 Sep 2017.
24. Culp SH, Schellhammer PF, Williams MB. Might men diagnosed with metastatic prostate cancer benefit from definitive treatment of the primary tumor? A SEER-based study. Eur Urol. 2014;65(6):1058–66.
25. Leyh-Bannurah SR, Gazdovich S, Budaus L, Zaffuto E, Briganti A, Abdollah F, et al. Local therapy improves survival in metastatic prostate cancer. Eur Urol. 2017;72(1):118–24.
26. Satkunasivam R, Kim AE, Desai M, Nguyen MM, Quinn DI, Ballas L, et al. Radical prostatectomy or external beam radiation therapy vs no local therapy for survival benefit in metastatic prostate cancer: a SEER-medicare analysis. J Urol. 2015;194(2):378–85.
27. Rusthoven CG, Jones BL, Flaig TW, Crawford ED, Koshy M, Sher DJ, et al. Improved survival with prostate radiation in addition to androgen deprivation therapy for men with newly diagnosed metastatic prostate cancer. J Clin Oncol. 2016;34(24):2835–42.
28. Chow E, Harris K, Fan G, Tsao M, Sze WM. Palliative radiotherapy trials for bone metastases: a systematic review. J Clin Oncol. 2007;25(11):1423–36.
29. Bekelman JE, Epstein AJ, Emanuel EJ. Single- vs multiple-fraction radiotherapy for bone metastases from prostate cancer. JAMA. 2013;310(14):1501–2.
30. Parker C, Nilsson S, Heinrich D, Helle SI, O'Sullivan JM, Fossa SD, et al. Alpha emitter radium-223 and survival in metastatic prostate cancer. N Engl J Med. 2013;369(3):213–23.

12 Adjuvant and Salvage Radiation Therapy for Prostate Cancer After Radical Prostatectomy

Joo Hwan Lee and Sung Hwan Kim

12.1 Introduction

Although radical prostatectomy (RP) provides excellent cancer control, tumor recurrence occurred in approximately 15–40% of patients within 5 years usually with elevated prostate-specific antigen (PSA) level [1, 2]. Postoperative radiation therapy is recommended for patients with adverse risk factors after complete surgical resection, subclinical disease detected by elevated postoperative serum PSA, or clinical tumor recurrence in prostatic fossa.

Postoperative radiation therapy (RT) includes adjuvant radiation therapy (ART) and salvage radiation therapy (SRT). ART is administered to the prostate bed with or without prophylactic pelvic lymph node in patients without evidence of recurrence (detectable PSA level, clinical evidence of local or distant recurrence). Salvage RT is given to patients with any evidence of residual or recurrent disease including biochemical failure [3].

J. H. Lee · S. H. Kim (✉)
Department of Radiation Oncology, St. Vincent Hospital, College of Medicine, The Catholic University of Korea, Seoul, South Korea
e-mail: rainonly@catholic.ac.kr; kimandre@catholic.ac.kr

12.2 Adjuvant Radiation Therapy

The rationale for ART is based on three randomized trials (Table 12.1). Southwest Oncology Group (SWOG) trial 8794 [4, 10] was conducted among patients with pT3N0 prostate cancer if they had risk factors of recurrence such as positive surgical margin (PSM), extraprostatic extension (EPE), and seminal vesicle invasion (SVI). A total of 425 patients were randomized into ART group with 60–64 Gy or observation group. ART group showed better 10-year metastasis-free survival (71 vs. 61%; HR, 0.71; 95% CI, 0.54–0.94; $p = 0.016$) and overall survival (74 vs. 66%; HR, 0.72; 95% CI, 0.55–0.96; $p = 0.023$). ART extended median survival duration by nearly 2 years.

European Organisation for Research and Treatment of Cancer (EORTC) trial 22911 [6, 7] evaluated biochemical progression-free survival of 1005 pT2-3N0 prostate cancer patients who had same risk factors as those of SWOG 8794 [4, 10]. Eligible patients were randomly assigned to ART group (60 Gy of conventional irradiation to the surgical bed for 6 weeks, $n = 502$) or observation group ($n = 503$) until biochemical progression. ART significantly improved 10-year biochemical failure-free survival (60.6 vs. 41.4%; HR, 0.49; 95% CI, 0.41–0.59; $p < 0.0001$) and locoregional control rate (92.7 vs. 83.4%; HR, 0.45; 95% CI, 0.32–0.68; $p < 0.0001$) at median follow-up of 10.6 years. However, overall, clinical progression-free or metastasis-free survival did not show significant differences between the two groups.

C. S. Kim (ed.), *Management of Advanced Prostate Cancer*,
https://doi.org/10.1007/978-981-10-6943-7_12

Table 12.1 Clinical trials of adjuvant radiation therapy after radical prostatectomy

Trial	Accrual	Inclusion criteria	Patients	Group	Median follow-up, years	PSA control rate, %	Local control rate, %	Clinical PFS, %	Metastasis-free survival, %	OS, %	Remarks
SWOG 8794 [4, 5]	1988–1997	pT3N0M0 with EPE, SVI, or PSM	425	ART ($n = 214$)	12.7	52[a]	92	68[a]	71[a]	74[a]	34% patients with detectable PSA
				Observation ($n = 211$)		26	78	52	61	66	
EORTC 22911 [6, 7]	1992–2001	pT2-3N0M0 with EPE, SVI, or PSM	1005	ART ($n = 502$)	10.6	60.6[a,b]	92.7[a,b]	70.3[b,c]	89.9	76.9	29% patients with detectable PSA
				Observation ($n = 503$)		41.4	83.4	64.8	89	80.7	
ARO 9602 [8, 9]	1997–2004	pT3-4aN0M0	307	ART ($n = 148$)	10	56[a,c]	NR	NR	NS	NS	Small sample size to address survival

PSA prostate-specific antigen, *PFS* progression-free survival, *OS* overall survival, *EPE* extraprostatic extension, *SVI* seminal vesicle invasion, *PSM* positive surgical margin, *ART* adjuvant radiation therapy, *NR* not reported, *NS* nonspecific

[a]Statistically significant improvement with adjuvant RT

[b]Benefit restricted to younger patients

[c]Benefit restricted to patients with PSM

German Cancer Society Arbeitsgemeinschaft Radiologische Onkologie (ARO) trial 9602 [8, 9] was the only trial that did not include patients with detectable PSA level, contrary to SWOG 8794 (34%) and EORTC 22911 (29%) trials. A total of 307 patients with pT3-4N0 prostate cancer were randomized to 60Gy ART group or observation group. Primary endpoint of that study was progression-free survival. Definition of progression included biochemical failure, local or distant clinical recurrence, or death from any cause. ART improved 10-year progression-free survival (57 vs. 27%; HR, 0.49; 95% CI, 0.35–0.67; $p < 0.0001$) in patients with PSM. Otherwise, ART showed no benefit for overall or metastasis-free survival.

Meta-analysis of these three randomized trials has been reported by Daly et al. [11]. ART improved 10-year overall survival (risk difference (RD), −0.11; 95% CI, −0.20 to −0.02), biochemical progression-free survival (RD, −0.29; 95% CI, −0.39 to −0.19), local control (RD, −0.14; 95% CI, −0.21 to −0.07), and metastatic-free survival (RD, −0.11; 95% CI, −0.20 to −0.01). However, this meta-analysis did not include 10 years of follow-up of ARO or EORTC trial. Shaikh et al. have reported another meta-analysis [12]. ART resulted in better 10-year biochemical progression-free survival (HR, 0.48; 95% CI, 0.42–0.55; $p < 0.00001$) and clinical progression-free survival (HR, 0.73; 95% CI, 0.62–0.87; $p = 0.0003$). Metastasis-free survival was significantly improved in ART group (OR, 0.77; 95% CI, 0.62–0.96; $p = 0.02$). However, ART showed no benefit for overall survival (HR, 0.97; 95% CI, 0.79–1.14; $p = 0.89$).

In summary, ART after RP reduced biochemical failure and locoregional or clinical progression in patients with adverse pathologic features including PSM, EPE, and SVI. ART reduced approximately 50–60% of the risk of biochemical failure. However, its impact on metastases or overall survival is uncertain.

There is no optimal timing for ART. In clinical practice, ART is usually administrated within 4 months after RT, after urinary incontinence cause by the surgery has resolved because of the potential to deter recovery. In the three randomized clinical trials, ART was administrated within 3–6 months after RP [4, 6–10].

The radiation dose for ART is also unclear. Higher dose increases not only tumor control rate but also the toxicity. In practice, 65–70.2 Gy is delivered at most institutions. In some reports, with the conformal radiation therapy, doses of more than 70.2 Gy improved biochemical control without increasing toxicity [13–15].

12.3 Salvage Radiation Therapy

Prostate-specific antigen is a very sensitive tumor marker for recurrence of prostate cancer. PSA should be undetectable at 4 weeks after RP considering its half-life. Rise of PSA is usually detected before detecting clinical disease progression. This is called biochemical failure or recurrence. AUA/ASTRO Guideline 2013 has suggested the definition of biochemical recurrence to be detectable or rising PSA value after surgery of >0.2 ng/mL with a second confirmatory level >0.2 ng/mL [5]. In case of biochemical recurrence, SRT should be recommended because biochemical recurrence is associated with increased metastasis or death from prostate cancer [16, 17].

Although no randomized trial has been conducted to evaluate the effect of salvage radiotherapy, there were patients with detectable PSA levels after RT in two trials. In SWOG 8794, SRT showed significant reduction of metastatic recurrence in the patients with detectable PSA level after RP [10]. In EORTC 22911, SRT showed significant reduction of biochemical failure risk in the patients with detectable PSA level after RP. SRT also reduced the clinical progression rate in this group, which did not reach statistical significance [6].

There are several retrospective studies which support the efficacy of SRT in the patients with detectable PSA or local recurrence after RT. At a median of 9 years after RP, SRT significantly increased the prostate cancer-specific survival rate compared to the group without salvage treatment (22 vs. 11%; HR, 0.32; 95% CI, 0.19–0.54; $p < 0.001$) [18]. Boorjian et al. [19] have reported that salvage radiotherapy can decrease the risk of local recurrence (HR, 0.13; 95% CI, 0.06–0.28; $p < 0.001$). It can also delay androgen deprivation therapy (ADT, HR, 0.81; 95% CI, 0.71–0.93; $p = 0.003$) and systemic progression (HR, 0.24;

95% CI, 0.13–0.45; $p < 0.001$). However, it has no significant ($p = 0.48$) effect on mortality at a median follow-up of 11.5 years after RP. Cotter et al. [20] have reported that SRT can improve overall survival of patients with biochemical recurrence after RP.

Stephenson et al. [21] have evaluated oncologic outcome and risk factors in 1540 patients who received SRT after RP. At a median follow-up duration of 53 months after completion of SRT, 866 patients experienced disease progression. The 6-year progression-free probability after SRT was 32% (95% CI, 28–35%). Risk factors for progression-free survival were PSA level before SRT ($p < 0.001$), Gleason grade after RP ($p < 0.001$), PSADT ($p < 0.001$), resection margins ($p < 0.001$), ADT administered before or during SRT ($p < 0.001$), and lymph node involvement ($p = 0$ 0.019). With these significant risk factors and previously known factors, they have proposed a pretreatment nomogram to predict 6-year progression-free probability after SRT (Fig. 12.1).

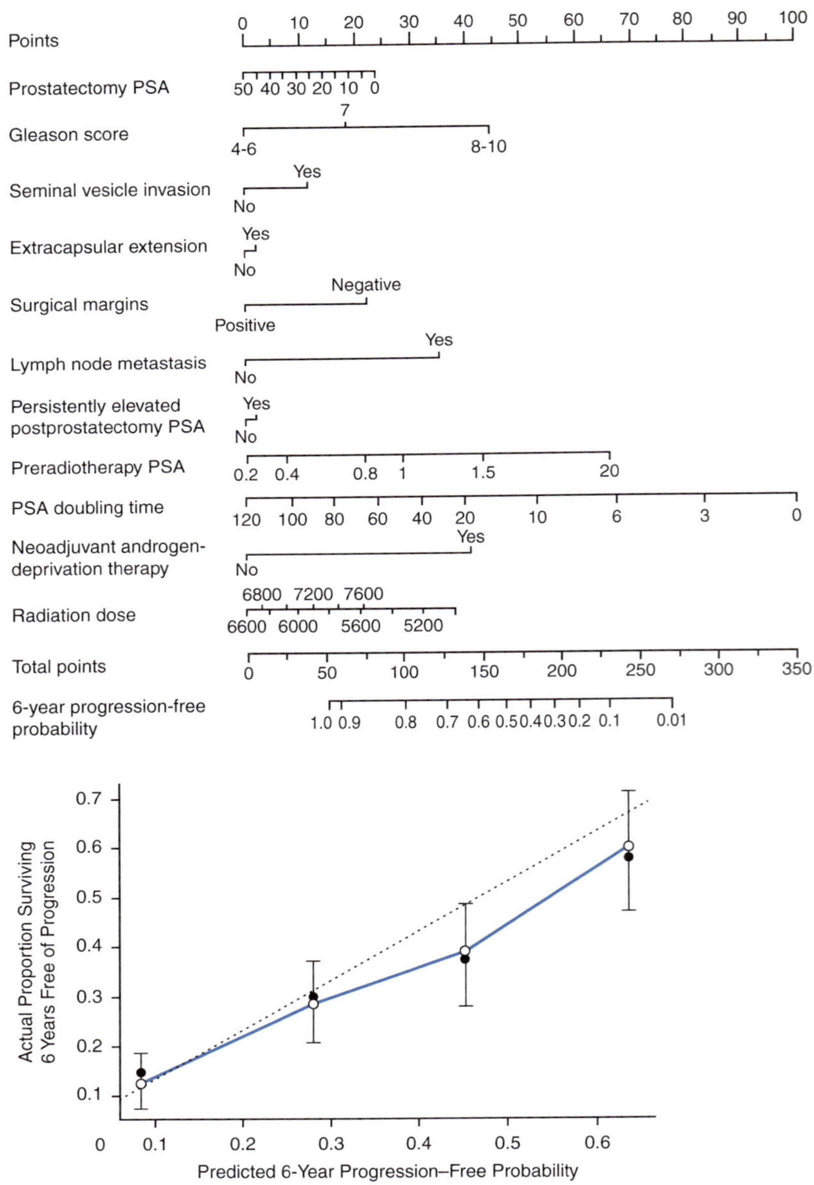

Fig. 12.1 Pretreatment nomogram predicting 6-year progression-free probability after salvage radiotherapy for prostate-specific antigen (PSA) recurrence after radical prostatectomy. Figures from Stephenson AJ, et al.: Predicting the outcome of salvage radiation therapy for recurrent prostate cancer after radical prostatectomy [21]. Instructions: Locate the patient's Gleason score on the respective axis. Draw a straight line up to the points axis to determine how many points toward disease recurrence that the patient receives for his or her Gleason score. Repeat this process for the other ten disease and treatment parameters. Sum the points and locate this number on the total points axis. Draw a straight line down to find the patient's probability of remaining free of disease progression at 6 years after salvage radiotherapy, provided the patient does not die of another cause first

King [22] has conducted a systemic review for 5587 SRT patients from 41 studies. RFS decreased by approximately 2.6% per each 0.1 ng/mL of PSA increase at the time of SRT (95% CI, 2.2–3.1; Fig. 12.2). Therefore, he concluded that SRT should be initiated at the lowest possible PSA level.

Though there was no prospective trial for optimal dose of SRT, high dose over 65Gy seemed to improve tumor control based on reduction in biochemical progression without severe toxicity increase. King [23] has conducted a meta-analysis of dose-response correlation after including 10,034 patients from 71 studies. The dose-response showed a sigmoid curve (p = 0.0001), and TCD50 was 65.8Gy. Recurrence-free survival was 58.4 vs. 38.5% at dose of 70Gy and 60Gy, respectively (Fig. 12.3). RFS was improved by 2.0% for each Gy (95% CI, 1.1–3.2).

The need for elective pelvic lymph node irradiation is another concern. Spiotto et al. [24] have evaluated 160 patients who received RP and SRT. In that study, 72 patients received elective pelvic irradiation, while 42 did not. Pelvic RT resulted in superior 5-year biochemical recurrence-free survival in patients with high-risk factors (47 vs. 21%; p = 0.008), including Gleason score ≥ 8, preoperative PSA level >20 ng/mL, prostatic capsule involvement, SVI, or pathologic lymph node metastasis. Moghanaki et al. [25] have performed a retrospective study to compare biochemical progression-free survival after SRT between whole pelvic irradiation (n = 112) and prostate bed only irradiation (n = 135). At a median follow-up of 4 years, elective pelvic irradiation did not increase biochemical progression-free survival for all patients. However, it did improve biochemical progression-free survival for patients with high pre-SRT PSA levels ≥0.4 ng/mL (adjusted HR, 0.47; 95% CI, 0.236–0.935; p = 0.031).

12.4 Androgen Deprivation Therapy with Salvage Radiation Therapy

Applying ADT to SRT is supported by two RCT. Radiation therapy oncology group (RTOG) 9601 [26] is a randomized, double-blind, and placebo-controlled trial that evaluates whether the addition of ADT for 24 months during and after SRT could prolong overall survival compared to radiation therapy plus placebo. They enrolled 771 patients with prostate cancer whose PSA level was increased to 0.2–4.0 ng/mL at least 8 weeks after surgery. Patients were randomly assigned to SRT with

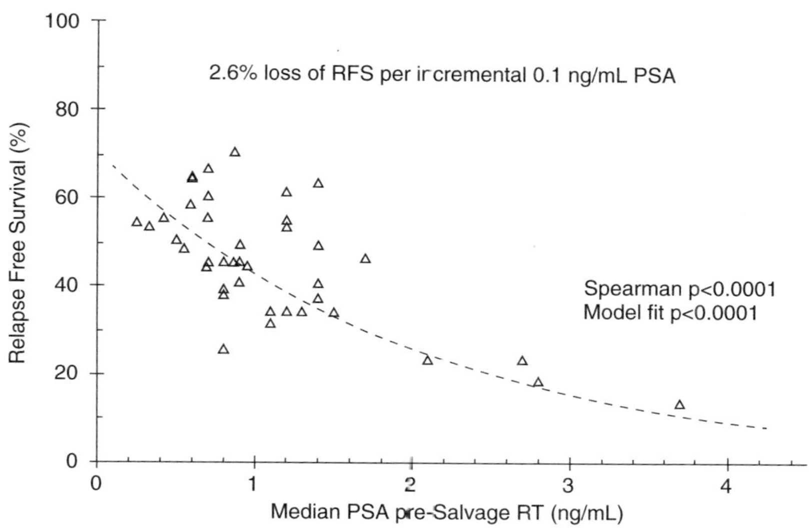

Fig. 12.2 Relapse-free survival vs. PSA level before salvage radiotherapy. Figure from Christopher R. King: The Timing of Salvage Radiotherapy After Radical Prostatectomy: A Systematic Review [22]

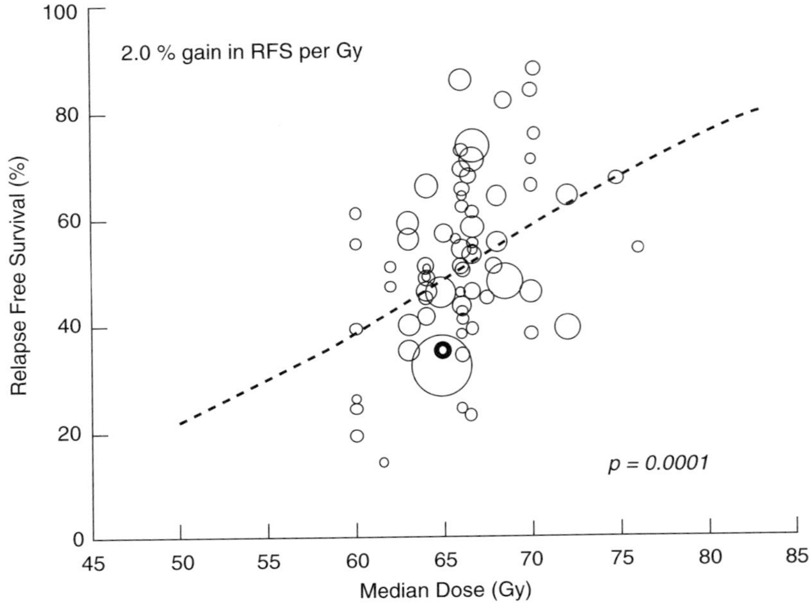

Fig. 12.3 PSA relapse-free survival vs. SRT dose for all eligible salvage RT studies. Data from Christopher R. King: The dose-response of salvage radiotherapy following radical prostatectomy: A systematic review and meta-analysis [23]

64.8Gy in 36 fractions or SRT with long-term ADT. Bicalutamide was administrated 150 mg daily for 2 years in ADT arm. At follow-up of 13 years, ADT arm showed better 12-year overall survival (76.3 vs. 71.3%; HR, 0.77; 95% CI, 0.59–0.99; p = 0.04), mortality rate from prostate cancer (5.8 vs. 13.4%; $p < 0.001$), and metastasis rate (14.5 vs. 23.0%; $p = 0.005$). The incidence of late complications induced by radiation therapy was similar in both groups. However, the incidence of gynecomastia was increased in ADT arm (69.7 vs. 10.9%; $p < 0.001$). Since RTOG 9601 trial was conducted in 1998, high-dose bicalutamide was used as ADT. Since then, it has been superseded by gonadotropin-releasing hormone (GnRH) agonists. ART with GnRH agonist was investigated in GETUG-AFU 16 phase III trial after enrolling 743 prostate cancer patients with biochemical failure (rising of PSA by 0.2–2.0 μg/L) after RP [27]. Enrolled patients were randomly assigned to standard SRT of 66 Gy in 33 fractions arm or SRT with short-term ADT arm. As an ADT, goserelin was subcutaneously injected on the first day of radiation therapy and 3 months later. Addition of ADT increased 5-year progression-free survival (80 vs. 62%; HR, 0.50; 95% CI, 0.38–0.66; $p < 0.0001$) without increasing complications. Ongoing RADICALS (Radiotherapy and Androgen Deprivation in Combination After Local Surgery) trial is a phase III trial that evaluates the effect of adding short-term or long-term ADT to SRT [28].

12.5 ART or SRT

Nowadays, ultrasensitive PSA assays make early SRT possible by detecting PSA levels as low as 0.01 ng/mL. As a result, there have been controversies about whether ART or SRT is better. The answer of this question is still uncertain.

Ku et al. [29] have performed a meta-analysis after analyzing 2380 patients from seven published reports (three RCTs, three retrospective observational studies, one matched-control analysis). Patients who received ART showed better 10-year biochemical failure-free survival compared to the patients who received SRT (risk ratio/RR, 0.70; 95% CI, 0.63–0.76). However, there were no significant differences in 10-year progression-free survival (RR, 0.88; 95% CI, 0.72–1.08) or overall survival (RR, 0.94; 95% CI, 0.80–1.11) between ART and SRT.

Fossati et al. [30] have performed a retrospective evaluation for 510 pT3N0 patients with undetectable PSA after RP. ART was performed in 243 patients, while early SRT was given to 267 patients. They were performed after PSA rose in two subsequent examinations without exceeding 0.5 ng/mL. At a median follow-up of 94 months, metastasis-free survival (92 vs. 91%; $p = 0.9$) or overall survival (89 vs. 92%; $p = 0.9$) did not significantly differ between the two groups.

There are ongoing randomized control trials that compare immediate RT with early SRT, including RADICAL trial [28] and RAVES (Radiotherapy Adjuvant Versus Early Salvage) trial [31]. Once results of these trials are published, we will know the appropriate timing for postoperative RT.

At present, AUA/ASTRO guideline [5] recommends ART to patients with adverse pathologic findings including PSM, SVI, and EPE while it recommends SRT to patients with biochemical failure, which was defined as detectable PSA level more than 0.2 ng/mL with a second confirmation over 0.2 ng/mL after RP.

12.6 Toxicity of Radiation Therapy

Toxicity of postoperative RT is similar to that of primary RT. Acute toxicity occurs during RT and within 2–3 months after completion of RT. Most acute toxicities are genitourinary (GI) or gastrointestinal (GU) toxicities. Nearly 40–60% of patients will experience acute complications such as diarrhea, nausea, vomiting, urinary frequency, dysuria, or hematuria while less than 10% of patients will experience grade 3 or 4 complications [6].

Feng et al. [32] have reported 5-year late complications of 959 patients who received postoperative RT. Grade ≥ 2 GU toxicity developed in 16% of patients who received ART. It also developed in 11% of patients treated with SRT. Of those patients on androgen deprivation therapy (ADT), Grade ≥ 2 toxicity occurred in 19%, compared to 11% in the patients without ADT.

Of the grade 2 GI toxicity, rectal bleeding was most common (4%), followed by frequency and proctitis. All other toxicities occurred in 1% of cases.

Intensity-modulated radiation therapy (IMRT) is used in more than 80% of all patients currently [33]. Goenak et al. [34] have reported that IMRT can reduce late grade >2 gastrointestinal complications from 10.2 to 1.9% compared to conformal radiation therapy. Rate of late grade 2 or more complication is about 10%. Ghadjar et al. [35] have conducted late toxicity evaluation in SAKK 09/10 randomized trial. Grade 2 late GU toxicity was observed in 13% of patients who received 64 Gy and 16.6% in patients who received 70 Gy. Grade 3 or more complication rates were 0.6 or 1.7%, respectively. Grade 2 late GI toxicity was found in 16% of patients who received 64 Gy and 15.4% of patients who received 70 Gy. Grade 3 or more complication rate was 0.6 or 2.3%, respectively.

12.7 Summary

Postoperative RT includes ART and SRT. ART should be administrated in patients with adverse pathologic features including PSM, EPE, and SVI after RP and SRT are recommended to patients with biochemical recurrence defined as PSA level which is detectable or rising over 0.2 ng/mL on at least two successive evaluations after surgery. The comparison between ART and early SRT is unclear; we will know the appropriate timing for postoperative RT with the results of ongoing RCTs. Applying ADH with SRT improved oncologic outcome in two RCTs, and the efficacy of long-term use of GnRH agonist is under investigation.

References

1. Lepor H. Radical retropubic prostatectomy. Urol Clin North Am. 2001;28(3):509–19, viii
2. Ward JF, Moul JW. Rising prostate-specific antigen after primary prostate cancer therapy. Nat Clin Pract Urol. 2005;2(4):174–82.
3. Valicenti RK, Thompson I Jr, Albertsen P, Davis BJ, Goldenberg SL, Wolf JS, et al. Adjuvant and salvage radiation therapy after prostatectomy: American

Society for Radiation Oncology/American Urological Association guidelines. Int J Radiat Oncol Biol Phys. 2013;86(5):822–8.
4. Thompson IM Jr, Tangen CM, Paradelo J, Lucia MS, Miller G, Troyer D, et al. Adjuvant radiotherapy for pathologically advanced prostate cancer: a randomized clinical trial. JAMA. 2006;296(19):2329–35.
5. Thompson IM, Valicenti RK, Albertsen P, Davis BJ, Goldenberg SL, Hahn C, et al. Adjuvant and salvage radiotherapy after prostatectomy: AUA/ASTRO Guideline. J Urol. 2013;190(2):441–9.
6. Bolla M, van Poppel H, Tombal B, Vekemans K, Da Pozzo L, de Reijke TM, et al. Postoperative radiotherapy after radical prostatectomy for high-risk prostate cancer: long-term results of a randomised controlled trial (EORTC trial 22911). Lancet. 2012;380(9858):2018–27.
7. Bolla M, van Poppel H, Collette L, van Cangh P, Vekemans K, Da Pozzo L, et al. Postoperative radiotherapy after radical prostatectomy: a randomised controlled trial (EORTC trial 22911). Lancet. 2005;366(9485):572–8.
8. Wiegel T, Bartkowiak D, Bottke D, Bronner C, Steiner U, Siegmann A, et al. Adjuvant radiotherapy versus wait-and-see after radical prostatectomy: 10-year follow-up of the ARO 96-02/AUO AP 09/95 trial. Eur Urol. 2014;66(2):243–50.
9. Wiegel T, Bottke D, Steiner U, Siegmann A, Golz R, Storkel S, et al. Phase III postoperative adjuvant radiotherapy after radical prostatectomy compared with radical prostatectomy alone in pT3 prostate cancer with postoperative undetectable prostate-specific antigen: ARO 96-02/AUO AP 09/95. J Clin Oncol. 2009;27(18):2924–30.
10. Thompson IM, Tangen CM, Paradelo J, Lucia MS, Miller G, Troyer D, et al. Adjuvant radiotherapy for pathological T3N0M0 prostate cancer significantly reduces risk of metastases and improves survival: long-term followup of a randomized clinical trial. J Urol. 2009;181(3):956–62.
11. Daly T, Hickey BE, Lehman M, Francis DP, See AM. Adjuvant radiotherapy following radical prostatectomy for prostate cancer. Cochrane Database Syst Rev. 2011(12):Cd007234.
12. Shaikh MP, Alite F, Wu MJ, Solanki AA, Harkenrider MM. Adjuvant radiotherapy versus wait-and-see strategy for pathologic T3 or margin-positive prostate cancer: a meta-analysis. Am J Clin Oncol. 2017.
13. Ost P, Fonteyne V, Villeirs G, Lumen N, Oosterlinck W, De Meerleer G. Adjuvant high-dose intensity-modulated radiotherapy after radical prostatectomy for prostate cancer: clinical results in 104 patients. Eur Urol. 2009;56(4):669–75.
14. Cozzarini C, Montorsi F, Fiorino C, Alongi F, Bolognesi A, Da Pozzo LF, et al. Need for high radiation dose (>or=70 gy) in early postoperative irradiation after radical prostatectomy: a single-institution analysis of 334 high-risk, node-negative patients. Int J Radiat Oncol Biol Phys. 2009;75(4):966–74.
15. De Meerleer G, Fonteyne V, Meersschout S, Van den Broecke C, Villeirs G, Lumen N, et al. Salvage intensity-modulated radiotherapy for rising PSA after radical prostatectomy. Radiother Oncol. 2008;89(2):205–13.
16. Albertsen PC, Hanley JA, Penson DF, Fine J. Validation of increasing prostate specific antigen as a predictor of prostate cancer death after treatment of localized prostate cancer with surgery or radiation. J Urol. 2004;171(6 Pt 1):2221–5.
17. Pound CR, Partin AW, Eisenberger MA, Chan DW, Pearson JD, Walsh PC. Natural history of progression after PSA elevation following radical prostatectomy. JAMA. 1999;281(17):1591–7.
18. Trock BJ, Han M, Freedland SJ, Humphreys EB, DeWeese TL, Partin AW, et al. Prostate cancer-specific survival following salvage radiotherapy vs observation in men with biochemical recurrence after radical prostatectomy. JAMA. 2008;299(23):2760–9.
19. Boorjian SA, Karnes RJ, Crispen PL, Rangel LJ, Bergstralh EJ, Blute ML. Radiation therapy after radical prostatectomy: impact on metastasis and survival. J Urol. 2009;182(6):2708–14.
20. Cotter SE, Chen MH, Moul JW, Lee WR, Koontz BF, Anscher MS, et al. Salvage radiation in men after prostate-specific antigen failure and the risk of death. Cancer. 2011;117(17):3925–32.
21. Stephenson AJ, Scardino PT, Kattan MW, Pisansky TM, Slawin KM, Klein EA, et al. Predicting the outcome of salvage radiation therapy for recurrent prostate cancer after radical prostatectomy. J Clin Oncol. 2007;25(15):2035–41.
22. King CR. The timing of salvage radiotherapy after radical prostatectomy: a systematic review. Int J Radiat Oncol Biol Phys. 2012;84(1):104–11.
23. King CR. The dose-response of salvage radiotherapy following radical prostatectomy: A systematic review and meta-analysis. Radiother Oncol. 2016;121(2):199–203.
24. Spiotto MT, Hancock SL, King CR. Radiotherapy after prostatectomy: improved biochemical relapse-free survival with whole pelvic compared with prostate bed only for high-risk patients. Int J Radiat Oncol Biol Phys. 2007;69(1):54–61.
25. Moghanaki D, Koontz BF, Karlin JD, Wan W, Mukhopadhay N, Hagan MP, et al. Elective irradiation of pelvic lymph nodes during post-prostatectomy salvage radiotherapy. Cancer. 2013;119(1):52–60.
26. Shipley WU, Seiferheld W, Lukka HR, Major PP, Heney NM, Grignon DJ, et al. Radiation with or without Antiandrogen Therapy in Recurrent Prostate Cancer. N Engl J Med. 2017;376(5):417–28.
27. Carrie C, Hasbini A, de Laroche G, Richaud P, Guerif S, Latorzeff I, et al. Salvage radiotherapy with or without short-term hormone therapy for rising prostate-specific antigen concentration after radical prostatectomy (GETUG-AFU 16): a randomised, multicentre, open-label phase 3 trial. Lancet Oncol. 2016;17(6):747–56.

28. Parker C, Sydes MR, Catton C, Kynaston H, Logue J, Murphy C, et al. Radiotherapy and androgen deprivation in combination after local surgery (RADICALS): a new Medical Research Council/ National Cancer Institute of Canada phase III trial of adjuvant treatment after radical prostatectomy. BJU Int. 2007;99(6):1376–9.
29. Ku JY, Lee CH, Ha HK. Long-term oncologic outcomes of postoperative adjuvant versus salvage radiotherapy in prostate cancer: Systemic review and meta-analysis of 5-year and 10-year follow-up data. Korean J Urol. 2015;56(11):735–41.
30. Fossati N, Karnes RJ, Boorjian SA, Moschini M, Morlacco A, Bossi A, et al. Long-term impact of adjuvant versus early salvage radiation therapy in pT3N0 prostate cancer patients treated with radical prostatectomy: results from a multi-institutional series. Eur Urol. 2017;71(6):886–93.
31. Pearse M, Fraser-Browne C, Davis ID, Duchesne GM, Fisher R, Frydenberg M, et al. A Phase III trial to investigate the timing of radiotherapy for prostate cancer with high-risk features: background and rationale of the Radiotherapy -- Adjuvant Versus Early Salvage (RAVES) trial. BJU Int. 2014;113(Suppl 2):7–12.
32. Feng M, Hanlon AL, Pisansky TM, Kuban D, Catton CN, Michalski JM, et al. Predictive factors for late genitourinary and gastrointestinal toxicity in patients with prostate cancer treated with adjuvant or salvage radiotherapy. Int J Radiat Oncol Biol Phys. 2007;68(5):1417–23.
33. Goldin GH, Sheets NC, Meyer AM, Kuo TM, Wu Y, Sturmer T, et al. Comparative effectiveness of intensity-modulated radiotherapy and conventional conformal radiotherapy in the treatment of prostate cancer after radical prostatectomy. JAMA Intern Med. 2013;173(12):1136–43.
34. Goenka A, Magsanoc JM, Pei X, Schechter M, Kollmeier M, Cox B, et al. Improved toxicity profile following high-dose postprostatectomy salvage radiation therapy with intensity-modulated radiation therapy. Eur Urol. 2011;60(6):1142–8.
35. Ghadjar P, Hayoz S, Bernhard J, Zwahlen DR, Holscher T, Gut P, et al. Acute toxicity and quality of life after dose-intensified salvage radiation therapy for biochemically recurrent prostate cancer after prostatectomy: first results of the randomized trial SAKK 09/10. J Clin Oncol. 2015;33(35):4158–66.

Part III

Androgen Deprivation Therapy for Advanced Prostate Cancer

Ji Youl Lee

Immediate vs. Delayed ADT for Recurrent Prostate Cancer

13

Tae Heon Kim and Seong Il Seo

13.1 Introduction

Despite high cure rates with radical prostatectomy or radiation therapy for localized prostate cancer, approximately 30% of men experience a rising prostate-specific antigen (PSA) level, a condition known as biochemical recurrence (BCR) [1–3]. Elevations in PSA may indicate local or distant recurrence. Thus, once BCR occurs the patient is presumed to have recurrent prostate cancer. Among patients who develop BCR, approximately one-third will develop clinical recurrence within 8 years from BCR [4]. Depending on the type of initial local therapy, reasonable options for BCR patients include observation with close surveillance, salvage radical prostatectomy, salvage radiation therapy, androgen deprivation therapy (ADT), and enrollment in investigational clinical trials. Of these options, ADT has long been accepted and widely used as an effective treatment for patients with advanced, recurrent, and disseminated prostate cancer, but it is associated with disadvantages including side effects as well as substantial cost. Not all patients with recurrent prostate cancer have the same prognosis, and understanding clinical factors that affect developing metastatic disease is crucial. Clinicians must balance a patient's competing benefit of survival gain and potential risk of an increased morbidity and impair quality of life. The trade-off between the relative benefits and harms of ADT in patients with recurrent prostate cancer is essential for consideration regarding in whom, how, and when it should be used. One of the most prominent questions in the treatment of patient with recurrent prostate cancer is that whether to initiate ADT immediately upon an increasing PSA level or to delay its use until the development of symptomatic or radiographic progression occurs. Despite the proven efficacy of ADT in recurrent prostate cancer, consensus as to the optimal time to initiate ADT remains in debate because results from clinical trials are mixed.

In this chapter, we review the relevant clinical trial data that may guide clinicians with respect to timing of ADT for treatment of recurrent prostate cancer.

13.2 Defining Recurrent Prostate Cancer

Among men treated with radical prostatectomy or radiation therapy for localized prostate cancer, the state of an increasing PSA level is known as BCR. A standard PSA cut point to define BCR has yet to be established. The definition of BCR is usually dependent upon the type of initial local treatment received. There are more than 50 dif-

T. H. Kim · S. I. Seo (✉)
Department of Urology, Samsung Medical Center, Sungkyunkwan University School of Medicine, Seoul, South Korea
e-mail: siseo@skku.edu

C. S. Kim (ed.), *Management of Advanced Prostate Cancer*,
https://doi.org/10.1007/978-981-10-6943-7_13

ferent definitions of BCR after radical prostatectomy. The American Urological Association Guidelines Panel defined BCR after radical prostatectomy as a value of 0.2 ng/mL or greater with a second confirmatory level of greater than 0.2 ng/mL [5]. This definition also has been adopted by the European Guidelines on Prostate Cancer [6]. For patients who receive radiation therapy, the PSA levels typically do not fall to undetectable level, and the kinetics of PSA decline are different from that in patients who receive radical prostatectomy. There have been several definitions offered to indicate BCR after radiation therapy. The American Urological Association Guidelines Panel found 99 different definitions of BCR following radiation therapy [5]. Among them, the American Society of Therapeutic Radiology and Oncology Consensus has defined BCR after radiation therapy as three successive PSA rises after the nadir, with the date of relapse backdated to midpoint between the nadir PSA and the fist rise [7]. Although the American Urological Association Guidelines Panel recommends that the American Society of Therapeutic Radiology and Oncology definition be adopted, it has several weaknesses, including this definition was not linked to any clinically significant outcomes such as clinical failure or cancer-specific or overall survival. As an alternative definition, the Radiation Therapy Oncology Group and American Society for Radiation Oncology Phoenix Consensus Conference defined BCR following radiation therapy as a rise of 2 ng/mL or higher than the nadir PSA, regardless of the serum concentration of the nadir PSA (Phoenix definition) [8]. It is now clear that the Phoenix definition of BCR after radiation therapy is more robust in predicting clinical outcomes.

13.3 Hormonal Therapy for Recurrent Prostate Cancer

Not all patients with recurrent prostate cancer have the same prognosis, and stratification of patients into appropriate risk groups is essential. ADT is one standard of care for patient with BCR after definite local therapy. ADT can be achieved via bilateral orchiectomy or via gonadotropin-releasing hormone agonists and antagonists. For patients with recurrent prostate cancer, however, the impact of ADT on overall survival and quality of life remains unestablished primarily due to the lack of data derived from well-designed controlled trials [9, 10]. ADT for patients with BCR after radical prostatectomy or radiation therapy is associated with a decline of PSA and deferred time to development of clinical or radiographic progression. On the other hand, ADT is known to affect patient's quality of life related to potential adverse events [11]. These potential adverse events include reduced energy, loss of libido, poor sexual function, memory loss, poor metabolic health, cardiovascular disease, bone loss, and fracture risk [12–14]. Therefore, the trade-offs between survival gain and risk of potential adverse events are important considerations in the decision-making process on timing and duration of ADT.

13.4 Timing of ADT

There is no overall and complete consensus about the appropriate timing of ADT for patient with recurrent prostate cancer after radical prostatectomy or radiation therapy. A decision to adopt immediate ADT or delayed ADT in standard clinical practice depends on consideration of pretreatment prognostic factors including absolute baseline PSA, PSA kinetics, tumor T stage, Gleason score, surgical margin status, and lymph node status. While some advocate delaying ADT until the development of clinical or radiographic progression, others recommend immediate ADT initiation. Uncertainty about the overall survival benefits of starting ADT immediately, combined with serious side effects and quality of life that may accompany ADT, has led many patients to delay ADT initiation.

For patients with BCR and clinical or radiographic metastatic disease, it is acknowledged that immediate initiation of ADT can improve symptoms (e.g., pain) and reduces further metastatic progression or the development of skeletal-related events, thus improving the patient's overall quality of life with respect to complications from the disease itself. However, one must remember that immediate ADT has not been shown to improve overall survival in these patients. There are a moderate decrease of 17% in relative risk for cancer-specific mortality, a moderate increase of 15% in relative risk for non-prostate cancer-specific mortality, and no overall survival advantage for immediate initiation of ADT versus withholding until symptomatic progression [9].

Appropriate timing of ADT for BCR without metastatic disease is controversial. Garcia-Albeniz et al. [15] evaluated patients with PSA-only recurrence after primary radical prostatectomy or radiotherapy in order to determine the optimal timing of ADT. They found that there was no overall or cancer-specific survival benefit of immediate ADT initiation (within 3 months after BCR) compared with delayed ADT initiation (at clinical progression or short PSA doubling time). Siddiqui et al. [16] found that patients who received ADT at the moment of BCR with different thresholds of PSA after radical prostatectomy did not have improved cancer-specific survival or systemic progression-free survival compared with patients who received delayed ADT after BCR. Duchesne et al. in the TOAD trial [17] reported the results of a multicenter, randomized trial comparing immediate ADT with delayed ADT by about 2 years. In this study, patients who received immediate ADT seemed to be slightly better than did those who had delayed ADT. The primary end point of overall survival was significantly improved with immediate receipt of ADT compared with delayed ADT. Five-year overall survival was 91.2% (84.2–95.2) in patients with immediate ADT versus 86.4% (95% CI 78.5–91.5) in patients with delayed ADT (log-rank $p = 0.047$). The unadjusted hazard ratio for overall survival for immediate ADT versus delayed ADT assignment was 0.55 (95% CI 0.30–1.00; $p = 0.050$). In subset analysis, however, immediate ADT did not lead to more favorable overall survival compared with delayed ADT in patients with PSA-only recurrence. The estimated 5-year overall survival rates were 84.3% (73.9–90.8) in the immediate ADT group and 78.2% (95% CI 67.2–85.8) in the delayed ADT group (log-rank $p = 0.10$). Furthermore, immediate use of ADT was associated with early detriments in specific hormone treatment-related symptoms, but with no other demonstrable effect on overall functioning or health-related quality of life [18]. In retrospective study from the Department of Defense Center for Prostate Disease Research Database, Moul et al. [19] reported that there was no beneficial effect of immediate ADT in terms of development of clinical metastasis for patients who have experienced BCR after radical prostatectomy. A subset analysis revealed, however, immediate ADT in those who have experienced BCR has been found to decrease the rates of distant metastasis in patients with high-risk features defined as Gleason sum greater than 7 or PSA doubling time less than 12 months. Another retrospective review of patients who had experienced BCR after undergoing radiation therapy, the use of immediate ADT prolonged metastasis-free survival in those with PSA doubling time <12 months [20]. However, no benefit was seen in those with PSA doubling time ≥12 months. Similarly, Klayton et al. [21] found a significant improvement of cancer-specific survival for patients receiving immediate ADT, but not in the group with a PSA doubling time >6 months.

13.5 Summary

Despite definitive local therapy, such as radical prostatectomy or radiation therapy, a significant number of patients will experience BCR of their disease. When planning the optimal course of ADT for a patient with recurrent prostate cancer, multiple clinical factors must be taken into consideration, especially in the known side effects and the impact on survival gain. The potential benefits of ADT should be discreetly considered and balanced against its potential harms. In terms of optimal timing of ADT, immediate initiation of ADT is a reasonable option for patients with high-risk features of clinical or radiologic progression, defined mainly by a short PSA doubling time, high absolute PSA, and high Gleason score.

References

1. Roehl KA, Han M, Ramos CG, Antenor JA, Catalona WJ. Cancer progression and survival rates following anatomical radical retropubic prostatectomy in 3,478 consecutive patients: long-term results. J Urol. 2004;172(3):910–4.
2. Freedland SJ, Humphreys EB, Mangold LA, Eisenberger M, Dorey FJ, Walsh PC, et al. Risk of prostate cancer-specific mortality following biochemical recurrence after radical prostatectomy. JAMA. 2005;294(4):433–9.
3. Kupelian PA, Mahadevan A, Reddy CA, Reuther AM, Klein EA. Use of different definitions of biochemical failure after external beam radiotherapy changes conclusions about relative treatment efficacy for localized prostate cancer. Urology. 2006;68(3):593–8.
4. Pound CR, Partin AW, Eisenberger MA, Chan DW, Pearson JD, Walsh PC. Natural history of progression after PSA elevation following radical prostatectomy. JAMA. 1999;281(17):1591–7.
5. Cookson MS, Aus G, Burnett AL, Canby-Hagino ED, D'Amico AV, Dmochowski RR, et al. Variation in the definition of biochemical recurrence in patients treated for localized prostate cancer: the American Urological Association Prostate Guidelines for Localized Prostate Cancer Update Panel report and recommendations for a standard in the reporting of surgical outcomes. J Urol. 2007;177(2):540–5.
6. Cornford P, Bellmunt J, Bolla M, Briers E, De Santis M, Gross T, et al. EAU-ESTRO-SIOG Guidelines on prostate cancer. Part II: Treatment of relapsing, metastatic, and castration-resistant prostate cancer. Eur Urol. 2017;71(4):630–42.
7. Consensus statement: guidelines for PSA following radiation therapy. American Society for Therapeutic Radiology and Oncology Consensus Panel. Int J Radiat Oncol Biol Phys. 1997;37(5):1035–41.
8. Roach M 3rd, Hanks G, Thames H Jr, Schellhammer P, Shipley WU, Sokol GH, et al. Defining biochemical failure following radiotherapy with or without hormonal therapy in men with clinically localized prostate cancer: recommendations of the RTOG-ASTRO Phoenix Consensus Conference. Int J Radiat Oncol Biol Phys. 2006;65(4):965–74.
9. Loblaw DA, Virgo KS, Nam R, Somerfield MR, Ben-Josef E, Mendelson DS, et al. Initial hormonal management of androgen-sensitive metastatic, recurrent, or progressive prostate cancer: 2006 update of an American Society of Clinical Oncology practice guideline. J Clin Oncol. 2007;25(12):1596–605.
10. Paller CJ, Antonarakis ES, Eisenberger MA, Carducci MA. Management of patients with biochemical recurrence after local therapy for prostate cancer. Hematol Oncol Clin North Am. 2013;27(6):1205–19, viii
11. Lubeck DP, Grossfeld GD, Carroll PR. The effect of androgen deprivation therapy on health-related quality of life in men with prostate cancer. Urology. 2001;58(2 Suppl 1):94–100.
12. Braga-Basaria M, Dobs AS, Muller DC, Carducci MA, John M, Egan J, et al. Metabolic syndrome in men with prostate cancer undergoing long-term androgen-deprivation therapy. J Clin Oncol. 2006;24(24):3979–83.
13. Smith MR, Lee H, McGovern F, Fallon MA, Goode M, Zietman AL, et al. Metabolic changes during gonadotropin-releasing hormone agonist therapy for prostate cancer: differences from the classic metabolic syndrome. Cancer. 2008;112(10):2188–94.
14. Shahinian VB, Kuo YF, Freeman JL, Goodwin JS. Risk of fracture after androgen deprivation for prostate cancer. N Engl J Med. 2005;352(2):154–64.
15. Garcia-Albeniz X, Chan JM, Paciorek A, Logan RW, Kenfield SA, Cooperberg MR, et al. Immediate versus deferred initiation of androgen deprivation therapy in prostate cancer patients with PSA-only relapse. An observational follow-up study. Eur J Cancer. 2015;51(7):817–24.
16. Siddiqui SA, Boorjian SA, Inman B, Bagniewski S, Bergstralh EJ, Blute ML. Timing of androgen deprivation therapy and its impact on survival after radical prostatectomy: a matched cohort study. J Urol. 2008;179(5):1830–7, discussion 7
17. Duchesne GM, Woo HH, Bassett JK, Bowe SJ, D'Este C, Frydenberg M, et al. Timing of androgen-deprivation therapy in patients with prostate cancer with a rising PSA (TROG 03.06 and VCOG PR 01-03 [TOAD]): a randomised, multicentre, non-blinded, phase 3 trial. Lancet Oncol. 2016;17(6):727–37.
18. Duchesne GM, Woo HH, King M, Bowe SJ, Stockler MR, Ames A, et al. Health-related quality of life for immediate versus delayed androgen-deprivation therapy in patients with asymptomatic, non-curable prostate cancer (TROG 03.06 and VCOG PR 01-03 [TOAD]): a randomised, multicentre, non-blinded, phase 3 trial. Lancet Oncol. 2017;18(9):1192–201.
19. Moul JW, Wu H, Sun L, McLeod DG, Amling C, Donahue T, et al. Early versus delayed hormonal therapy for prostate specific antigen only recurrence of prostate cancer after radical prostatectomy. J Urol. 2004;171(3):1141–7.
20. Pinover WH, Horwitz EM, Hanlon AL, Uzzo RG, Hanks GE. Validation of a treatment policy for patients with prostate specific antigen failure after three-dimensional conformal prostate radiation therapy. Cancer. 2003;97(4):1127–33.
21. Klayton TL, Ruth K, Buyyounouski MK, Uzzo RG, Wong YN, Chen DY, et al. PSA doubling time predicts for the development of distant metastases for patients who fail 3DCRT Or IMRT using the phoenix definition. Pract Radiat Oncol. 2011;1(4):235–42.

14 Intermittent Versus Continuous ADT for Advanced Prostate Cancer

Kyu Won Lee and Ji Youl Lee

14.1 Introduction

Androgen deprivation therapy (ADT) is the main systemic treatment of metastatic prostate cancer. However, the indications for ADT have been expanded to locally advanced disease with development of medical castration. Reversible medical androgen deprivation has facilitated adjuvant ADT in men with high-risk features treated with radiation or surgery. Considering the toxic effects of androgen deprivation and deterioration in quality of life, permanent androgen deprivation in patients with symptom-free biochemical recurrence seems unsuitable.

Intermittent androgen deprivation therapy (intermittent ADT) has been studied in an attempt to delay the development of castration resistance and reduce adverse events associated with ADT. Appropriate intermittent ADT protocol and patient selection are important to balance effective cancer treatment with minimal adverse events.

K. W. Lee · J. Y. Lee (✉)
Department of Urology, College of Medicine, The Catholic University of Korea,
Seoul, Republic of Korea
e-mail: firss@catholic.ac.kr; uroljy@catholic.ac.kr

14.2 Two Complementary Ideas: Rationale for Intermittent Androgen Deprivation Therapy

14.2.1 Development of Castration-Resistant Prostate Cancer

Progression to castration resistance should be delayed since it is the major cause of death in patients treated with ADT. An androgen-dependent tumor model suggests that androgen deprivation therapy initially eliminates the differentiated cells, but if the disease progresses, the proportion of androgen-independent stem cells increases [1]. It can be assumed that, if androgen is supplemented prior to disease progression, surviving stem cells will differentiate into androgen-dependent tumors, which can be responsive to subsequent androgen withdrawal. Thus, the concept for intermittent ADT is to allow recovery of testosterone during a period of treatment cessation after androgen deprivation, restoring the apoptotic potential and helping tumor cells remain sensitive to treatment [2].

In an androgen-dependent model, the time to castration resistance almost tripled when intermittent ADT was applied [3]. In a small clinical trial, the 3-year risk of progression rate was lower in the intermittent ADT group than in the continuous ADT group [4]. However, in large clinical trials such as SWOG 9346 and CIC-CTG

C. S. Kim (ed.), *Management of Advanced Prostate Cancer*,
https://doi.org/10.1007/978-981-10-6943-7_14

PR.7, it was concluded that intermittent ADT had no survival benefit compared to continuous ADT [5, 6].

14.2.2 Negative Impact of Continuous Androgen Deprivation Therapy

Adverse events associated with ADT include hot flush, reduced muscle and bone mass, sexual dysfunction, cognitive dysfunction, changes in body habitus, gynecomastia, anemia, and metabolic syndrome. Furthermore, cardiovascular-related morbidity associated with metabolic syndrome is a common cause of death in patients treated with ADT. To reduce adverse events, deterioration in health-related quality of life, and cardiovascular mortality, discontinuation of ADT and recovery of testosterone during the off-treatment period of ADT should be considered in patients with poor compliance with ADT.

Crook et al. reported that intermittent ADT was associated with better quality of life, assessed with the use of questionnaire (QLQ-C30), especially in terms of frequency of hot flush, desire for sexual activity, and urinary symptoms. However, for the functional domains (physical, role, and global health), the intermittent therapy arm was comparable to continuous arm [5]. Secondary analysis of the SWOG 9346 trial showed that intermittent ADT did not reduce the incidence of long-term adverse events, and older men assigned to intermittent ADT had no apparent reduction in bone, endocrine, or cognitive events, but rather experienced increased ischemic and thrombotic events [7]. In a meta-analysis comparing intermittent ADT and continuous ADT, Botrel et al. concluded that the impact in QoL was similar for both groups, but sexual activity scores were higher and the incidence of hot flashes was lower in patients treated with intermittent ADT [8].

In a meta-analysis of the association between intermittent ADT and cardiovascular events, Jin et al. reported that intermittent therapy did not reduce cardiovascular events or thromboembolic events, but did reduce cardiovascular-related mortality [9].

14.3 Patient Selection for Intermittent Androgen Deprivation Therapy

14.3.1 Clinical Application of Intermittent Androgen Deprivation Therapy

Since its introduction in 1987 by Klotz et al., intermittent ADT has been clinically applied with the development of PSA monitoring. Although many clinical trials for intermittent ADT have been performed, it is still unclear which patients are suitable candidates for intermittent ADT. Recent large-scale clinical trials provide information on how to make decisions based on the extent of disease progression [5, 6].

14.3.2 Nonmetastatic Prostate Cancer

In a clinical trial of patients with elevated PSA after radiotherapy, Crook et al. performed an interim analysis of overall survival for non-inferiority of intermittent ADT compared to continuous ADT [5]. Intermittent ADT consisted of 8-month treatment cycles, with a nontreatment interval based on PSA level. At a median follow-up of 6.9 years, 268 patients treated with intermittent ADT and 256 treated with continuous ADT had died. The median overall survival was 8.8 years in the continuous ADT group and 9.1 years in the intermittent ADT group. The hazard ratio for intermittent ADT was 1.03 (95% CI, 0.86–1.23), and the P-value for non-inferiority was 0.009 (Fig. 14.1).

The disease-specific hazard ratio was 1.23 (95% CI, 0.94–1.60; $P = 0.13$), showing favorable outcome in the continuous ADT group. The risk of progression to castration resistance in the intermittent ADT group seems to be low (HR 0.81; 95% CI, 0.68–0.98; $P = 0.03$), but this might be due to the bias caused by the definition of castration resistance (disease progression with castrate range of testosterone level). In the intermittent ADT group, even if PSA is increased, the treatment should be restarted, and the testosterone is reduced to the castration level before it can be judged as castration resistance prostate cancer.

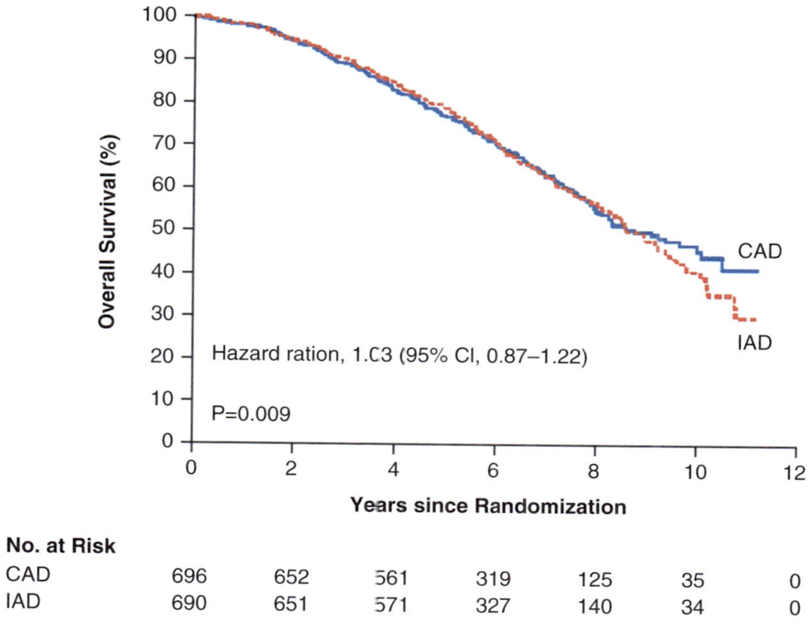

Fig. 14.1 Overall survival in patients treated with intermittent androgen deprivation therapy compared to those treated with continuous androgen deprivation therapy in a cohort of men after radiotherapy (N Engl J Med 2012;367:895–903)

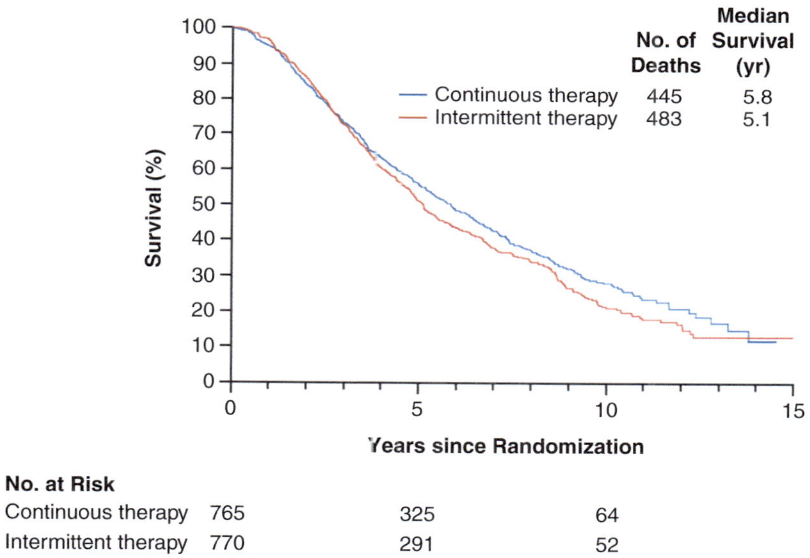

Fig. 14.2 Median survival in patients treated with intermittent androgen deprivation therapy compared to those treated with continuous androgen deprivation therapy in a cohort of metastatic hormone-sensitive prostate cancer patients (N Engl J Med 2013;368:1314–25)

14.3.3 Metastatic Prostate Cancer

The largest clinical trial of intermittent ADT, SWOG 9346, was conducted in metastatic hormone-sensitive prostate cancer patients [6]. The objectives of that study were to assess the non-inferiority of intermittent ADT for survival and quality of life 3 months after randomization. Among 3040 enrolled patients, 1535 were randomly assigned to continuous ADT ($N = 765$) and intermittent ADT ($N = 770$). The median survival was 5.8 years in the continuous ADT group and 5.1 years in the intermittent ADT group (HR 1.10; 90% CI, 0.99–1.23) (Fig. 14.2).

This study was designed to demonstrate the non-inferiority of intermittent ADT based on a hazard ratio of 1.20. In the results, the relative risk was 10%, but it was statistically inconclusive because the confidence interval included 1.00 and 1.20 (0.99–1.23). Therefore, lower survival of the intermittent ADT group could not be ruled out.

14.3.4 Candidates for Intermittent Androgen Deprivation Therapy

Previous studies have shown that intermittent ADT in locally advanced prostate cancer reduces adverse events associated with ADT and maintains better quality of life without affecting survival, but intermittent ADT in metastatic prostate cancer might compromise survival without improving quality of life [5, 6]. Therefore, factors such as stage and grade of tumor, life expectancy, comorbidities, and sexual activity should be considered when selecting patients to be treated with intermittent ADT.

14.4 Appropriate Regimen for Intermittent Androgen Deprivation Therapy

14.4.1 PSA Level and Schedules for Intermittent Androgen Deprivation Therapy

Intermittent ADT has been studied in many clinical trials, but there is still no consensus on PSA threshold or cycle length for intermittent ADT. The high heterogeneity in the current meta-analysis of clinical trials for intermittent ADT reflects this problem [8, 10].

Definite criteria for PSA level for selection and monitoring of intermittent ADT patients and standardization of measurement is required. It was recently reported that a PSA level higher than 4 ng/mL after 7 months of ADT is a strong predictor of survival in patients with metastatic prostate cancer, and patients with a PSA level lower than 0.2 ng/mL had a better chance of survival [11]. On the other hand, in a recent study that evaluated the combination of radiotherapy plus ADT in patients with localized or locally advanced prostate cancer, posttreatment PSA level higher than 5 ng/mL was associated with a decreased risk of cancer-specific survival [12].

The CIC-CTG PR.7 trial included patients who underwent definitive radiotherapy at least 12 months before enrollment and had a PSA level higher than 3 ng/mL and no metastasis [5]. After an induction period of 8 months, the nontreatment period was initiated in the intermittent ADT group if there was no progression of disease and if the PSA level was less than 4 ng/mL and not elevated more than 1 ng/mL above the previously measured level. The PSA level was monitored every 2 months during the nontreatment period, and treatment was reinitiated at a PSA level higher than 10 ng/mL.

In contrast, Hussain et al. enrolled metastatic prostate cancer patients with PSA level higher than 5 ng/mL before treatment in the SWOG 9346 study [6]. Patients with a PSA level lower than 4 ng/mL after a 7-month induction period with combined androgen blockade were randomly assigned to the continuous ADT or intermittent ADT group. Both groups underwent clinical assessment every 3 months, and the treatment was resumed when the PSA level rose to baseline or 20 ng/mL in the intermittent ADT group.

14.4.2 Recommendations for Intermittent Androgen Deprivation Therapy

Based on previous studies, Wolff et al. recommended the principles for intermittent ADT as follows [10]:

1. Induction period of ADT should last 3–6 months.
2. For men with metastatic disease, the PSA level should fall to <4.0 ng/mL.
3. For men with recurrent disease, the PSA level should fall to <0.5 ng/mL.
4. Reinitiation of the treatment:
   (a) Clinical progression of disease.
   (b) PSA doubling time <6 months.
   (c) PSA level increases to between 10 and 15 ng/mL in men with metastatic disease.

   (d) PSA level increases to between 4 and 10 ng/mL in men with nonmetastatic disease.
5. When treatment is reinitiated, it should be continued for ≥6 months.
6. PSA tests and clinical examinations should be conducted every 3 or 6 months.

Intermittent ADT can improve patient compliance by minimizing adverse events from ADT and improving quality of life. However, intermittent therapy in advanced prostate cancer patient can increase the risk of recurrence and mortality. Therefore, patients should be informed of the benefits and risks of intermittent ADT before treatment. Patients should also be informed that the beginning of the off-treatment period is not a permanent disruption of therapy and that frequent assessment of PSA level and monitoring of cancer progression are required.

14.5 Summary

- Intermittent ADT has been studied in an attempt to delay the development of castration resistance and reduce adverse events associated with ADT.
- Intermittent ADT can improve patient compliance by minimizing adverse events from ADT and improving quality of life, but it is not related to prolonged survival.
- Selection of eligible patients for intermittent ADT is important because intermittent therapy in advanced prostate cancer patient can increase the risk of recurrence and mortality.
- Although many clinical trials for intermittent ADT have been performed, it is still unclear which patients are suitable for the treatment.
- It is necessary to establish guidelines for intermittent ADT through evidence synthesis of previous studies.
- Patients should be informed of the benefits and risks of intermittent ADT before treatment.

References

1. Bruchovsky N, Rennie PS, Coldman AJ, Goldenberg SL, To M, Lawson D. Effects of androgen withdrawal on the stem cell composition of the Shionogi carcinoma. Cancer Res. 1990;50(8):2275–82.
2. Abrahamsson PA. Potential benefits of intermittent androgen suppression therapy in the treatment of prostate cancer: a systematic review of the literature. Eur Urol. 2010;57(1):49–59.
3. Akakura K, Bruchovsky N, Goldenberg SL, Rennie PS, Buckley AR, Sullivan LD. Effects of intermittent androgen suppression on androgen-dependent tumors. Apoptosis and serum prostate-specific antigen. Cancer. 1993;71(9):2782–90.
4. de Leval J, Boca P, Yousef E, Nicolas H, Jeukenne M, Seidel L, et al. Intermittent versus continuous total androgen blockade in the treatment of patients with advanced hormone-naive prostate cancer: results of a prospective randomized multicenter trial. Clin Prostate Cancer. 2002;1(3):163–71.
5. Crook JM, O'Callaghan CJ, Duncan G, Dearnaley DP, Higano CS, Horwitz EM, et al. Intermittent androgen suppression for rising PSA level after radiotherapy. N Engl J Med. 2012;367(10):895–903.
6. Hussain M, Tangen CM, Berry DL, Higano CS, Crawford ED, Liu G, et al. Intermittent versus continuous androgen deprivation in prostate cancer. N Engl J Med. 2013;368(14):1314–25.
7. Hershman DL, Unger JM, Wright JD, Ramsey S, Till C, Tangen CM, et al. Adverse health events following intermittent and continuous androgen deprivation in patients with metastatic prostate cancer. JAMA Oncol. 2016;2(4):453–61.
8. Botrel TE, Clark O, dos Reis RB, Pompeo AC, Ferreira U, Sadi MV, et al. Intermittent versus continuous androgen deprivation for locally advanced, recurrent or metastatic prostate cancer: a systematic review and meta-analysis. BMC Urol. 2014;14:9.
9. Jin C, Fan Y, Meng Y, Shen C, Wang Y, Hu S, et al. A meta-analysis of cardiovascular events in intermittent androgen-deprivation therapy versus continuous androgen-deprivation therapy for prostate cancer patients. Prostate Cancer Prostatic Dis. 2016;19(4):333–9.
10. Wolff JM, Abrahamsson PA, Irani J, da Silva FC. Is intermittent androgen-deprivation therapy beneficial for patients with advanced prostate cancer? BJU Int. 2014;114(4):476–83.
11. Hussain M, Tangen CM, Higano C, Schelhammer PF, Faulkner J, Crawford ED, et al. Absolute prostate-specific antigen value after androgen deprivation is a strong independent predictor of survival in new metastatic prostate cancer: data from Southwest Oncology Group Trial 9346 (INT-0162). J Clin Oncol. 2006;24(24):3984–90.
12. D'Amico AV, Chen MH, de Castro M, Loffredo M, Lamb DS, Steigler A, et al. Surrogate endpoints for prostate cancer-specific mortality after radiotherapy and androgen suppression therapy in men with localised or locally advanced prostate cancer: an analysis of two randomised trials. Lancet Oncol. 2012;13(2):189–95.

LHRH Agonist and Antagonist for Prostate Cancer

15

Jin Bong Choi and Jun Sung Koh

15.1 Introduction

ADT is the main treatment for advanced prostate cancer. Combination therapy with radiotherapy in early stage prostate cancer is increasing. LHRH agonists are the most frequently used type of ADT for several years, and they have suppressed the serum testosterone to castration level in almost all patients. Furthermore, LHRH antagonist was developed recently as an alternative form of ADT with direct and immediate suppression of testosterone without initial testosterone flare phenomenon. Therefore, in this chapter, we will describe the comparative efficacy and safety between LHRH agonists and LHRH antagonists for prostate cancer.

15.2 LHRH Agonist

15.2.1 Mechanism of LHRH Agonist

The secretion of LHRH is pulsatile. An intermittent LHRH release is necessary for a physiologic stimulation of gonadotropin secretion. A sustained stimulation of the pituitary by repeated injections of LHRH agonists or periodic administration of microcapsules of LHRH agonists induces suppression of the hypophyseal-gonadal axis through a reduction of pituitary receptors for LHRH, decrease in the expression of mRNA for LHRH receptor, rapid homologous desensitization of LHRH receptors, and inhibition of blood levels of luteinizing hormone (LH), follicle-stimulating hormone (FSH), and other sex steroids. This downregulation of pituitary receptors creates a state of reversible medical castration.

Because daily injections of LHRH agonists are inconvenient and produce compliance problems, long-acting delivery systems were developed. The microcapsules are formulated to release a dose of about 100 μg peptide per day over a 30–90-day period. These microcapsules are composed of 2–6% of LHRH agonists dispersed in poly (lactide-co-glycolide) polymer which is biodegradable and biocompatible.

15.2.2 LHRH Agonists for Treatment of Prostate Cancer

15.2.2.1 Clinical Efficacy of LHRH Agonists

The efficacy of therapy with LHRH agonists in advanced prostate cancer patients was first demonstrated in 1981 [1]. Ten patients with stage III

J. B. Choi · J. S. Koh (✉)
Department of Urology, College of Medicine, The Catholic University of Korea, Seoul, South Korea
e-mail: cjb0812@catholic.ac.kr; gostraight@catholic.ac.kr

C. S. Kim (ed.), *Management of Advanced Prostate Cancer*, https://doi.org/10.1007/978-981-10-6943-7_15

and IV prostate cancer were treated with two LHRH agonists for 6 weeks to 12 months. [D-Trp6] LHRH was given subcutaneously at a dose of 100 μg/day, and [D-Ser(But)6] Des-Gly-NH2 10-LHRH ethylamide was also used subcutaneously at a dose of 50 μg once daily or intranasally (500 μg twice daily). Plasma testosterone levels declined 75% by the third week of treatment in all patients. Normalization or decrease of acid phosphatase (ACP) levels occurred at 2 months and 47% decrease in alkaline phosphatase (ALP) at 10 weeks. There was relief of bone pain in stage IV patients with bone metastases and was the radiologically improvement in one patient. It was concluded that LHRH agonists were effective for prostatic cancer with fewer side effects than estrogen treatment.

In other clinical trial, 81 prostate cancer patients were treated daily for 3 months with decapeptyl. The outcomes were compared to those treated with other hormones. Prostatic size was normal in 26% of patients and was reduced to more than half in an additional 18%. Bone scan showed improvements of bone lesions in 15% [2]. LHRH agonists avoid the psychological side effects or the cardiovascular, hepatic, and mammotropic effects of estrogen. The responses of tumors after 3–19 months of therapy were similar to surgical castration. Long-term therapy with LHRH agonist is preferred as an alternative to surgical castration or estrogen treatment.

15.2.2.2 Flare Phenomenon of LHRH Agonists

The initial exposure to LHRH agonists results in the flare phenomenon of LH and testosterone level. This phenomenon is observed in all LHRH agonists and occasionally can bring a life-threatening worsening of symptoms. Fortunately, the co-administration of an antiandrogen can block the increase of testosterone levels. Although it had been said that the antiandrogen administration should precede the LHRH agonist treatment about 1 week, someone has reported that there were no differences in PSA levels with the administration simultaneously [3]. Usually, antiandrogen co-administration is required for about 1 month.

15.2.2.3 Safety of LHRH Agonists

Androgen deprivation produced by LHRH agonists may lead to worsening of clinical symptoms in advanced disease like bone pain, spinal cord compression, and urethral compression. In general, use of LHRH agonists leads to impotence, hot flashes, nausea, sweating, muscle loss, osteoporosis, bone fractures, reduced insulin sensitivity, elevated serum cholesterol, anemia, gynecomastia, and declined cognitive performance [4].

In spite of that, LHRH agonists are still the preferred treatment for patients with advanced prostate cancer, and LHRH agonists are selected in 70% of patients for primary treatment. LHRH agonists can be also used with local treatments in localized prostate cancer patients. And LHRH agonists are also recommended in patients with an increasing PSA levels after radiotherapy or radical prostatectomy.

15.3 LHRH Antagonist

15.3.1 Mechanism of LHRH Antagonist

LHRH antagonist competes with endogenous LHRH for LHRH receptor site producing a competitive receptor block. Thus, LHRH antagonists cause a prompt inhibition of the release of sex steroids and gonadotropins in contrast to LHRH agonists which make this effect only after downregulation of LHRH receptors. A major advantage of LHRH antagonists over LHRH agonists is their capacity to induce a prompt inhibition of LH, FSH, and sex steroid secretion in a few hours after the administration. The therapy with antagonists also avoids a flare phenomenon caused by a transient release of LH and sex steroids, which occurs during administration of LHRH agonists.

15.3.2 LHRH Antagonists for Treatment of Prostate Cancer

15.3.2.1 Clinical Efficacy of LHRH Antagonists

Clinical trials showed persistent inhibition of testosterone levels in advanced prostatic cancer patients who treated subcutaneously with cetrorelix for several months. After the first week of therapy, a significant decrease of bone pain, bladder outlet obstruction relief, and improvement of LUTS were noted. After 6 weeks, the PSA level and serum alkaline phosphatases fell to normal values. In patients with stage III disease, there was a decrease in prostate size. An improvement in obstructive symptoms and prolonged inhibition of serum testosterone to castration levels were also obtained in benign prostatic hyperplasia patients. No side effects other than impotence were noted [5].

The response to cetrorelix was also evaluated in five advanced prostatic cancer patients with paraplegia due to compression of the spinal cord or cauda equina. They could not be treated with LHRH agonists because of the flare phenomenon. After treatment, the neurologic symptoms regressed in all patients. In one patient, myelography demonstrated that the disappearance of the spinal cord compression and ultrasonography showed a significant decrease in prostate size. Baseline levels of FSH, LH, and testosterone decreased markedly after the first day of therapy and remained low [6]. Abarelix was synthesized in 1998, developed over the last decade, and approved by the FDA in 2003. However, because of hypersensitivity reaction in some patients, its use was discontinued in the USA in 2005.

15.3.2.2 Clinical Efficacy of Degarelix

Unlike abarelix, degarelix has no systemic allergic reactions. Degarelix is a decapeptide with 5 D-amino acids and two other non-coded amino acids. Degarelix is the third generation LHRH antagonist and approved by the FDA in 2008. Degarelix was evaluated for safety and effectiveness in three phase II clinical trials. Degarelix was well tolerated in all trials, and yearlong treatment was associated with rapid, profound, and sustained inhibition of testosterone to castrate levels. There was also rapid PSA suppression. These three studies concluded that the most effective loading dose of degarelix was 240 mg with an 80 or 160 mg maintenance dose [7].

The phase III clinical trials demonstrated that both degarelix doses (80 or 160 mg) were statistically non-inferior to leuprolide in testosterone response. The primary end point was serum testosterone ≤0.5 ng/mL until day 364 at every monthly measurement. The median testosterone level rose from baseline after 3 days in leuprolide group and remained at ≤0.5 ng/mL until day 28. Also, surge of testosterone was observed in 80% of the leuprolide group but 0% in the degarelix group. The degarelix groups, both 240/80 mg and 240/160 mg, were significantly more rapid in suppression of PSA compared to the leuprolide group. Degarelix treatment produced a more rapid suppression of LH and FSH levels and remained suppressed until the end. In the leuprolide group, there was an initial increase in both gonadotropins, and FSH levels did not fall as much as in the degarelix group [8, 9].

15.3.2.3 Cardiovascular Advantage of LHRH Antagonists

Additionally, retrospective analysis from pooled data of phase III clinical trials suggests a lower risk of major cardiovascular events with degarelix in patients with a history of cardiovascular disease, although this remains a subject of debate. A mouse model of low-density lipoprotein receptor knockout mice demonstrated that those mice treated with LHRH antagonists develop less adiposity, atherosclerosis, and metabolic syndrome compared with mice that had undergone orchiectomy or LHRH agonist therapy [10]. Another possible biologic explanation may lie in the presence of FSH receptors within the endothelial surface of blood vessel. FSH receptors would be stimulated by LHRH agonist therapy but would presumably be less stimulated through LHRH antagonist therapy which also suppresses FSH [11].

15.3.2.4 Disadvantage of Delivery System

Degarelix has the disadvantage of needing monthly depot injections, while LHRH agonists are available in 3-, 4-, or even 6-month depot formulations. And the large volume and need for two injections for the starting dose lead to common injection site reactions at therapy initiation.

15.4 LHRH Agonist vs. LHRH Antagonist for Prostate Cancer

15.4.1 Biochemical Markers

Sciarra et al. reported a meta-analysis and systematic review of five randomized controlled trials with degarelix versus LHRH agonists for advanced prostate cancer [12–18]. Both treatments were able to maintain testosterone suppression to ≤0.5 ng/mL from day 28 to 364. Castration testosterone levels were maintained for all the follow-up period in 98 and 96% of groups, respectively. In the first 1 month, treatment with degarelix made castration testosterone level in a significantly higher when compared to LHRH agonists (97 vs. 45%). The difference in PSA reduction from baseline at 1 month was not statistically significant between degarelix and LHRH agonists.

15.4.2 Oncological Outcomes

Oncological outcomes were studied in one randomized phase III clinical trial, CS21 trial (www.clinicaltrial.gov), though the primary end point was castration with testosterone level of ≤0.5 ng/mL from days 28 to 364 [8, 14]. The overall survival was significantly higher in patients receiving degarelix compared to LHRH agonist at 12 months (97.4% (CI, 93.8–98.9) vs. 95.1% (CI, 90.7–97.4); *p* value, 0.05). PSA progression-free survival was also analyzed at 12 months. The results from CS21 trial suggested that PSA progression occurred more frequently in patients receiving LHRH agonist compared to degarelix (12.9 vs. 7.7%, *p* value is not determined). However, the results of this study were mainly focused on PSA progression-free survival, and the numbers of death were very low in both groups. In addition, it did not analyze the data about prostate cancer-specific survival and clinical progression-free survival. Therefore, the comparison of the oncological outcome between LHRH agonist and LHRH antagonist was not fully evaluated yet.

15.4.3 Adverse Events and Symptoms

Adverse events were reported to 61 and 59% in the degarelix and LHRH agonists group, respectively. Flushing was the most frequently reported side effects in both group, and most reported adverse events were mild to moderate. Degarelix had a higher rate of injection site reactions than LHRH agonists. Cardiovascular events were reported to 1.6 and 3.6% in the degarelix and LHRH agonists group, respectively. And lower urinary tract symptoms showed a higher decrease in the degarelix than in the LHRH agonists group [18].

15.4.4 Cost-Effectiveness

Fisher et al. reported that degarelix was the dominant strategy over goserelin. However, Lu et al. reported that degarelix did not appear to be cost-effective compared to triptorelin plus short-term antiandrogen in the management of advanced prostate cancer with incremental cost-effectiveness ratio of US$ 69,832/quality-adjusted life years for degarelix versus triptorelin [19]. Hatoum et al. performed cost-effectiveness analysis using a data from CS21 comparing monthly degarelix with leuprolide. Markov model and a 20-year time horizon found the increasing cost-effectiveness ratio for degarelix to be US$ 245/quality-adjusted life years. They concluded that degarelix provides a cost-effective

Table 15.1 LHRH agonist vs. LHRH antagonist for prostate cancer

	LHRH agonists	LHRH antagonists
Testosterone suppression		
Long-term suppression	Maintain testosterone to castration levels	
Short-term suppression	Prolonged suppression	Rapid suppression
PSA level	No significant difference	
Oncological outcome		
Respective effects	Effective	Effective
Comparative analysis	Limited yet	
FSH suppression	Partial suppression	Complete suppression
Injection cycle	Every 3-month injection	Monthly injection
Adverse events		
General side effects	Comparable	
Initial testosterone flare	Yes	No
Injection site reactions	More in LHRH antagonist	
Prostate size change	No significant difference	
LUTS	More improved in LHRH antagonist	
Cost-effectiveness	Controversy	

treatment for ADT among patients with locally advanced prostate cancer. The above characteristics of LHRH agonists and LHRH antagonists are summarized in Table 15.1.

15.5 The Switch from LHRH Antagonist to LHRH Agonist

Garnick and Mottet reported this theory in 2012 through a multicenter, open-label design study [20]. A total of 176 patients with localized prostate cancer and a PSA level <10 ng/mL were enrolled into the study. After administration of abarelix for 3 months, subjects were switched to administration of leuprolide or goserelin monthly. The primary end point was obtaining and maintaining serum testosterone levels until day 141 at ≤50 ng/dL. Ninety four percent of patients had obtained the castration levels of testosterone at day 85. During the switch over period, the percentage of patients obtaining the castrate levels of testosterone decreased to 87% at day 7 but increased again to 93% after injection of the LHRH agonist.

Miyazawa et al. reported this theory about degarelix [21]. They enrolled 40 prostate cancer patients who were treated initially with degarelix and were switched to leuprolide later. The patients were divided into three groups according to the time of conversion to leuprolide: 3-month, 2-month, and 1-month group. A mild and short period testosterone surge was reported in 8.3%. FSH and LH levels were significantly higher in 1-month group compared with 2- or 3-month group. The clinical symptoms were not worsening around switching time in any patients.

Degarelix is available only as 1-month depot and requires monthly dosing. This has been a problem for doctors and patients. In contrast, the present LHRH agonists can be administered every 3 months. Three-month formulation can reduce the number of visits, as well as the number of injections. Therefore, switching from LHRH antagonist to LHRH agonist appears to be a reasonable therapeutic option in prostate cancer patients without metastatic. Besides, there is no need to treat with antiandrogens additionally.

15.6 Summary

- The comparison of the oncological outcome between LHRH agonist and LHRH antagonist is not fully evaluated yet.
- Both LHRH agonist and LHRH antagonist were able to maintain testosterone to castration levels, and no significant differences were found regarding PSA level.
- LHRH antagonists suppress testosterone to castration level in a higher percentage in the beginning compared to LHRH agonist.
- General side effects were comparable between LHRH agonist and LHRH antagonist.
- LHRH agonists result in an initial flare of LH and testosterone levels.
- LHRH antagonists induce more injection site reactions than LHRH agonists and lack of long-acting delivery systems.

- Prostate volume reduction was similar between LHRH agonist and LHRH antagonist though lower urinary tract symptoms improved more in LHRH antagonist.

References

1. Tolis G, Ackman D, Stellos A, Mehta A, Labrie F, Fazekas AT, et al. Tumor growth inhibition in patients with prostatic carcinoma treated with luteinizing hormone-releasing hormone agonists. Proc Natl Acad Sci U S A. 1982;79(5):1658–62.
2. Mathe G, Schally AV, Comaru-Schally AM, Mauvernay RY, Vovan ML, Machover D, et al. Phase II trial with D-Trp-6-LH-RH in prostatic carcinoma: comparison with other hormonal agents. Prostate. 1986;9(4):327–42.
3. Tsushima T, Nasu Y, Saika T, Maki Y, Noda M, Suyama B, et al. Optimal starting time for flutamide to prevent disease flare in prostate cancer patients treated with a gonadotropin-releasing hormone agonist. Urol Int. 2001;66(3):135–9.
4. Rick FG, Block NL, Schally AV. Agonists of luteinizing hormone-releasing hormone in prostate cancer. Expert Opin Pharmacother. 2013;14(16):2237–47.
5. Gonzalez-Barcena D, Vadillo-Buenfil M, Gomez-Orta F, Fuentes Garcia M, Cardenas-Cornejo I, Graef-Sanchez A, et al. Responses to the antagonistic analog of LH-RH (SB-75, Cetrorelix) in patients with benign prostatic hyperplasia and prostatic cancer. Prostate. 1994;24(2):84–92.
6. Gonzalez-Barcena D, Vadillo-Buenfil M, Cortez-Morales A, Fuentes-Garcia M, Cardenas-Cornejo I, Comaru-Schally AM, et al. Luteinizing hormone-releasing hormone antagonist cetrorelix as primary single therapy in patients with advanced prostatic cancer and paraplegia due to metastatic invasion of spinal cord. Urology. 1995;45(2):275–81.
7. Rick FG, Block NL, Schally AV. An update on the use of degarelix in the treatment of advanced hormone-dependent prostate cancer. Onco Targets Ther. 2013;6:391–402.
8. Klotz L, Boccon-Gibod L, Shore ND, Andreou C, Persson BE, Cantor P, et al. The efficacy and safety of degarelix: a 12-month, comparative, randomized, open-label, parallel-group phase III study in patients with prostate cancer. BJU Int. 2008;102(11):1531–8.
9. Clinton TN, Woldu SL, Raj GV. Degarelix versus luteinizing hormone-releasing hormone agonists for the treatment of prostate cancer. Expert Opin Pharmacother. 2017;18(8):825–32.
10. Albertsen PC, Klotz L, Tombal B, Grady J, Olesen TK, Nilsson J. Cardiovascular morbidity associated with gonadotropin releasing hormone agonists and an antagonist. Eur Urol. 2014;65(3):565–73.
11. Radu A, Pichon C, Camparo P, Antoine M, Allory Y, Couvelard A, et al. Expression of follicle-stimulating hormone receptor in tumor blood vessels. N Engl J Med. 2010;363(17):1621–30.
12. Klotz L, Miller K, Crawford ED, Shore N, Tombal B, Karup C, et al. Disease control outcomes from analysis of pooled individual patient data from five comparative randomised clinical trials of degarelix versus luteinising hormone-releasing hormone agonists. Eur Urol. 2014;66(6):1101–8.
13. Lee D, Nielsen SK, van Keep M, Andersson F, Greene D. Quality of life improvement in patients treated with degarelix versus leuprorelin for advanced prostate cancer. J Urol. 2015;193(3):839–46.
14. Tombal B, Miller K, Boccon-Gibod L, Schroder F, Shore N, Crawford ED, et al. Additional analysis of the secondary end point of biochemical recurrence rate in a phase 3 trial (CS21) comparing degarelix 80 mg versus leuprolide in prostate cancer patients segmented by baseline characteristics. Eur Urol. 2010;57(5):836–42.
15. Mason M, Maldonado Pijoan X, Steidle C, Guerif S, Wiegel T, van der Meulen E, et al. Neoadjuvant androgen deprivation therapy for prostate volume reduction, lower urinary tract symptom relief and quality of life improvement in men with intermediate- to high-risk prostate cancer: a randomised non-inferiority trial of degarelix versus goserelin plus bicalutamide. Clin Oncol. 2013;25(3):190–6.
16. Anderson J, Al-Ali G, Wirth M, Gual JB, Gomez Veiga F, Colli E, et al. Degarelix versus goserelin (+ antiandrogen flare protection) in the relief of lower urinary tract symptoms secondary to prostate cancer: results from a phase IIIb study (NCT00831233). Urol Int. 2013;90(3):321–8.
17. Axcrona K, Aaltomaa S, da Silva CM, Ozen H, Damber JE, Tanko LB, et al. Androgen deprivation therapy for volume reduction, lower urinary tract symptom relief and quality of life improvement in patients with prostate cancer: degarelix vs goserelin plus bicalutamide. BJU Int. 2012;110(11):1721–8.
18. Sciarra A, Fasulo A, Ciardi A, Petrangeli E, Gentilucci A, Maggi M, et al. A meta-analysis and systematic review of randomized controlled trials with degarelix versus gonadotropin-releasing hormone agonists for advanced prostate cancer. Medicine. 2016;95(27):e3845.
19. Lu L, Peters J, Roome C, Stein K. Cost-effectiveness analysis of degarelix for advanced hormone-dependent prostate cancer. BJU Int. 2012;109(8):1183–92.
20. Garnick MB, Mottet N. New treatment paradigm for prostate cancer: abarelix initiation therapy for immediate testosterone suppression followed by a luteinizing hormone-releasing hormone agonist. BJU Int. 2012;110(4):499–504.
21. Miyazawa Y, Kato H, Arai S, Furuya Y, Sekine Y, Nomura M, et al. Clinical endocrinological evaluation of the gonadal axis (testosterone, LH and FSH) in prostate cancer patients switched from a GnRH antagonist to a LHRH agonist. Basic Clin Androl. 2015;25:7.

Abiraterone or Enzalutamide in Chemotherapy-Naïve Metastatic CRPC

16

Ho Seok Chung and Taek Won Kang

16.1 Introduction

The current standard of care for metastatic prostate cancer is androgen deprivation therapy (ADT); however, after 5 years, significant patients undergo disease progression despite hormonal manipulation and castrate testosterone levels [1, 2]. Multiple new treatment agents have been developed for men with metastatic castration-resistant prostate cancer (mCRPC) including chemotherapeutic agents, such as docetaxel and cabazitaxel [3–5]. Docetaxel and cabazitaxel are the only US Food and Drug Administration (FDA)-approved chemotherapeutic agents for the mCRPC treatment, decrease PSA levels, and palliate symptoms, but survival benefits are limited. Also, use of systemic chemotherapy generally be reserved for men with symptomatic mCRPC and may be limited by the presence of pre-existing medical conditions and the risk of developing adverse effects [6]. Because the androgen receptor (AR) activates PSA gene expression, more understanding of the role of the AR in prostate cancer progression has led to the improvement of treatment strategies to further suppress AR signaling in mCRPC [7]. Both abiraterone acetate and enzalutamide have been studied and shown to prolong overall survival in large phase III trials in the chemotherapy-naïve mCRPC settings.

H. S. Chung · T. W. Kang (✉)
Department of Urology, Chonnam National University Medical School, Gwangju, South Korea

16.2 Abiraterone in Chemotherapy-Naïve mCRPC

Abiraterone acetate is an inhibitor of cytochrome P-450 c17, a critical enzyme in extragonadal and testicular androgen synthesis, thereby stopping the testes and the tissues in the body from making androgen [8–10]. Until recently, only one study (COU-AA-302) was identified for the treatment of abiraterone in patients with chemotherapy-naïve mCRPC. This study compared abiraterone plus prednisone with placebo plus prednisone (referred to as "abiraterone" or "prednisone," respectively) in chemotherapy-naïve mCRPC [11–16]. In the COU-AA-302 study, 1088 chemotherapy-naive asymptomatic or mildly symptomatic mCRPC patients without visceral metastases were randomized in a 1:1 ratio (546 were assigned to abiraterone and 542 to prednisone). Patients received abiraterone acetate 1 g (four 250-mg tablets) or four placebo tablets orally once daily at least 1 h before and 2 h after a meal and prednisone 5 mg orally twice daily [15]. The median follow-up duration was 49.2 months (Table 16.1).

Median overall survival (OS) in the abiraterone group was significantly longer than in

C. S. Kim (ed.), *Management of Advanced Prostate Cancer*,
https://doi.org/10.1007/978-981-10-6943-7_16

Table 16.1 Study characteristics of abiraterone or enzalutamide in chemotherapy-naïve metastatic CRPC

Study name	Experiment (*n*)	Control (*n*)	Median/mean age, years		Medical PSA level (ng/mL)	Sites of metastasis, *n*	Median follow-up duration, months
			Treatment	Control			
COU-AA-302 [4–9]	Abiraterone acetate 1000 mg daily plus PD 5 mg twice a day	Prednisone 5 mg twice daily plus placebo	71.0 (44–95)	70.0 (44–90)	42.0/37.7	Bone only: 274 (51%)/267 (49%) Soft tissue or node: 267 (49%)/271 (50%) No visceral metastasis	49.2
PREVAIL [12, 13]	Enzalutamide 160 mg daily	Placebo	72 (43–93)	71 (42–93)	54.1/44.2	Bone: 741 (85.0%)/690 (81.7%) Lymph node: 437(50.1%)/434 (51.4%) Visceral disease (lung or liver): 98 (11.2%)/106(12.5%)	~22
TERRAIN [14]	Bicalutamide 50 mg daily	Enzalutamide 160 mg daily	71 (48–91)	71 (50–96)	22/21	Bone only: 83(45%)/92(48%) Soft tissue only: 36(20%)/29 (15%) Bone and soft tissue: 64(35%)/69 (36%)	16.7/20.0

the prednisone group (34.7 months [95% CI 32.7–36.8] vs. 30.3 months [28.7–33.3]; HR 0.81 [95% CI 0.70–0.93]; $p = 0.0033$) [12]. Patients receiving abiraterone compared with prednisone had statistically significant improvement in radiographic progression-free survival (rPFS) ($p < 0.0001$), with a median time to disease progression or death of 16.5 vs. 8.2 months, respectively (HR 0.52 [95% CI, 0.45–0.61]; $p < 0.0001$) [14]. Health-related quality of life (HRQoL) was assessed with the Functional Assessment of Cancer Therapy-Prostate (FACT-P) questionnaire. Median time to HRQoL deterioration (i.e., a decrease from baseline in the FACT-P total score by ten points or more) was longer in patients assigned to abiraterone group than prednisone group as assessed by the FACT-P total score (12.7 months [95% CI 11.1–14.0] vs. 8.3 months [7.4–10.6]; HR 0.78 [95% CI 0.66–0.92]; $p = 0.003$) [16]. More adverse events (AEs) were observed in the abiraterone group. In all, grade 3 or 4 AEs were observed in 290 patients (54%) in the abiraterone group and 236 patients (44%) in the prednisone group [12]. The most common grade 3–4 adverse events of special interest were cardiovascular disorders (8% in the abiraterone group vs. 4% in the placebo group), increased alanine aminotransferase (6 vs. <1%), and hypertension (5 vs. 3%) [12]. Elderly patients ($n = 350$) treated with abiraterone-prednisone showed significant improvements in OS and rPFS than prednisone alone (HR 0.71 [95% CI 0.53–0.96] and HR 0.63 [95% CI 0.48–0.83], respectively), similar to younger patients ($n = 738$, HR 0.81 [95% CI 0.63–1.03] and HR 0.49 [95% CI 0.40–0.59], respectively) [11].

16.3 Enzalutamide in Chemotherapy-Naïve mCRPC

Enzalutamide (formerly known as MDV3100) is a targeted AR inhibitor that overcomes resistance to conventional antiandrogens that competitively binds to the ligand-binding domain of the androgen receptor and inhibits androgen receptor translocation to the cell nucleus, recruitment of androgen receptor cofactors, and androgen receptor binding to DNA [17, 18].

One study (PREVAIL) compared enzalutamide with placebo in chemotherapy-naïve mCRPC [19, 20]. In this study, a total of 1717 patients (12% of the included patients had visceral metastases) were enrolled with randomly assigned to receive either oral enzalutamide (at a dose of 160 mg) or placebo once daily with or without food (872 in the enzalutamide group and 845 in the placebo group). Continued ADT was required. Previous antiandrogen therapy and concurrent use of glucocorticoids were permitted but not required. This study was stopped after the planned interim analysis, because of the observed benefit of the active treatment in the two co-primary outcomes rPFS and OS. The median follow-up duration was approximately 22 months.

The rate of rPFS at 12 months was 65% in the enzalutamide group, as compared with 14% in the placebo group (81% risk reduction; HR 0.19 [95% CI, 0.15–0.23]; $P < 0.001$) [20]. A total of 626 patients (72%) in the enzalutamide group, as compared with 532 patients (63%) in the placebo group, were alive at the data cutoff date (HR 0.71 [95% CI, 0.60–0.84]; $p < 0.001$) [20]. HRQoL was assessed at baseline and during treatment using the FACT-P and EuroQol-5 Dimension (EQ-5D) questionnaires. Median time to deterioration in FACT-P total score was 11.3 months (95% CI 11.1–13.9) in patients with enzalutamide and 5·6 months (5.5–5.6) in patients with placebo (HR 0.62 [95% CI 0.54–0.72]; $p < 0.0001$) [19]. The enzalutamide group showed clinically meaningful improvements than the placebo group in FACT-P total score (327 [40%] of 826 vs. 181 [23%] of 790) and in EQ-5D utility index (224 [28%] of 812 vs. 99 [16%] of 623) [19]. AEs grade 3 or higher was reported in 43% in the enzalutamide group, as compared with 37% in the placebo group [20]. In enzalutamide group, the most common grade 3 or higher event and cardiac event was hypertension (7%) and atrial fibrillation (2%), respectively [20]. One patient in each group had a seizure. In patients with visceral metastases, an increase OS was observed in patients treated with enzalutamide compared to placebo with a HR of 0.82 (95% CI 0.55–1.23) [20].

One study (TERRAIN) compared bicalutamide with enzalutamide in patients with chemotherapy-naïve mCRPC [21]. Another study (STRIVE) evaluated enzalutamide compared with bicalutamide in chemotherapy-naïve prostate cancer patients, but this study included non-metastatic patients [22]. In the TERRAIN study, 375 asymptomatic or mildly symptomatic patients with at least two bone lesions or soft tissue metastases were randomly assigned to receive enzalutamide 160 mg/day or bicalutamide 50 mg/day in addition to ADT, both taken orally until disease progression (184 to enzalutamide and 191 to bicalutamide) [21]. Median follow-up time was 20.0 months (IQR 15.0–25.6) in the enzalutamide group and 16.7 months (10.2–21.9) in the bicalutamide group.

OS was not reported in this study. Patients in the enzalutamide group had significantly improved median PFS (15.7 months [95% CI 11.5–19 4]) compared with patients in the bicalutamide group (5.8 months [4.8–8.1]; HR 0.44 [95% CI 0.34–0.57]; $p < 0{\cdot}0001$) [21]. Time to FACT-P total score deterioration was longer for patients in the enzalutamide group than for those in the bicalutamide group (median 13.8 months [95% CI 11.1–22] for patients in the enzalutamide group vs. 8.5 months [5.8–11.3] for patients in the bicalutamide group; $p = 0.0067$) [21]. The grade 3 or more AEs were observed in 40% (73/183) of the enzalutamide group and 38% (72/189) of the bicalutamide group had AEs. Serious AEs were reported by 31% (57/183) and 23% (44/189) in the enzalutamide and bicalutamide groups, respectively [21]. One of the nine deaths in the enzalutamide group was regarded as to be possibly related to treatment (due to systemic inflammatory response syndrome) compared with none of the three deaths in the bicalutamide group.

Differences in the patient selection and dividing subgroups in these studies can inform treatment options indirectly to the physicians. The previously stated studies with abiraterone or enzalutamide restricted inclusion to asymptomatic and minimally symptomatic chemotherapy-naïve mCRPC patients, to verify the role in the pre-chemotherapy setting. The phase III ALLIANCE study (NCT01949337), adding abiraterone in patients treated with enzalutamide, is currently under investigation. Because of these novel agents developed within a short period of time, prospective data of their effective sequential use are insufficient. The clinical challenge now is to reach a consensus on the ideal way to sequence effective treatments, by the individual use to specific patient subgroups [23].

16.4 Summary

So far, the evidence for optimal treatment of OS and PFS in chemotherapy-naïve patient with mCRPC was verified as abiraterone plus prednisone and enzalutamide. Treatment options excluding abiraterone plus enzalutamide would be considered for individual situation by considering the quality of studies, patient selection, and both HRQoL and AEs. These new agents may provide an effective, convenient, less toxic treatment for chemotherapy-naïve mCRPC. The sequence and combination of treatment options in chemotherapy-naïve patients with mCRPC is still a clinical challenge. Novel AR-targeting agents especially abiraterone and enzalutamide comparted with each other in head to head clinical trials could help to the selection for the patients with chemotherapy-naïve mCRPC.

References

1. Sridhar SS, Freedland SJ, Gleave ME, Higano C, Mulders P, Parker C, et al. Castration-resistant prostate cancer: from new pathophysiology to new treatment. Eur Urol. 2014;65(2):289–99.
2. Akram ON, Mushtaq G, Kamal MA. An overview of current screening and management approaches for prostate cancer. Curr Drug Metab. 2015;16(8):713–8.
3. Petrylak DP, Tangen CM, Hussain MH, Lara PN Jr, Jones JA, Taplin ME, et al. Docetaxel and estramustine compared with mitoxantrone and prednisone for advanced refractory prostate cancer. N Engl J Med. 2004;351(15):1513–20.
4. Tannock IF, de Wit R, Berry WR, Horti J, Pluzanska A, Chi KN, et al. Docetaxel plus prednisone or mitoxantrone plus prednisone for advanced prostate cancer. N Engl J Med. 2004;351(15):1502–12.
5. de Bono JS, Oudard S, Ozguroglu M, Hansen S, Machiels JP, Kocak I, et al. Prednisone plus cabazitaxel or mitoxantrone for metastatic castration-resistant prostate cancer progressing after docetaxel treatment: a randomised open-label trial. Lancet. 2010;376(9747):1147–54.
6. Chandrasekar T, Yang JC, Gao AC, Evans CP. Mechanisms of resistance in castration-resistant prostate cancer (CRPC). Transl Androl Urol. 2015;4(3):365–80.
7. Coutinho I, Day TK, Tilley WD, Selth LA. Androgen receptor signaling in castration-resistant prostate cancer: a lesson in persistence. Endocr Relat Cancer. 2016;23(12):T179–t97.
8. Attard G, Belldegrun AS, de Bono JS. Selective blockade of androgenic steroid synthesis by novel lyase inhibitors as a therapeutic strategy for treating metastatic prostate cancer. BJU Int. 2005;96(9):1241–6.
9. Molina A, Belldegrun A. Novel therapeutic strategies for castration resistant prostate cancer: inhibition of persistent androgen production and androgen receptor mediated signaling. J Urol. 2011;185(3):787–94.
10. Montgomery RB, Mostaghel EA, Vessella R, Hess DL, Kalhorn TF, Higano CS, et al. Maintenance of intratumoral androgens in metastatic prostate cancer: a mechanism for castration-resistant tumor growth. Cancer Res. 2008;68(11):4447–54.
11. Smith MR, Rathkopf DE, Mulders PF, Carles J, Van Poppel H, Li J, et al. Efficacy and safety of abiraterone acetate in elderly (75 years or older) chemotherapy naive patients with metastatic castration resistant prostate cancer. J Urol. 2015;194(5):1277–84.
12. Ryan CJ, Smith MR, Fizazi K, Saad F, Mulders PF, Sternberg CN, et al. Abiraterone acetate plus prednisone versus placebo plus prednisone in chemotherapy-naive men with metastatic castration-resistant prostate cancer (COU-AA-302): final overall survival analysis of a randomised, double-blind, placebo-controlled phase 3 study. Lancet Oncol. 2015;16(2):152–60.
13. Morris MJ, Molina A, Small EJ, de Bono JS, Logothetis CJ, Fizazi K, et al. Radiographic progression-free survival as a response biomarker in metastatic castration-resistant prostate cancer: COU-AA-302 results. J Clin Oncol. 2015;33(12):1356–63.
14. Rathkopf DE, Smith MR, de Bono JS, Logothetis CJ, Shore ND, de Souza P, et al. Updated interim efficacy analysis and long-term safety of abiraterone acetate in metastatic castration-resistant prostate cancer patients without prior chemotherapy (COU-AA-302). Eur Urol. 2014;66(5):815–25.
15. Ryan CJ, Smith MR, de Bono JS, Molina A, Logothetis CJ, de Souza P, et al. Abiraterone in metastatic prostate cancer without previous chemotherapy. N Engl J Med. 2013;368(2):138–48.
16. Basch E, Autio K, Ryan CJ, Mulders P, Shore N, Kheoh T, et al. Abiraterone acetate plus prednisone versus prednisone alone in chemotherapy-naive men

with metastatic castration-resistant prostate cancer: patient-reported outcome results of a randomised phase 3 trial. Lancet Oncol. 2013;14(12):1193–9.
17. Tran C, Ouk S, Clegg NJ, Chen Y, Watson PA, Arora V, et al. Development of a second-generation antiandrogen for treatment of advanced prostate cancer. Science. 2009;324(5928):787–90.
18. Attard G, Swennenhuis JF, Olmos D, Reid AH, Vickers E, A'Hern R, et al. Characterization of ERG, AR and PTEN gene status in circulating tumor cells from patients with castration-resistant prostate cancer. Cancer Res. 2009;69(7):2912–8.
19. Loriot Y, Miller K, Sternberg CN, Fizazi K, De Bono JS, Chowdhury S, et al. Effect of enzalutamide on health-related quality of life, pain, and skeletal-related events in asymptomatic and minimally symptomatic, chemotherapy-naive patients with metastatic castration-resistant prostate cancer (PREVAIL): results from a randomised, phase 3 trial. Lancet Oncol. 2015;16(5):509–21.
20. Beer TM, Armstrong AJ, Rathkopf DE, Loriot Y, Sternberg CN, Higano CS, et al. Enzalutamide in metastatic prostate cancer before chemotherapy. N Engl J Med. 2014;371(5):424–33.
21. Shore ND, Chowdhury S, Villers A, Klotz L, Siemens DR, Phung, et al. Efficacy and safety of enzalutamide versus bicalutamide for patients with metastatic prostate cancer (TERRAIN): a randomised, double-blind, phase 2 study. Lancet Oncol. 2016;17(2):153–63.
22. Penson DF, Armstrong AJ, Concepcion R, Agarwal N, Olsson C, Karsh L, et al. Enzalutamide versus bicalutamide in castration-resistant prostate cancer: the STRIVE trial. J Clin Oncol. 2016;34(18):2098–106.
23. Lorente D, Mateo J, Perez-Lopez R, de Bono JS, Attard G. Sequencing of agents in castration-resistant prostate cancer. Lancet Oncol. 2015;16(6):e279–92.

17 Abiraterone or Enzalutamide in CRPC After Chemotherapy

U-Syn Ha

17.1 Introduction

Most prostate cancer patients treated with androgen deprivation therapy (ADT) as systemic therapy will develop castration-resistant prostate cancer (CRPC). CRPC is most frequently characterized by a rise in serum prostate-specific antigen (PSA) levels over time in the context of low (< 50 ng/mL) serum testosterone levels. Expression of PSA is typically regulated by the androgen receptor (AR), supporting a role for AR in CRPC. The biological significance of CRPC is that an important mechanism of CRPC is the upregulation of intracellular androgen and/or androgen receptor (AR), leading to sustained AR-directed growth of prostate cancer despite a castrate level of serum androgens [1]. Thus, patients with CRPC are usually sensitive to sequential "secondary" hormonal therapies directed at AR inhibition. The treatment landscape for CRPC has expanded in the past decade to include several novel agents. These novel therapies have been directed specifically against CRPC, including abiraterone acetate (AA) and enzalutamide [2, 3]. The recent US Food and Drug Administration (FDA)-approved enzalutamide (Xtandi) and abiraterone (Xytiga) based on researches showed improvement of survival in the treatment for CRPC after chemotherapy. The present article reviews recent advances of the novel AR-targeted therapeutic agents for CRPC.

U.-S. Ha
Department of Urology, College of Medicine, The Catholic University of Korea, Seoul, South Korea
e-mail: ushamd@catholic.ac.kr

17.2 Enzalutamide

17.2.1 Understanding for Mechanism of Actions

The new AR antagonist, enzalutamide is a second-generation AR antagonist, found in in vitro and murine models. It has ability to inhibit AR signaling in the cells of overexpressed ARs with high binding affinity to the androgen [4, 5]. Unlike former antiandrogens, enzalutamide targets multiple stages of the androgen-signaling pathway (Fig. 17.1). In a LNCaP/AR castration-resistant human prostate cancer cell model, enzalutamide bound to the AR showed an eightfold greater affinity than bicalutamide. AR binds with high affinity to enzalutamide and translocates much less efficiently into the nucleus, and important AR fractions remain in the cytoplasm. Enzalutamide induced regression of established LNCaP/AR xenograft tumor cells, which overexpressed ARs, in castrated male mice model [6]. On the other hand, bicalutamide treatment was shown to only retard the growth of tumor. Enzalutamide blocked induction of PSA and transmembrane serine protease 2, leading a lack of agonist activity. Furthermore, cancer

C. S. Kim (ed.), *Management of Advanced Prostate Cancer*,
https://doi.org/10.1007/978-981-10-6943-7_17

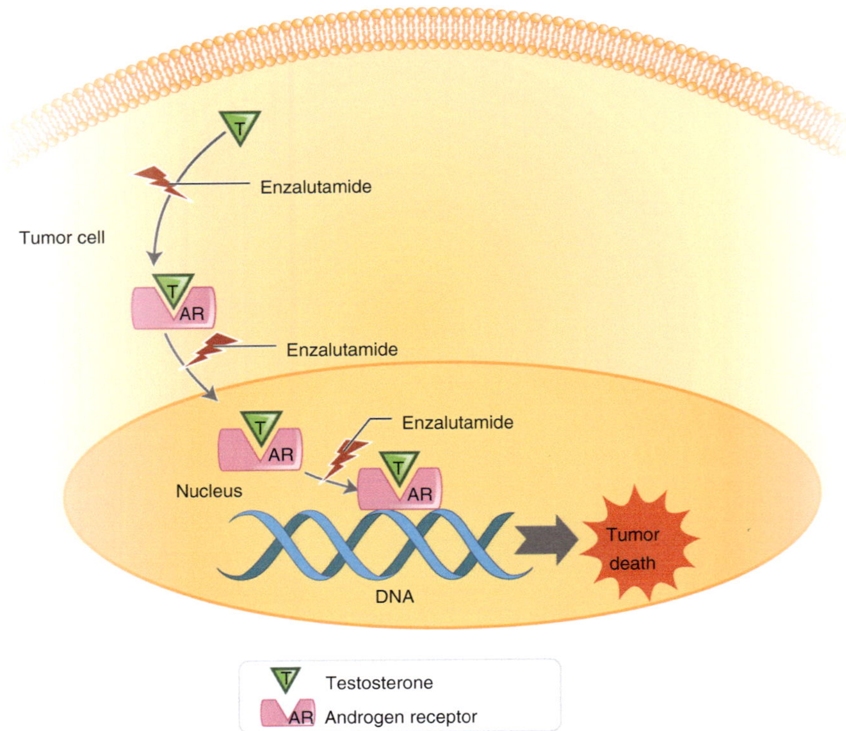

Fig. 17.1 Mechanism of action of enzalutamide. Enzalutamide has multiple targets in the androgen-signaling pathway and mainly blocks androgen receptor (AR)

regression in the patient treated with enzalutamide is also associated with the evidence of cancer cell apoptosis [6].

17.2.2 Clinical Study of Enzalutamide

Based on the encouraging results of the phase I/II trial, results of the phase I/II study, a phase III double-blinded, placebo-controlled trial (AFFIRM—A Study Evaluating the Efficacy and Safety of the Investigational Drug MDV3100) was performed. A total of 1199 men with mCRPC from 166 sites were randomized in a 2:1 manner to be treated with either enzalutamide 160 mg daily ($n = 800$) or placebo ($n = 399$) [7]. The primary end point was overall survival (OS). Patients receiving placebo were able to cross over with enzalutamide. After 14 months, the median OS was significantly improved in the enzalutamide arm versus the placebo arm, which found a median OS of 18.4 months in the enzalutamide arm and 13.6 months in the placebo arm (hazard ratio [HR]: 0.63; 95% CI 0.53–0.75; $p < 0.001$).

Enzalutamide also outperformed placebo in all of the predetermined secondary end points with statistical significance: PSA reduction of more than 50% (54 in the enzalutamide arm vs. 2% in the placebo arm; $p < 0.001$), soft-tissue response rate (29 in the enzalutamide arm vs. 4% in the placebo arm; $p < 0.001$), quality-of-life response rate (43 in the enzalutamide arm vs. 18% in the placebo arm; $p < 0.001$), time to PSA elevation (8.3 in the enzalutamide arm vs. 3.0 months in the placebo arm; HR, 0.25; 95% CI 0.20–0.30; $p < 0.001$), radiographic progression-free survival (PFS) (8.3 in the enzalutamide arm vs. 2.9 months in the placebo arm; HR, 0.40; 95% CI 0.35–0.47; $p < 0.001$), and the time to the first skeletal-related event (16.7 in the enzalutamide arm vs. 13.3 months in the placebo arm; HR, 0.69; 95% CI 0.57–0.84; $p < 0.001$). The patients treated with enzalutamide were well tolerated in this trial, with the most common adverse events being fatigue, diarrhea, and hot flashes. Five of the 800 patients had seizures—several of whom had predisposing conditions such as brain metastases or concomitant medications that lower the seizure threshold, with one additional patient having a seizure after data lock (<1% risk) [7, 8].

17.3 Abiraterone Acetate

17.3.1 Understanding for Mechanism of Actions

Adrenal androgen is converted and uptake in patients treated with ADT, resulting in residual intratumoral androgen. And de novo synthesis from cholesterol or progesterone precursors within the tumor is the cause of the production of residual androgen [9, 10]. The critical enzyme required for androgen synthesis from cholesterol is CYP17A. Expression of CYP17A in the adrenal gland accounts for existing circulating adrenal androgens, as well as dehydroepiandrosterone (DHEA) and androstenedione (AED), and the results of several studies have supported the expression of CYP17A in castration-resistant prostate tumors [11]. Abiraterone acetate blocks androgen biosynthesis via inhibiting of 17α-hydroxylase/C17, 20-lyase (CYP17). These enzymes, which are required for androgen biosynthesis, are expressed in the testis, adrenal gland, and prostate. CYP17A has arisen as a main target of novel therapeutics.

Another suggested mechanism of action is that abiraterone inhibits AR itself, as well as other AR pathway targets including the enzyme named 3β-hydroxysteroid dehydrogenase (3β-HSD), which is required for androgen biosynthesis. Regarding its activity against 3β-HSD type I, abiraterone was demonstrated that it inhibits two key reactions mediated by 3β-HSD type I, the conversion of DHEA to AED and of 5α-androstanediol to testosterone, inhibiting AR-regulated gene expression [12] (Fig. 17.2).

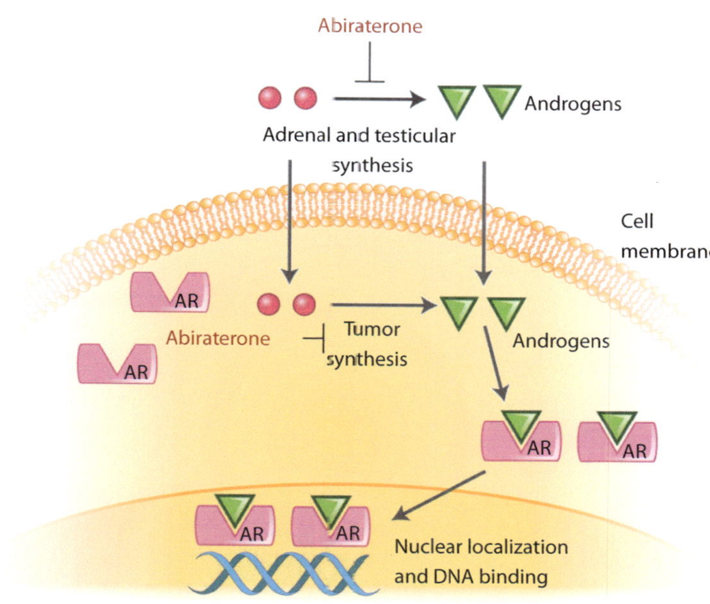

Fig. 17.2 Mechanism of action of Abiraterone acetate inhibits androgen synthesis in testicular, adrenal, and prostatic tumor tissues

17.3.2 Clinical Study for CRPC Following Chemotherapy

In men with metastatic CRPC following chemotherapy, a phase II single-agent study of abiraterone, in which only 17% of patients were treated with prior ketoconazole, reported that PSA decreased by more than 50% in 51% of patients, with partial radiographic responses in 27% of patients and a median time to progression of 24 weeks [13]. In a phase II study of abiraterone combined with prednisone, PSA declines of more than 50% were observed in 36% of patients (47% of patients were treated with prior ketoconazole) with a median time to progression of 24 weeks [14].

Based on the positive results of phase I/II, phase III studies were conducted with the 1195 eligible patients. Of these, 797 were randomly assigned to abiraterone arm (abiraterone acetate with prednisone) and 398 to placebo arm (placebo with prednisone). At median follow-up (20.2 months, interquartile range [IQR] 18.4–22.1), median OS for the abiraterone arm was longer than in the placebo arm (15.8 months, in the abiraterone arm vs. 11.2 months in the placebo arm; HR 0·74, 95% CI 0.64–0.86; $p < 0{\cdot}0001$). Median time to PSA progression (8.5 months in the abiraterone arm vs. 6.6 months in the placebo arm; HR 0.63, 95% CI 0.52–0.78; $p < 0{\cdot}0001$), median radiologic PFS (5.6 months in the abiraterone arm vs. 3.6 months in the placebo arm; HR 0·66, 95% CI 0·58–0·76; $p < 0{\cdot}0001$), and proportion of patients who had a PSA response (29.5% in the abiraterone arm vs. 5.5% in the placebo arm; $p < 0{\cdot}0001$) were all improved in the abiraterone arm compared with the placebo arm. Fatigue (9% in the abiraterone arm vs. 10% in the placebo arm), anemia (8% in the abiraterone arm vs. 8% in the placebo arm), back pain (7% in the abiraterone arm vs. 10% in the placebo arm), and bone pain (6% in the abiraterone arm vs. 8% in the placebo arm) are the most common adverse events. These results confirm that abiraterone acetate significantly prolongs overall survival in patients with CRPC following docetaxel treatment [15].

17.4 Selection for the Treatment of CRPC

Both enzalutamide and abiraterone acetate have now been approved by FDA for the post-chemotherapy mCRPC. Current NCCN guidelines suggest that either enzalutamide or abiraterone acetate is a reasonable choice in this setting. However there is currently a paucity of evidence with regards to the first-line treatment of choice, as well as to the optimal sequencing for these therapies. Importantly, no randomized head-to-head trials of enzalutamide and abiraterone acetate have been conducted to date.

Recently published one meta-analysis suggested remarkable results [16]. Pairwise meta-analysis was conducted to gain direct evidence, and network meta-analysis to gain indirect evidence. Remarkably, enzalutamide and abiraterone were both significantly improve OS, compared to control group. Enzalutamide was the most effective agent in improvement of OS ($HR = 0.71$), and abiraterone seemed to be less effective compared with enzalutamide ($HR = 0.78$). Enzalutamide improved PFS ($HR = 0.36$), but abiraterone did not significantly improve PFS compared with control groups. Enzalutamide ($HR = 0.20$) and abiraterone ($HR = 0.56$) both significantly extend times to PSA progression [16].

Both drugs are effective for CRPC patients, but two drugs have cross-resistance mechanism. If the disease progresses while using one of the two drugs, it may not be effective changing to another drug due to resistance. Further prospective studies about sequential treatment or combination therapy of enzalutamide and abiraterone needed.

17.5 Summary

- The recent US Food and Drug Administration (FDA)-approved enzalutamide (Xtandi) and abiraterone (Xytiga) based on researches showed improvement of survival in the treatment for CRPC after chemotherapy.

- Enzalutamide is a second-generation AR antagonist, found to have ability to inhibit multiple steps in the androgen-signaling pathway with high binding affinity to the AR targets
- Abiraterone acetate blocks androgen biosynthesis via inhibiting of 17α-hydroxylase/C17, 20-lyase (CYP17). These enzymes, which are required for androgen biosynthesis, are expressed in the testis, adrenal gland, and prostate.
- In randomized phase III clinical trial, the enzalutamide and abiraterone extended survival in men with metastatic CRPC after chemotherapy.
- Until now, no consensus has been reached regarding the agent that provides the best oncological outcomes among the two agents for the treatment of metastatic CRPC after chemotherapy.
- Enzalutamide and abiraterone are effective for CRPC patients, but two drugs have cross-resistance mechanism. If the disease progresses while using one of the two drugs, it may not be effective changing to another drug due to resistance.

References

1. Montgomery RB, Mostaghel EA, Vessella R, Hess DL, Kalhorn TF, Higano CS, et al. Maintenance of intratumoral androgens in metastatic prostate cancer: a mechanism for castration-resistant tumor growth. Cancer Res. 2008;68(11):4447–54.
2. de Bono JS, Logothetis CJ, Molina A, Fizazi K, North S, Chu L, et al. Abiraterone and increased survival in metastatic prostate cancer. N Engl J Med. 2011;364(21):1995–2005.
3. Ryan CJ, Smith MR, de Bono JS, Molina A, Logothetis CJ, de Souza P, et al. Abiraterone in metastatic prostate cancer without previous chemotherapy. N Engl J Med. 2013;368(2):138–48.
4. Tran C, Ouk S, Clegg NJ, Chen Y, Watson PA, Arora V, et al. Development of a second-generation antiandrogen for treatment of advanced prostate cancer. Science (New York, NY). 2009;324(5928):787–90.
5. Guerrero J, Alfaro IE, Gomez F, Protter AA, Bernales S. Enzalutamide, an androgen receptor signaling inhibitor, induces tumor regression in a mouse model of castration-resistant prostate cancer. Prostate. 2013;73(12):1291–305.
6. El-Amm J, Patel N, Freeman A, Aragon-Ching JB. Metastatic castration-resistant prostate cancer: critical review of enzalutamide. Clin Med Insights Oncol. 2013;7:235–45.
7. Scher HI, Fizazi K, Saad F, Taplin ME, Sternberg CN, Miller K, et al. Increased survival with enzalutamide in prostate cancer after chemotherapy. N Engl J Med. 2012;367(13):1187–97.
8. Zhang T, Zhu J, George DJ, Armstrong AJ. Enzalutamide versus abiraterone acetate for the treatment of men with metastatic castration-resistant prostate cancer. Expert Opin Pharmacother. 2015;16(4):473–85.
9. Mostaghel EA. Abiraterone in the treatment of metastatic castration-resistant prostate cancer. Cancer Manag Res. 2014;6:39–51.
10. Locke JA, Wasan KM, Nelson CC, Guns ES, Leon CG. Androgen-mediated cholesterol metabolism in LNCaP and PC-3 cell lines is regulated through two different isoforms of acyl-coenzyme A:Cholesterol Acyltransferase (ACAT). Prostate. 2008;68(1):20–33.
11. Efstathiou E, Titus M, Tsavachidou D, Tzelepi V, Wen S, Hoang A, et al. Effects of abiraterone acetate on androgen signaling in castrate-resistant prostate cancer in bone. J Clin Oncol Off J Am Soc Clin Oncol. 2012;30(6):637–43.
12. Li R, Evaul K, Sharma KK, Chang KH, Yoshimoto J, Liu J, et al. Abiraterone inhibits 3beta-hydroxysteroid dehydrogenase: a rationale for increasing drug exposure in castration-resistant prostate cancer. Clin Cancer Res. 2012;18(13):3571–9.
13. Reid AH, Attard G, Danila DC, Oommen NB, Olmos D, Fong PC, et al. Significant and sustained antitumor activity in post-docetaxel, castration-resistant prostate cancer with the CYP17 inhibitor abiraterone acetate. J Clin Oncol Off J Am Soc Clin Oncol. 2010;28(9):1489–95.
14. Danila DC, Morris MJ, de Bono JS, Ryan CJ, Denmeade SR, Smith MR, et al. Phase II multicenter study of abiraterone acetate plus prednisone therapy in patients with docetaxel-treated castration-resistant prostate cancer. J Clin Oncol Off J Am Soc Clin Oncol. 2010;28(9):1496–501.
15. Fizazi K, Scher HI, Molina A, Logothetis CJ, Chi KN, Jones RJ, et al. Abiraterone acetate for treatment of metastatic castration-resistant prostate cancer: final overall survival analysis of the COU-AA-301 randomised, double-blind, placebo-controlled phase 3 study Lancet Oncol. 2012;13(10):983–92.
16. Kang M, Jeong CW, Kwak C, Ku JH, Kim HH. Comparing the clinical efficacy of abiraterone acetate, enzalutamide, and orteronel in patients with metastatic castration-resistant prostate cancer by performing a network meta-analysis of eight randomized controlled trials. Oncotarget. 2017;8(35):59690–7.

Clinical Results of Secondary Hormonal Treatment

18

Jae Young Park

18.1 Introduction

Prostate cancer (PCa) is one of the leading malignant causes of death in men globally, with an incidence of 1,095,000 new cases diagnosed each year causing 307,000 cancer-specific deaths in 2012 [1]. Many patients with PCa can be cured with local treatments, but approximately one-third of them will ultimately become a progressive disease, which will be characterized by increasing prostate-specific antigen (PSA) levels. Androgen deprivation therapy (ADT) including surgical or medical castration has been regarded as primary systemic therapy for metastatic PCa for more than 50 years. Surgical castration is the traditional treatment option which means bilateral orchiectomy. Nowadays, medical castration with gonadotropin-releasing hormone (GnRH) analogues and/or antiandrogen which suppresses testosterone production is the most common option in primary ADT.

However, despite initial treatment shows efficacy in most patients with PCa at first, the further progression which is indicated by either increasing PSA levels or new sites of metastasis is usually detectable within 18–24 months [2]. Treatment options for patients are limited when PCa becomes refractory to primary ADT, and the patients complain of bone pain, general weakness, or cachexia, and accordingly the life expectancy is shortened, with a median overall survival of 2 years [2–4].

Interestingly, in many cases, after experiencing disease progression on primary ADT, the patients with further secondary hormonal manipulations demonstrate biochemical and/or clinical responses. Recently many articles have been published demonstrating that PCa showing clinical progression during ADT is not truly resistant to the androgen effects. As a result of molecular adaptations after ADT, hypersensitivity PCa cell to low androgen levels induces persistent signaling-mediated growth through the androgen receptor (AR) [5]. Therefore, "hormone refractory" PCa seems to be inappropriate, and it would be more accurate to name these cancers as the castration-resistant PCa (CRPC). Second-line hormonal maneuvers traditionally include combined androgen blockade (CAB), antiandrogens alone, antiandrogen withdrawal, glucocorticoids, ketoconazole, and estrogens. Although these agents could not show definite improvement in cancer-specific survival, these secondary hormonal maneuvers consistently demonstrate biochemical/clinical benefits in most CRPC patients. However, the duration of response is short, therapeutic result is limited, and the mechanisms of action are generally nonspecific except for antiandrogens [6]. Herein, this review summarizes the current secondary hormone therapies in the management of CRPC.

J. Y. Park, M.D., Ph.D.
Department of Urology, Korea University Ansan Hospital, Korea University College of Medicine, Ansan, South Korea
e-mail: jaeyoungpark@korea.ac.kr

C. S. Kim (ed.), *Management of Advanced Prostate Cancer*,
https://doi.org/10.1007/978-981-10-6943-7_18

18.1.1 Second-Line Antiandrogens and Antiandrogen Withdrawal

Several antiandrogen therapy regimens when initial ADT becomes ineffective are the following: CAB, antiandrogens alone, or antiandrogen withdrawal. Deferred use of antiandrogens after PCa progression has shown a 50% or greater decrease in PSA in 80% of patients with localized disease and 54% of those with metastatic disease [7]. Fossa et al. showed that deferred flutamide resulted in 50% or greater PSA decrease in 23% of symptomatic CRPC patients [8].

Second-line antiandrogen monotherapy can lead to a PSA response of 50% or greater in 4–50% of patients. The response duration of treatment is 4.0–11.0 months. The adverse effects of antiandrogen monotherapy include breast pain/tenderness and gynecomastia. These symptoms can be prevented with prophylactic breast irradiation [9–14]. Particularly, 20–40% of the patients who received prior flutamide therapy have PSA decreases of 50% or greater after being treated with high doses of bicalutamide (150–200 mg) [2]. Joyce et al. reported a similar result regarding nilutamide, with a PSA decrease of 50% or greater in 29% of PCa [12].

Antiandrogens often begin to have AR agonist activity partially after its prolonged use. Accordingly, antiandrogen discontinuation in CRPC leads to antiandrogen withdrawal syndrome (AAWD), which means PSA declines after antiandrogen discontinuation with symptomatic improvement [15–17]. AAWD results in a PSA decline of 50% or greater in 10–15% of cases, with responses lasting a median of 6 months [17, 18]. Notably, however, survival benefits in these patients are very low despite a significant decrease in the PSA level [18].

18.1.2 Steroid Hormone Manipulation

Ketoconazole which is an oral antifungal agent was first described to have activity in PCa over 30 years ago and has long been used off-label in the treatment of CRPC prior to docetaxel. It blocks androgen synthesis by inhibiting the C17, 20-desmolase enzyme which is a key microsomal cytochrome P450-dependent enzyme. C17, 20-desmolase enzyme is necessary for adrenal androgen and testosterone biosynthesis. Accordingly, ketoconazole suppresses the production of testosterone, glucocorticoids, mineralocorticoids, and estrogens. It is also reported that ketoconazole has direct cytotoxic effects on PCa cells by inhibiting DNA synthesis in vitro and possibly inducing G0/G1 cell cycle arrest in other cancers [19, 20]. High-dose ketoconazole therapy with 400 mg three times daily and replacement hydrocortisone has become the standard dose schedule [21]. Aminoglutethimide has the pharmacologic action inhibiting the steroid biosynthesis from cholesterol to pregnenolone. For the most part, ketoconazole took the place of aminoglutethimide because of its several side effects [6]. Thirty to sixty percent of CRPC cases showed clinical benefit from ketoconazole, with a median response duration of 7 months [6, 18, 22, 23]. It has been shown that ketoconazole induces a 50% or greater decrease in PSA in 32% of the patients [18]. Very recently, the study investigating the clinical efficacy of ketoconazole was performed. It showed that the median progression-free survival of the patients treated also increased with the number of HSD3B1 variant alleles inherited: 5.4 months for 0 variant alleles, 9.7 months for 1, and 15.2 months for 2 [24]. However, ketoconazole is often associated with moderate-to-severe adverse effects such as hepatotoxicity, lethargy, skin rash, abdominal pain, nausea, mucositis, and diarrhea. Additionally, it can result in adverse drug interactions through inhibition of the cytochromes p450 in the liver. Another recent study regarding low-dose ketoconazole (200 mg PO three times daily) reported that the median progression-free survival was 138 days, and 3 out of 29 patients experienced treatment-related grade 3 side effects [21].

Corticosteroids may act in a variety of ways in men with prostate cancer. As a treatment strategy, corticosteroids represent a minimally toxic, low-cost therapy with some activity against prostate cancer and with an apparent beneficial effect on quality of life [25]. Therefore, it has been used widely in second-line hormonal treatment while the duration of treatment response is only a few months. Some studies reported a PSA decline of 50% or higher in 20% of patients for prednisone or hydrocortisone and in up to 60% for dexamethasone [26–28]. The hypothesis of this response is assumed that the continuous administration of glucocorticoid leads to adrenal insufficiency, which suppresses androgen production from adrenal gland. Glucocorticoids have another palliative effect including pain control, preventing nausea and vomiting even if duration of its treatment is short.

18.1.3 Estrogen-Based Treatment

Diethylstilbestrol (DES) is known as being able to decrease androgen production by inhibiting hypothalamic GnRH and pituitary LH production. DES has been shown to be an active inhibitor against PCa cell lines [29]. Several studies reported that DES decreases PSA level by 50% or more in 20–40% of patients, with a median duration of 4 months. However, this therapeutic success is often accompanied by a substantially increased risk of vascular side effects such as cerebrovascular accidents, myocardial infarction, and pulmonary embolism [2, 6]. Therefore, concomitant anticoagulation agent such as warfarin or aspirin is generally recommended when DES is prescribed due to these side effects [6]. However, estrogen therapy such as DES has been reported to decrease osteoporosis and bone resorption and has potential benefits on cognitive function [30].

18.2 Summary

When PCa becomes a progressive disease despite ADT, there are several treatment options; if the patients receive only GnRH, CAB would be recommended. If the patients receive CAB, antiandrogens alone or antiandrogen withdrawal can be recommended. Ketoconazole and glucocorticoids are other agents which interfere with androgen synthesis in adrenal gland. DES suppresses androgen production by inhibiting hypothalamic and pituitary pathway. It can increase cardiovascular side effect but is also known to decrease osteoporosis and bone resorption.

Many new drugs come to the clinical field now. However, the response rates and durations are still limited. The secondary hormonal treatment which can result in PSA response for several months can be beneficial to CRPC patients although this response has a limited efficacy.

References

1. IARC: GLOBOCAN. In: http://globocan.iarc.fr/Pages/fact_sheets_cancer.aspx International Agency for Research on Cancer, 2012.
2. Lam JS, Leppert JT, Vemulapalli SN, Shvarts O, Belldegrun AS. Secondary hormonal therapy for advanced prostate cancer. J Urol. 2006;175(1):27–34.
3. Petrylak DP, Tangen CM, Hussain MH, Lara PN Jr, Jones JA, Taplin ME, et al. Docetaxel and estramustine compared with mitoxantrone and prednisone for advanced refractory prostate cancer. N Engl J Med. 2004;351(15):1513–20.
4. Tannock IF, de Wit R, Berry WR, Horti J, Pluzanska A, Chi KN, et al. Docetaxel plus prednisone or mitoxantrone plus prednisone for advanced prostate cancer. N Engl J Med. 2004;351(15):1502–12.
5. Gregory CW, Johnson RT, Mohler JL, French FS, Wilson EM. Androgen receptor stabilization in recurrent prostate cancer is associated with hypersensitivity to low androgen. Cancer Res. 2001;61(7):2892–8.
6. Molina A, Belldegrun A. Novel therapeutic strategies for castration resistant prostate cancer: inhibition of persistent androgen production and androgen receptor mediated signaling. J Urol. 2011;185(3):787–94.
7. Jackson E Jr, Pandey P, Seaver LE, Feliz TP. Prostate specific antigen after gonadal androgen withdrawal and deferred flutamide treatment. J Urol. 1995;154(2):448–53.
8. Fossa S, Slee PT, Brausi M, Horenblas S, Hall R, Hetherington J, et al. Flutamide versus prednisone in patients with prostate cancer symptomatically progressing after androgen-ablative therapy: a phase III study of the European organization for research and treatment of cancer genitourinary group. J Clin Oncol. 2001;19(1):62–71.
9. Debruyne FJ, Murray R, Fradet Y, Johansson JE, Tyrrell C, Boccardo F, et al. Liarozole—a novel treatment approach for advanced prostate cancer: results of a large randomized trial versus cyproterone acetate. Urology. 1998;52(1):72–81.
10. Desai A, Stadler WM, Vogelzang NJ. Nilutamide: possible utility as a second-line hormonal agent. Urology. 2001;58(6):1016–20.

11. Joyce R, Fenton MA, Rode P, Constantine M, Gaynes L, Kolvenbag G, et al. High dose bicalutamide for androgen independent prostate cancer: effect of prior hormonal therapy. J Urol. 1998;159(1):149–53.
12. Kassouf W, Tanguay S, Aprikian AG. Nilutamide as second line hormone therapy for prostate cancer after androgen ablation fails. J Urol. 2003;169(5):1742–4.
13. Kucuk O, Fisher E, Moinpour CM, Coleman D, Hussain MH, Sartor AO, et al. Phase II trial of bicalutamide in patients with advanced prostate cancer in whom conventional hormonal therapy failed: a Southwest Oncology Group study (SWOG 9235). Urology. 2001;58(1):53–8.
14. Scher HI, Liebertz C, Kelly WK, Mazumdar M, Brett C, Schwartz L, et al. Bicalutamide for advanced prostate cancer: the natural versus treated history of disease. J Clin Oncol. 1997;15(8):2928–38.
15. Kelly WK, Scher HI. Prostate specific antigen decline after antiandrogen withdrawal: the flutamide withdrawal syndrome. J Urol. 1993;149(3):607–9.
16. Scher HI, Kelly WK. Flutamide withdrawal syndrome: its impact on clinical trials in hormone-refractory prostate cancer. J Clin Oncol. 1993;11(8):1566–72.
17. Suzuki H, Okihara K, Miyake H, Fujisawa M, Miyoshi S, Matsumoto T, et al. Alternative nonsteroidal antiandrogen therapy for advanced prostate cancer that relapsed after initial maximum androgen blockade. J Urol. 2008;180(3):921–7.
18. Small EJ, Halabi S, Dawson NA, Stadler WM, Rini BI, Picus J, et al. Antiandrogen withdrawal alone or in combination with ketoconazole in androgen-independent prostate cancer patients: a phase III trial (CALGB 9583). J Clin Oncol. 2004;22(6):1025–33.
19. Chen R-J, Lee W-S, Liang Y-C, Lin J-K, Wang Y-J, Lin C-H, et al. Ketoconazole induces G0/G1 arrest in human colorectal and hepatocellular carcinoma cell lines. Toxicol Appl Pharmacol. 2000;169(2):132–41.
20. Rochlitz C, Damon L, Russi M, Geddes A, Cadman E. Cytotoxicity of ketoconazole in malignant cell lines. Cancer Chemother Pharmacol. 1988;21(4):319–22.
21. Lo EN, Beckett LA, Pan C-X, Robles D, Suga JM, Sands JM, et al. Prospective evaluation of low-dose ketoconazole plus hydrocortisone in docetaxel pretreated castration-resistant prostate cancer patients. Prostate Cancer Prostatic Dis. 2015;18(2):144–8.
22. Figg WD, Liu Y, Arlen P, Gulley J, Steinberg SM, Liewehr DJ, et al. A randomized, phase II trial of ketoconazole plus alendronate versus ketoconazole alone in patients with androgen independent prostate cancer and bone metastases. J Urol. 2005;173(3):790–6.
23. Kruit W, Stoter G, Klijn J. Effect of combination therapy with aminoglutethimide and hydrocortisone on prostate-specific antigen response in metastatic prostate cancer refractory to standard endocrine therapy. Anti-Cancer Drugs. 2004;15(9):843–7.
24. Almassi N, Reichard C, Li J, Russell C, Perry J, Ryan CJ, et al. HSD3B1 and response to a nonsteroidal CYP17A1 inhibitor in castration-resistant prostate cancer. JAMA Oncol. 2017;
25. Tannock I, Gospodarowicz M, Meakin W, Panzarella T, Stewart L, Rider W. Treatment of metastatic prostatic cancer with low-dose prednisone: evaluation of pain and quality of life as pragmatic indices of response. J Clin Oncol. 1989;7(5):590–7.
26. Kantoff PW, Halabi S, Conaway M, Picus J, Kirshner J, Hars V, et al. Hydrocortisone with or without mitoxantrone in men with hormone-refractory prostate cancer: results of the cancer and leukemia group B 9182 study. J Clin Oncol. 1999;17(8):2506–13.
27. Small EJ, Meyer M, Marshall ME, Reyno LM, Meyers FJ, Natale RB, et al. Suramin therapy for patients with symptomatic hormone-refractory prostate cancer: results of a randomized phase III trial comparing suramin plus hydrocortisone to placebo plus hydrocortisone. J Clin Oncol. 2000;18(7):1440–50.
28. Storlie JA, Buckner JC, Wiseman GA, Burch PA, Hartmann LC, Richardson RL. Prostate specific antigen levels and clinical response to low dose dexamethasone for hormone-refractory metastatic prostate carcinoma. Cancer. 1995;76(1):96–100.
29. Robertson CN, Roberson KM, Padilla GM, O'Brien ET, Cook JM, Kim C-S, et al. Induction of apoptosis by diethylstilbestrol in hormone-insensitive prostate cancer cells. JNCI. 1996;88(13):908–17.
30. Scherr DS, Pitts WR. The nonsteroidal effects of diethylstilbestrol: the rationale for androgen deprivation therapy without estrogen deprivation in the treatment of prostate cancer. J Urol. 2003;170(5):1703–8.

19 Side Effects and Management of ADT for Prostate Cancer

Mun Su Chung and Seung Hwan Lee

19.1 Introduction

Androgen deprivation therapy (ADT) is the main treatment for advanced prostate cancer and is increasingly used in combination with radiotherapy in patients with earlier stages of prostate cancer. For many years, gonadotropin-releasing hormone (GnRH) agonists have been the ADT standard of treatment. There are, however, several drawbacks related to the mechanism of action of GnRH agonists. In particular, the initial testosterone surge associated with these agents delays the achievement of castration levels of testosterone and can produce a flare in clinical symptoms in patients with advanced disease [1, 2]. Furthermore, microsurges in testosterone levels occur with repeated agonist administration [3]. In this context, it is interesting to note that increases in testosterone above 1.1 nmol/L (32 ng/dL) during agonist treatment were associated with a significantly shorter survival free of androgen-independent progression than patients who had increases <32 ng/dL [4]. Despite the proven success of hormonal therapy, most patients showing an initial response will eventually experience disease progression [5]. Cancer that relapses after initial ADT is termed androgen-independent or castration-resistant prostate cancer (CRPC) [6]. The precise definition of CPRC is, however, controversial. Recent European Association of Urology guidelines define CRPC as castration levels of testosterone (<1.7 nmol/L [50 ng/dL]) and three consecutive rises of PSA, 1 week apart, resulting in two 50% increases over the nadir, with a PSA > 2 ng/mL, despite consecutive hormonal manipulations [7]. However, other definitions of progression have been used. Sharifi et al., for example, defined androgen independence as the first sustained increase in PSA level from the PSA nadir after starting ADT [8]. Based on this definition, they found that the median time to androgen independence was 13–19 months after starting ADT, depending on the disease stage at initiation. In patients with metastatic disease, it is estimated that >90% will progress to androgen independence within 18–24 months [9]. As CRPC carries a much poorer prognosis [10] and might signal the need for chemotherapy [11], any delay in the onset of castration resistance is clearly desirable. GnRH antagonists represent an alternative form of ADT, with a direct and immediate action that allows castration without an initial testosterone surge or subsequent microsurges.

M. S. Chung
Department of Urology, Catholic Kwandong University, International St. Mary's Hospital, Incheon, South Korea
e-mail: skidms@catholic.ac.kr

S. H. Lee (✉)
Department of Urology, Urological Science Institute, Yonsei University College of Medicine, Seoul, Korea
e-mail: leeseh@yuhs.ac

C. S. Kim (ed.), *Management of Advanced Prostate Cancer*,
https://doi.org/10.1007/978-981-10-6943-7_19

19.2 Osteoporosis

Widespread androgen ablation therapy applied to an increasing aging population, already predisposed to loss of bone mineral density (BMD), has caused an epidemic of osteopenia and osteoporosis. More than half of men meet the BMD criteria for osteopenia or osteoporosis before the initiation of ADT [12]. It has been estimated that 4 years of ADT will place the average man in the osteopenic range. Treatment of osteoporosis begins with recognition. Daily supplementation of calcium and vitamin D is recommended by the National Institutes of Health at doses of 1200–1500 mg/day and 400 IU/day, respectively [13].

19.3 Hot Flashes

Hot flashes are not life-threatening but are among the most common side effects of androgen ablation, affecting between 50% and 80% of patients [14]. They are a result of the abrupt withdrawal of sex hormones from the circulation, which lowers the temperature set point in the preoptic area of the anterior hypothalamus thus causing the peripheral thermoregulatory mechanisms to be activated inappropriately. Noted triggers include increased ambient temperature, stress, anxiety, and alcohol. Treatment of hot flashes should be reserved for those who suffer from them.

19.4 Sexual Dysfunction (Erectile Dysfunction and Loss of Libido)

The effects of ADT on sexual function were reported to be profound. Loss of sexual functioning is not inevitable, however, with up to 20% of men on ADT able to maintain some sexual activity [15]. Libido is more severely compromised, with approximately 5% of men maintaining a high level of sexual interest with ADT [16]. Treatment for loss of libido is extremely difficult—if not impossible—for those on ADT. Likewise, medical treatments, such as oral phosphodiesterase type 5 inhibitors, or local treatments, such as intracavernosal injections of alprostadil, can still be effective in selected patients but may not be used over the long term.

19.5 Cognitive Function

There is a high suggestion that ADT is linked to subtle but significant cognitive declines in men with prostate cancer. In a study of ADT on cognitive function [17], after 12 months of ADT, there was a reduction in scores pertaining to immediate span of attention, working memory, and visual–spatial function when compared with a control group. A review of nine studies (but with the largest cohort including only 57 men receiving ADT and 51 controls) [18] found that 47–69% of men on ADT experienced a decline in at least one cognitive domain, most commonly in visual–spatial abilities and executive functioning; however, the individual study findings were inconsistent [19].

19.6 Changes in Body Habitus

A loss of muscle mass and increase in body fat are common in men treated with ADT, and these changes are most pronounced with the initiation of ADT. After 1 year of ADT, the mean overall weight increases from 1.8% to 3.8%, which translates into about 2 kg for a 90 kg man [20]. Regular exercise may help patients limit the accumulation of fat and even prevent prostate cancer progression.

19.7 Diabetes and Metabolic Syndrome

It is well established today that low testosterone levels in men are associated with insulin resistance and type 2 diabetes mellitus. In fact, there is a complex and multiparametric correlation between testosterone deficiency and obesity, which represents a risk factor for cardiovascular disease [21, 22]. Furthermore, studies have shown that testosterone replacement treatment improves insulin sensitivity and glycemic profiles in hypogonadal men.

Evidence regarding insulin sensitivity in patients treating ADT is limited, and the studies are quite heterogeneous as to design (different types of ADT, short and long duration, presence or absence of control group, etc.) and the results are controversial. Nevertheless, it seems that ADT decreases insulin sensitivity in nondiabetic men within 12 weeks of initiating treatment [23–26]. The exact mechanism by which ADT increases insulin resistance is not yet clearly understood. The observed increase in fat mass, and particularly in the abdomen, in these men is thought to contribute to the reduced insulin sensitivity. Moreover, it has been speculated that certain pro-inflammatory adipokines such as TNF-a, IL-6, and resistin are increased in patients on ADT and might play a role in insulin resistance [27, 28]. Although insulin resistance appears early in men undergoing ADT, it seems that fasting hyperglycemia and frank diabetes need a year or more to develop. However, randomized studies on this subject are lacking.

Data from the Surveillance, Epidemiology, and End Results (SEER) database including 73,196 men with local or locally advanced prostate cancer treated with LHRH agonists (36%) or orchiectomy (7%) reported a higher diabetes incidence (adjusted hazard ratio, 1.42) in these men [29]. The results from the Canadian database analysis of 20,000 men are similar [30]. Another observational study of 14,597 veterans also found that treatment with LHRH agonists was associated with a statistically significant increased incidence of diabetes [31]. Recently, a retrospective study of 12,191 men diagnosed with localized prostate cancer showed that ADT may increase diabetes risk by 60% [32]. Additionally, it has been found that ADT might worsen glycemic control and increase glycosylated hemoglobin levels in patients with diabetes [33, 34].

As the risk for diabetes development during ADT is high, the need for diabetes screening among men with prostate cancer under long-term treatment is obvious. In the absence of evidence-based recommendations, risk-adapted screening and intervention according to the guidelines from the ADA may be applied to this specific population [35]. Screening men at baseline and again in a year for those treated with long-term ADT and using fasting plasma glucose and hemoglobin A1c as screening tests seem reasonable. Individuals with hemoglobin A1c between 6.0% and 6.5% or impaired fasting glucose (fasting glucose, 100–125 mg/dL) should be considered to be at high-risk for developing diabetes and need to be counseled to lose weight and undertake moderate physical activity [36]. In those with preexisting diabetes, intensification of hypoglycemic treatment and a more frequent follow-up might be necessary, depending on their blood glucose and HbA1c levels.

19.8 Cardiovascular Morbidity and Mortality

The increased rates of obesity, insulin resistance, diabetes, hyperlipidemia, and metabolic syndrome observed in patients on ADT would support the hypothesis of a similar effect on cardiovascular disease (CVD). Moreover, this hypothesis might well be strengthened by recent findings indicating that several biological mechanisms induced by ADT, such as increased inflammation, atherogenic plaque formation, and plaque destabilization, could further promote CVD development in these patients [37].

Large randomized control trials are lacking, and the existing evidence regarding CVD morbidity and mortality for patients receiving ADT is somewhat controversial. Data from observational studies indicate overall a positive relationship between ADT and CVD. In a large population-based cohort study of 185,106 men, it was found that ADT was independently associated with an increased risk of myocardial infarction (MI) and diabetes [38]. A retrospective analysis, however, using data from the Cancer of the Prostate Strategic Urologic Research Endeavor (CaPSURE) and including men with prostate cancer treated with radical prostatectomy followed or not with ADT found a significant correlation of ADT with increased CV mortality, but only among patients over 65 years old ($p = 0.002$) [39]. Furthermore, a recent meta-analysis of randomized controlled trials showed that antiandrogen was associated with a 30% decreased risk for myocardial infarction compared to GnRH agonists, while maximal androgen blockade was associated with a 10% increased risk for stroke when compared to antiandrogen [40].

In the Radiation Therapy Oncology Group (RTOG) study protocol 85-31, 68 patients with advanced prostate cancer who had either radiotherapy alone or in combination with ADT were enrolled and demonstrated no statistically significant difference regarding mortality related to CVD between the two groups ($p = 0.17$). The RTOG trial 86-1069 involved patients with locally advanced prostate cancer who had received a 4-month scheme of ADT plus radiation treatment (RT) versus those who had RT alone. Again, there was no statistical difference between the treatment groups as regards CV mortality ($p = 0.32$). The RTOG protocol 92-0270 also included patients with locally advanced prostate cancer, but both groups received ADT in addition to RT (28 months and 4 months). As above, there was no significant difference in CV mortality between the two groups ($p = 0.58$). All these results were fully supported by a meta-analysis of eight randomized control trials of ADT versus no or delayed ADT in patients with nonmetastatic prostate cancer which showed that sudden death due to CVD in patients receiving ADT was not different to those with no or delayed therapy [41]. Similar findings were reported in the European Organization for Research and Treatment of Cancer (EORTC) analysis [42].

Preexisting comorbidities and different durations of the ADT could explain the observed result discrepancy among the studies. Comorbidities are important independent prognostic factors for patients with cancer, and the inclusion of the existing comorbidities in hospital-based cancer registries will increase the value and use of observational research [43].

Regarding LHRH antagonists, Smith et al. [44] found that the use of degarelix in ADT for prostate cancer did not affect the CV events in the overall population ($p = 0.45$), although in the subgroup of patients with underlying CV disease, the incidence of those events was increased significantly after the use of degarelix ($p = 0.0013$). In Albertsen's reanalysis of six RCTs, degarelix was shown to be superior to leuprolide, being associated with fewer CV events in patients with or without coexisting CVD ($p = 0.016$ and $p = 0.025$, respectively) [45]. These studies appear to point to LHRH antagonists as an ideal alternative in ADT for high-risk patients with CVD.

It is well known that in the general male population, individuals with reduced risk factors for CVD have a lower incidence of heart disease and stroke [46], and although strong data on ADT attributable risk for cardiovascular disease and mortality are inconsistent, the use of the American Heart Association guidelines can be considered in this population. According to these guidelines, primary prevention should feature total tobacco cessation and appropriate management of hypertension. Low-dose aspirin is recommended for men with a 10% or greater 10-year risk for coronary heart disease. Lifestyle modification should warrant weight control and low intake of saturated fat and cholesterol. If such modifications fail to achieve target LDL, statins should be used as first-line drug treatment of hyperlipidemia [47].

Regular physical activity could be an important factor for the prevention of CVD in prostate cancer patients. More specifically, exercise interventions that apply sound aerobic and resistance training principles should be suggested as being quite effective [48, 49]. In fact, all exercise programs are likely to reduce fatigue and enhance vitality, especially among patients with the highest levels of fatigue and lowest vitality. Men with prostate cancer could improve their strength, physical functioning, and cardiovascular health by increasing their physical activity [50, 51]. Finally, physical exercise improves quality of life, although it is not fully clear whether it affects metabolic risk factors in patients with ADT-treated prostate cancer [52].

19.9 Gynecomastia

Depending on the agents used in ADT, alterations in breast tissue are common. Gynecomastia, an increase in breast tissue, and mastodynia, or breast tenderness, may occur together or independently.

The peripheral conversion of testosterone to estradiol associated with the antiandrogens induces gynecomastia at high rates: 66.3% of men taking 150 mg bicalutamide developed gynecomastia and 72.7% developed mastodynia. Prophylactic RT (10 Gy) has been used to prevent or reduce painful gynecomastia, as a result of DES or antiandrogen therapy. The selective estrogen receptor modulator tamoxifen has been used to treat mastodynia [53].

19.10 Anemia

The anemia associated with ADT is very common: 90% of men receiving maximal androgen blockade experienced declines in hemoglobin concentration of at least 10% [54]. The etiology of anemia is thought to be secondary to lack of testosterone stimulation of erythroid precursors and a decrease in erythropoietin production. In an animal model, however, erythropoietin levels increased after ADT. Whatever the etiology, clinically, patients respond to recombinant human erythropoietin. The anemia is reversible after stopping ADT but may take up to a year.

19.10.1 Degarelix

Injection site reactions including pain, erythema, swelling, pruritus, and induration are the most frequent and important adverse events [55]. There are other rare adverse events which were reported in different studies: urinary tract infection and musculoskeletal and connective tissue adverse events. Other complications, including cardiovascular and cerebrovascular accidents, weight gain and arthralgia, and erectile dysfunction, were reported [55].

19.10.2 Enzalutamide

According to the results of the randomized, phase 3, placebo-controlled trial (AFFIRM) [56], quality of life measured using validated surveys was improved with enzalutamide compared with placebo. Adverse events were mild and included fatigue (34% vs. 29%), diarrhea (21% vs. 18%), hot flushes (20% vs. 10%), headache (12% vs. 6%), and seizures (0.63% vs. 0%). The incidence of cardiovascular diseases did not differ between the groups.

19.10.3 Abiraterone

The most common adverse events with abiraterone acetate/prednisone (>5%) were fatigue (39%); back or joint discomfort (28%–32%); peripheral edema (28%); diarrhea, nausea, or constipation (22%); hypokalemia (17%); hypophosphatemia (24%); atrial fibrillation (4%); muscle discomfort (14%); hot flushes (22%); urinary tract infection; cough; hypertension (22%, severe hypertension in 4%); urinary frequency and nocturia; dyspepsia; or upper respiratory tract infection [57]. The most common adverse drug reactions that resulted in drug discontinuation were increased impaired liver functions (11–12%) or cardiac diseases (19%, serious in 6%). Thus, monitoring of liver function, potassium and phosphate levels, and blood pressure readings on a monthly basis, at least initially is warranted during abiraterone acetate/prednisone therapy. Symptom-directed examination for cardiac disease also is warranted, particularly in patients with cardiovascular disease.

19.11 Summary

ADT is a valuable treatment for advanced prostate cancer in a variety of clinical situations. By being aware of the potential negative impact on quality of life, sexual function, cardio-metabolic health, and bone density and fracture risk, health professionals assisting men in making informed decisions about the role of ADT in their treatment regimen for prostate cancer are able to formulate comprehensive management and surveillance strategies. This is particularly important given the higher cardiovascular risk generally experienced by men in this age group. Although the clinical outcome data examining the effectiveness of managing CVD risk in men treating ADT are limited, extrapolating from the principals of monitoring and managing CVD risk in the general male population, and incorporating and extending these to men receiving ADT treatment, appears warranted. It is appropriate that physicians treating men with advanced prostate cancer take into account these additional potential psychosexual, bone, and cardio-metabolic morbidities and monitor accordingly. This could be done alone or in combination with any of the following—the urological team, the medical or radiation oncologist, and an endocrinologist—in addition to a cardiologist for men at high-risk for or with established CVD, to ensure the optimal quality of care for men with prostate cancer treated with ADT.

References

1. Van Poppel H, Nilsson S. Testosterone surge: rationale for gonadotropin-releasing hormone blockers? Urology. 2008;71(6):1001.
2. Thompson IM. Flare associated with LHRH-agonist therapy. Rev Urol. 2001;3(Suppl 3):S10–4.
3. Tombal B, Berges R. How good do current LHRH agonists control testosterone? Can this be improved with Eligard®? Eur Urol Suppl. 2005;4:30–6.
4. Morote J, Orsola A, Planas J, et al. Redefining clinically significant castration levels in patients with prostate cancer receiving continuous androgen deprivation therapy. J Urol. 2007;178:1290–5.
5. Hotte SJ, Saad F. Current management of castrate-resistant prostate cancer. Curr Oncol. 2010;17(Suppl 2):S72–9.
6. Chi KN, Bjartell A, Dearnaley D, et al. Castration-resistant prostate cancer: from new pathophysiology to new treatment targets. Eur Urol. 2009;56:594–605.
7. Heidenreich A, Bolla M, Joniau S et al.. Guidelines on prostate cancer. 2011. http://www.uroweb.org/gls/pdf/08_Prostate_Cancer.pdf. Accessed 8 Dec 2011.
8. Sharifi N, Dahut WL, Steinberg SM, et al. A retrospective study of the time to clinical endpoints for advanced prostate cancer. BJU Int. 2005;96:985–9.
9. Petrylak D. Therapeutic options in androgen-independent prostate cancer: building on docetaxel. BJU Int. 2005;96(Suppl 2):41–6.
10. Walczak JR, Carducci MA. Prostate cancer: a practical approach to current management of recurrent disease. Mayo Clin Proc. 2007;82:243–9.
11. Mahon KL, Henshall SM, Sutherland RL, et al. Pathways of chemotherapy resistance in castration-resistant prostate cancer. Endocr Relat Cancer. 2011;18:R103–23.
12. Wei JT, Gross M, Jaffe CA, Gravlin K, Lahaie M, Faerber GJ, al w. Androgen deprivation therapy for prostate cancer results in significant loss of bone density. Urology. 1999;54:607–11.
13. Michaelson MD, Cotter SE, Gargollo PC, Zietman AL, Dahl DM, Smith MR. Management of complications of prostate cancer treatment. CA Cancer J Clin. 2008;58:196–213.
14. Moyad MA. Complementary/alternative therapies for reducing hot flashes in prostate cancer patients: reevaluating the existing indirect data from studies of breast cancer and postmenopausal women. Urology. 2002;59:20–33.
15. Rousseau L, Dupont A, Labrie F, Couture M. Sexuality changes in prostate cancer patients receiving antihormonal therapy combining the antiandrogen flutamide with medical (LHRH agonist) or surgical castration. Arch Sex Behav. 1988;17:87–98.
16. Potosky AL, Knopf K, Clegg LX, Albertsen PC, Stanford JL, Hamilton AS, et al. Quality-of-life outcomes after primary androgen deprivation therapy: results from the Prostate Cancer Outcomes Study. J Clin Oncol. 2001;19:3750–7.
17. Alibhai SM, Breunis H, Timilshina N, Marzouk S, Stewart D, Tannock I, Naglie G, Tomlinson G, Fleshner N, Krahn M, et al. Impact of androgen-deprivation therapy on cognitive function in men with nonmetastatic prostate cancer. J Clin Oncol. 2010;28:5030–7.
18. Joly F, Alibhai SM, Galica J, Park A, Yi QL, Wagner L, Tannock IF. Impact of androgen deprivation therapy on physical and cognitive function, as well as quality of life of patients with nonmetastatic prostate cancer. J Urol. 2006;176:2443–7.
19. Nelson CJ, Lee JS, Gamboa MC, Roth AJ. Cognitive effects of hormone therapy in men with prostate cancer: a review. Cancer. 2008;113:1097–106.
20. Smith MR, Finkelstein JS, McGovern FJ, Zietman AL, Fallon MA, Schoenfeld DA, et al. Changes in body composition during androgen deprivation therapy for prostate cancer. J Clin Endocrinol Metab. 2002;87:599–603.
21. Traish AM, Zitzmann M. The complex and multifactorial relationship between testosterone deficiency (TD), obesity and vascular disease. Rev Endocr Metab Disord. 2015;16:249–68.
22. Ullah MI, Washington T, Kazi M, Tamanna S, Koch CA. Testosterone deficiency as a risk factor for cardiovascular disease. Horm Metab Res. 2011;43:153–64.

23. Zamboni M, Mazzali G, Fantin F, Rossi A, Di Francesco V. Sarcopenic obesity: a new category of obesity in the elderly. Nutr Metab Cardiovasc Dis. 2000;18:388–95.
24. Smith JC, Bennett S, Evans LM, et al. The effects of induced hypogonadism on arterial stiffness, body composition, and metabolic parameters in males with prostate cancer. J Clin Endocrinol Metab. 2001;86:4261–7.
25. Dockery F, Bulpitt CJ, Agarwal S, Donaldson M, Rajkumar C. Testosterone suppression in men with prostate cancer leads to an increase in arterial stiffness and hyperinsulinemia. Clin Sci (London). 2003;104:195–201.
26. Keating NL, O'Malley AJ, Smith MR. Diabetes and cardiovascular disease during androgen deprivation therapy for prostate cancer. J Clin Oncol. 2006;24:4448–56.
27. Hotamisligil GS, Spiegelman BM. Tumor necrosis factor α: a key component of the obesity-diabetes link. Diabetes. 1994;43:1271–8.
28. Cutolo M, Sulli A, Capellino S, et al. Sex hormones influence on the immune system: basic and clinical aspects in autoimmunity. Lupus. 2004;13:635–8.
29. Smith RM. Androgen deprivation therapy and risk for diabetes and cardiovascular disease in prostate cancer survivors. Curr Urol Rep. 2008;9:197–202.
30. Alibhai SM, Duong-Hua M, Sutradhar R, et al. Impact of androgen deprivation therapy on cardiovascular disease and diabetes. J Clin Oncol. 2009;27:3452–8.
31. Keating NL, O'Malley J, Stephen J, Smith MR. Diabetes and cardiovascular disease during androgen deprivation therapy: observational study of veterans with prostate cancer. J Natl Cancer Inst. 2010;102:39–46.
32. Tsai HT, Keating NL, Stephen K, et al. Risk of diabetes among patients receiving primary androgen deprivation therapy for clinically localized prostate cancer. J Urol. 2015;193:1956–62.
33. Keating N, Liu P, O'Malley A, Freedland S, Smith M. Androgen-deprivation therapy and diabetes control among diabetic men with prostate cancer. Eur Urol. 2014;65:816–24.
34. Morote J, Gomez-Caamano A, Alvarez-Ossorio J, et al. The metabolic syndrome and its components in patients with prostate cancer on androgen deprivation therapy. J Urol. 2015;193:1963–9.
35. American Diabetes Association. Standards of medical care in diabetes–2008. Diabetes Care. 2008;31(Suppl 1):12–54.
36. American Diabetes Association. Diagnosis and classification of diabetes mellitus. Diabetes Care. 2009;32(Suppl 1):62–7.
37. Berruti A, Dogliotti L, Terrone C, et al. Changes in bone mineral density, lean body mass and fat content as measured by dual energy x-ray absorptiometry in patients with prostate cancer without apparent bone metastases given androgen deprivation therapy. J Urol. 2002;167:2361–7.
38. Keating NL, O'Malley AJ, Freedland SJ, Smith MR. Does comorbidity influence the risk of myocardial infarction or diabetes during androgen-deprivation therapy for prostate cancer? Eur Urol. 2013;64:159–66.
39. Zareba P, Duivenvoorden W, Leong DP, Pinthus JH. Androgen deprivation therapy and cardiovascular disease: what is the linking mechanism? Ther Adv Urol. 2016;8:118–29.
40. Tsai HK, D'Amico AV, Sadetsky N, et al. Androgen deprivation therapy for localized prostate cancer and the risk of cardiovascular mortality. J Natl Cancer Inst. 2007;99:1516–24.
41. Nguyen PL, Je Y, Schutz FA, et al. Association of androgen deprivation therapy with cardiovascular death in patients with prostate cancer: a meta-analysis of randomized trials. JAMA. 2011;306:2359–66.
42. Bolla M, de Reijke TM, Van Tienhoven G, et al. Duration of androgen suppression in the treatment of prostate cancer. N Engl J Med. 2009;360:2516–27.
43. Piccirillo JF, Tierney RM, Costas I, et al. Prognostic importance of comorbidity in a hospital-based cancer registry. JAMA. 2004;291:2441–7.
44. Smith MR, Klotz L, van der Meulen E, et al. Gonadotropin-releasing hormone blockers and cardiovascular disease risk: analysis of prospective clinical trials of degarelix. J Urol. 2011;186:1835–42.
45. Albertsen PC, Klotz L, Tombal B, et al. Cardiovascular morbidity associated with gonadotropin releasing hormone agonists and an antagonist. Eur Urol. 2014;65:565–73.
46. Stamler J, Stamler R, Neaton JD, et al. Low risk-factor profile and long-term cardiovascular and noncardiovascular mortality and life expectancy: findings for 5 large cohorts of young adult and middle-aged men and women. JAMA. 1999;282:2012–8.
47. Lim TH, Orija IB, Pearlman BL. American College of Cardiology; American College of Cardiology. The new cholesterol treatment guidelines from the American College of Cardiology/American Heart Association, 2013: what clinicians need to know. Postgrad Med. 2014;126:35–44.
48. Wall BA. Androgen deprivation therapy and cardiovascular disease risk—The role of exercise in prostate cancer treatment. Front Oncol. 2016;6:200.
49. Galvão DA, Taaffe DR, Spry N. Combined resistance and aerobic exercise program reverses muscle loss in men undergoing androgen suppression therapy for prostate cancer without bone metastases: a randomized controlled trial. J Clin Oncol. 2010;28:340–7.
50. Taaffe DR, Newton RU, Spry N. Effects of different exercise modalities on fatigue in prostate cancer patients undergoing androgen deprivation therapy: A year-long randomised controlled trial. Eur Urol. 2017;72(2):293–9.
51. Gaskin CJ, Fraser SF, Owen PJ, Craike M, Orellana L, Livingston PM. Fitness outcomes from a randomised controlled trial of exercise training for men with prostate cancer: the ENGAGE study. J Cancer Surviv. 2016;10:972–80.

52. Teleni L, Chan RJ, Chan A. Exercise improves quality of life in androgen deprivation therapy-treated prostate cancer: systematic review of randomised controlled trials. Endocr Relat Cancer. 2016;23:101–12.
53. Serels S, Melman A. Tamoxifen as treatment for gynecomastia and mastodynia resulting from hormonal deprivation. J Urol. 1998;159:1309.
54. Strum SB, McDermed JE, Scholz MC, Johnson H, Tisman G. Anaemia associated with androgen deprivation in patients with prostate cancer receiving combined hormone blockade. Br J Urol. 1997;79:933–41.
55. Hosseini SA, Rajabi F, Akbari Sari A, Ayati M, Heidari S, Ghamary F. Degarelix for the treatment of advanced prostate cancer compared with GnRh-Agonists: a systematic review and meta-analysis. Med J Islam Repub Iran. 2016;30:317. eCollection 2016.
56. Scher HI, Fizazi K, Saad F, et al. Increased survival with enzalutamide in prostate cancer after chemotherapy. N Engl J Med. 2012;367:1187–97.
57. Ryan CJ, Smith MR, de Bono JS, et al. Abiraterone in metastatic prostate cancer without previous chemotherapy. N Engl J Med. 2013;368:138–48.

Part IV

Systemic Chemotherapy, Immunotherapy and Palliative Care for Advanced Prostate Cancer

Byung Ha Chung

Systemic Chemotherapy for Metastatic Hormone-Sensitive Prostate Cancer

20

Kyong Tae Moon and Tag Keun Yoo

20.1 Introduction

Traditionally, long-term androgen deprivation therapy (ADT) has been considered as the standard of care (SOC) for men with metastatic hormone-sensitive prostate cancer. But, unfortunately several months after the ADT, tumors become castration-resistant, and eventually all patients suffer from disease progression. In 2004, two randomized phase 3 trials demonstrated for the first time a survival benefit in patients with metastatic castration-resistant prostate cancer (mCRPC) utilizing docetaxel-based chemotherapy, setting a new standard of care for patients with mCRPC [1, 2]. The benefit of docetaxel-based chemotherapy in patients with mCRPC suggested that early chemotherapy might improve the prognosis of patients with metastatic hormone-sensitive prostate cancer (mHSPC). In bringing docetaxel into the hormone-sensitive setting, the rationale was to preemptively eradicate cancer cells inherently insensitive to ADT by acting on cellular targets outside of the androgen-signaling pathway, thus improving clinical outcomes. Recently, final results of three large, randomized, phase 3 trials (GETUG-AFU 15, CHAARTED, and STAMPEDE) evaluating the value of up-front docetaxel chemotherapy in mHSPC were reported.

20.2 GETUG-AFU 15 and CHAARTED Studies

The GETUG-AFU 15 and CHAARTED studies are summarized in Table 20.1. The GETUG-AFU 15 study randomized 385 men with mHSPC to receive hormone therapy plus docetaxel (75 mg/m^2 every 3 weeks, up to 9 cycles) or hormone therapy alone [3, 4]. After a median follow-up of 83.9 months, even though the biochemical progression-free survival and radiographic progression-free survival were significantly longer for patients randomized in the hormone therapy plus docetaxel group, the median overall survival was not significantly different between the two groups: 62.1 months (95% CI, 49.5–73.7) in the hormone therapy plus docetaxel group and 48.6 months (95% CI, 40.9–60.6) in the hormone therapy-alone group (HR, 0.88 [95% CI, 0.68–1.14]; $P = 0.3$). After CHAARTED study was published, GETUG-AFU 15 study performed post hoc analysis and updated survival analyses of all study cohorts. GETUG-AFU 15 study divided all patients into high-volume disease (HVD) and low-volume disease (LVD) on metastatic volume according to CHAARTED definition (discussed below). The post hoc analyses

K. T. Moon · T. K. Yoo (✉)
Department of Urology, Nowon Eulji Medical Center, Eulji University, Seoul, Korea
e-mail: ohmoon777@eulji.ac.kr; ytk5202@eulji.ac.kr

C. S. Kim (ed.), *Management of Advanced Prostate Cancer*,
https://doi.org/10.1007/978-981-10-6943-7_20

Table 20.1 Outcomes of GETUG-AFU 15 and CHAARTED studies

Study (ref.)	GETUG-AFU 15 [3, 4]			CHAARTED [5]		
Median follow-up (months)	83.9			28.9		
	All patients $n = 385$	HVD $n = 183$ (47.5%)	LVD $n = 202$ (52.5%)	All patients $n = 790$	HVD $n = 513$ (64.9%)	LVD $n = 277$ (35.1%)
Primary endpoint	*Overall survival (months)*					
ADT	48.6	35.1	83.4	44.0	32.2	NR
ADT+Doc	62.1	39.8	NR	57.6	49.2	NR
HR	0.88	0.78	1.02	0.61	0.6	0.6
p value	0.3	0.14	0.9	<0.001	<0.001	0.11
Secondary endpoint	*Biochemical PFS (months)*			*Time to clinical progression (months)*		
ADT	12.9	9.2	22.4	19.8		
ADT + Doc	22.9	15.2	40.9	33.0		
HR	0.7	0.6	0.7	0.61		
p value	0.0021	0.0039	0.0533	<0.001		

ADT androgen deprivation therapy, *Doc* docetaxel chemotherapy, *HR* hazard ratio, *HVD* high-volume disease, *LVD* low-volume disease, *NR* not reached, *PFS* progression-free survival

demonstrated a nonsignificant 20% reduction in the risk of death in the HVD subgroup, but, patients with LVD had no survival improvement with early docetaxel chemotherapy. No severe adverse events were reported in the ADT-alone group, but four treatment-related deaths occurred during the course of chemotherapy in the ADT plus docetaxel arm including two neutropenia-related deaths. If summarized, while the addition of docetaxel was associated with an improvement in biochemical and radiological progression-free survival, there was no significant improvement in overall survival with the addition of docetaxel, even with long-term follow-up.

The CHAARTED trial randomized 790 men with mHSPC to combination therapy (ADT plus docetaxel, 75 mg/m^2 every 3 weeks × 6 cycles) or ADT alone [5]. Patients were divided according to the extent of metastases (high volume [defined as the presence of visceral metastases or ≥4 bone lesions with ≥1 beyond the vertebral bodies and pelvis] vs. low volume). After a median follow-up of 28.9 months, the median overall survival was 13.6 months longer with combination therapy than with ADT alone (57.6 months vs. 44.0 months; HR, 0.61 [95% CI, 0.47–0.80]; $P < 0.001$). The proportion of patients who had a decrease in the PSA level to less than 0.2 ng/mL at 12 months was 27.7% in the combination group, as compared with 16.8% in the ADT-alone group ($P < 0.001$). The median time to the development of castration-resistant prostate cancer (biochemical, symptomatic, or radiographic) was 20.2 months with combination therapy, as compared with 11.7 months with ADT alone (HR, 0.61 [95% CI, 0.51–0.72]; $P < 0.001$). The benefit of combination therapy was more apparent in the subgroup with high-volume disease than in the overall study population, with a median overall survival that was 17.0 months longer in the combination group than in the ADT-alone group (49.2 months vs. 32.2 months; HR, 0.60 [95% CI, 0.45–0.81]; $P < 0.001$). In the low-volume disease, the median survival at the time of the analysis had not been reached in either study group, and the overall survival was not significantly different between two arms. When it comes to the toxicity, among the patients who received combination therapy, approximately 2% had a treatment-related grade 3 or 4 allergic reaction, and approximately 1% of the patients had a thromboembolic event. Approximately 6% of the patients in the combination group had neutropenic fever, and approximately 2% had grade 3 or 4 infection with neutropenia.

The population of patients included in the CHAARTED and GETUG-AFU-15 studies has some key differences including median follow-up periods, total patient number, and proportion of patients with high- versus low-risk disease.

The CHAARTED study was initially conceived as a trial for high-volume metastatic disease, defined as the presence of visceral metastases or ≥4 bone lesions with ≥1 beyond the vertebral bodies and pelvis. The protocol was later amended to allow enrollment of low-volume disease, as well as the end result being that the CHAARTED study cohort was enriched with high-volume patients (64.9%). On the other hand, only 22% of men in GETUG-AFU 15 were high-risk by the Glass criteria, but how this compares or correlates with the CHAARTED volume/risk criteria is unclear. To facilitate cross-comparison, GETUG-AFU 15 later retrospectively recategorized its patients to CHAARTED criteria, finding 47.5% to have high-volume disease. The large difference in median OS of the two control cohorts provides insight into the risk disparities that exist between the two study populations (54.2 vs. 44.0 months in GETUG-AFU 15 and CHAARTED, respectively). Enrichment of patients with high-volume disease in CHAARTED likely plays a large role in this discrepancy. Additionally, CHAARTED included a slightly higher proportion of patients with Gleason score 8–10 (60.8% vs. 56.1%). Consideration also should be paid to the availability of other therapeutic agents with proven survival benefits (i.e., cabazitaxel, abiraterone, and enzalutamide), as differences in posttrial treatment patterns are often a confounding variable. GETUG 15 had a much higher percentage of men who received salvage docetaxel therapy as compared with CHAARTED (45.2% vs. 22.5%), likely because no other drugs were approved for mCRPC until years after accrual closed for GETUG-AFU 15, whereas the availability of newer second-line agents overlapped considerably with the enrollment period for CHAARTED [6].

20.3 STAMPEDE Study

STAMPEDE (Systemic Therapy in Advancing or Metastatic Prostate Cancer: Evaluation of Drug Efficacy; NCT00268476), the largest of the three trials, is a randomized controlled trial using a multiarm, multistage platform design [7]. It accrued 2962 men with either high-risk localized (24%), node-positive (15%), or mHSPC (61%) to 4 separate treatment arms. Median age was 65 years (IQR 60–71). 165 (6%) men were previously treated with local therapy, and median prostate-specific antigen was 65 ng/mL (IQR 23–184). All patients were intended for long-term hormone therapy, started no longer than 12 weeks before randomization. Patients were randomly distributed 2:1:1:1 ratio to hormone therapy only, hormone therapy plus zoledronic acid, hormone therapy plus docetaxel, or hormone therapy with both zoledronic acid and docetaxel. Patients treated with zoledronic acid were given 4 mg of zoledronic acid at every 3 weeks for 6 times and then every 4 weeks until 2 years Patients treated with docetaxel were given 75 mg/m^2 of docetaxel at every 3 weeks and 10 mg prednisolone everyday. The definitive and intermediate primary outcome measures were overall survival and failure-free survival, respectively. Overall survival was defined as time from randomization to death from any cause. Failure-free survival was defined as time from randomization to first evidence of at least one of biochemical failure, progression either locally in lymph nodes or in distant metastases, or death from prostate cancer. Biochemical failure was defined as a rise of 50% above the within-24-week nadir and above 4 ng/mL and confirmed by retest or treatment. Median time to starting docetaxel was about 2 weeks after randomization and 9 weeks after starting hormone therapy. Of patients allocated to receive docetaxel as part of trial treatment, 456 (77%) patients assigned to hormone therapy plus docetaxel and 422 (71%) to hormone therapy with both zoledronic acid and docetaxel received the full six cycles. Most common reason for stopping docetaxel treatment was toxic effect and few patients were stopping docetaxel treatment for disease progression. Median follow-up was 43 months (IQR 30–60). Median overall survival was 71 months (IQR 32 to not reached) for hormone therapy only, not reached (32 to not reached) for hormone therapy plus zoledronic acid (HR, 0.94; 95% CI 0.79–1.11; $P = 0.450$), 81 months (41 to not reached) for hormone therapy plus docetaxel (HR, 0.78, 0.66–0.93; $P = 0.006$), and 76 months (39 to not reached) for hormone therapy with both zoledronic acid and docetaxel (HR, 0.82, 0.69–0.97; $P = 0.022$). There was also an improvement in failure-free survival both for hormone therapy plus docetaxel and for hormone therapy with both zoledronic acid and docetaxel.

In the hormone therapy-only group, median failure-free survival was 20 months and 5-year failure-free survival was 28%. On the other hand, in patients on for hormone therapy plus docetaxel, median failure-free survival was 37 months, and 5-year failure-free survival was 38%. And in patients on hormone therapy with both zoledronic acid and docetaxel, median failure-free survival was 36 months and 5-year failure-free survival was 34%. If summarized, docetaxel chemotherapy, given at the time of long-term hormone therapy initiation, improved survival, but zoledronic acid showed no evidence of survival benefit. The patients with docetaxel plus hormone therapy led to a survival advantage of 10 months, compared to the hormone therapy-only group (81 vs. 71 months; HR, 0.78; 95% CI 0.66–0.93; $P = 0.006$). In a subset analysis of 1817 patients with metastatic disease, an overall survival benefit of 15 months was observed for the docetaxel plus hormone therapy versus the hormone therapy-only group (60 vs. 45 months; HR, 0.76; 95% CI 0.62–0.92; $P = 0.005$).

The proportion of patients reporting worst adverse event ever as grade 3 or higher was highest with hormone therapy plus docetaxel (288 patients [52%]) and hormone therapy with both zoledronic acid and docetaxel (269 [52%]). This was mostly due to events during the first 6 months on trial, when the proportions were 17% ($n = 203$) for hormone therapy only group, 15% ($n = 91$) for hormone therapy plus zoledronic acid, 36% ($n = 198$) for hormone therapy plus docetaxel, and 39% ($n = 202$) for hormone therapy with both zoledronic acid and docetaxel, with docetaxel seeming to contribute the most toxicity. For 1998 patients with adverse event data around 1 year after randomization, the proportions of grade 3 or higher toxic effects were balanced, with 10% ($n = 76$) patients reporting a worst adverse event as grade 3 or higher with hormone therapy only, 10% ($n = 41$) with hormone therapy plus zoledronic acid, 10% with ($n = 43$) hormone therapy plus docetaxel, and 12% ($n = 49$) with hormone therapy with both zoledronic acid and docetaxel. The pattern and levels of adverse events were similar in the safety and intention-to-treat populations. There were eight deaths probably or possibly related to the research treatment: one on hormone therapy plus docetaxel (neutropenic sepsis) and seven on hormone therapy with both zoledronic acid and docetaxel (four neutropenic sepsis, one pneumocystic pneumonia, one interstitial pneumonitis, and one pneumonia).

20.4 Survival Benefit in High-Volume Disease

It is important to note that in which patients docetaxel chemotherapy is particularly effective. Which patients precisely benefit from six cycles of docetaxel? The most prominent of the clinical features is the tumor volume of the metastatic site. The CHAARTED study defined "high-volume disease" as the presence of visceral metastases or ≥4 bone lesions with ≥1 beyond the vertebral bodies and pelvis, and they did prospective stratification of high-volume versus low-volume disease. In both ADT-alone and ADT plus docetaxel group, approximately 65% had high-volume disease, and approximately 60% had a Gleason score of 8 or higher. CHAARTED subgroup analysis showed an unprecedented 17-month OS improvement with the addition of docetaxel in men with high-volume mHSPC (49.2 vs. 32.2 months; HR, 0.60; 95% CI, 0.45–0.81; $P < 0.001$). The benefit at the last analysis was more apparent in the subgroup with high-volume disease than in the overall CHAARTED study population. The GETUG-AFU 15 study first reported that the addition of docetaxel chemotherapy to ADT in patients with mHSPC did not improve the overall survival after a median follow-up of 49.9 months. After CHAARTED study was published, GETUG-AFU 15 study reported extended follow-up and retrospectively retrieved data on metastatic volume from medical files of all patients, applying the CHAARTED definition of high-volume and low-volume disease and updated survival analysis. After post hoc analysis, 47.5% patients of CHAARTED had high-volume disease, and the high-volume GETUG-AFU 15 cohort still did not show improvement in OS (39.0 vs. 35.1 months; HR, 0.8; 95% CI, 0.6–1.2; $P = 0.35$). The STAMPEDE trial, on the other hand, did not stratify for volume of metastatic disease and demonstrated clinical benefit for the entire patient population.

20.5 Availability in Low-Volume Disease

Both (GETUG-AFU 15 and CHAARTED) trials failed to show an OS advantage with docetaxel in low-volume subgroup, GETUG-AFU 15 study reported median OS was not reached in the ADT plus D arm and 83.4 months (95% CI, 61.8–NR) in the ADT arm (HR, 1.02 [95% CI, 0.67–1.55]; $P = 0.9$), and CHAARTED study reported the median survival at the time of the analysis had not been reached in either study group (HR with ADT + docetaxel, 0.60 [95% CI, 0.32–1.13]; $P = 0.11$). For men with low-volume disease, the number of events was too small at the time of reporting, and therefore longer follow-up is awaited. Until then, there is insufficient evidence to strongly recommend the routine use of early docetaxel therapy for low-volume mHSPC. However, this does not mean that we should not use docetaxel in low-volume disease at all. In the STAMPEDE trial, patients with non-metastatic disease did not experience a survival benefit, but they had a significant improvement in failure-free survival. The use of docetaxel in patients with high-risk cancer which is now a low-volume disease but will eventually progress to high-volume disease in the not-too-distant future will theoretically be of benefit to patients. Even though current data in this space is still in a state of immaturity, the use of chemotherapy in low-volume disease with features associated with poor prognosis or consistent with rapidly progressing disease can be justified. So, those patients with Gleason 8 or higher disease, poor PSA response to primary ADT, rapid PSA doubling time, disproportionately high or low PSA levels, bulky lymph node disease, and symptomatic disease can be seriously considered as candidates for up-front chemotherapy. Additionally, men with good performance status, who are young or have little to no medical comorbidities, should also be considered in order to maximally prolong time to disease progression and OS. At the same time, the potential toxicities of docetaxel treatment should be clearly discussed with patients.

20.6 Toxicity of Docetaxel Chemotherapy in mHSPC

Toxicity of docetaxel is a key consideration when using up-front chemotherapy for mHSPC. All of the three RCTs (GETUG-AFU 15, CHAARTED, and STEMPEDE) reported higher rates of febrile neutropenia (6–12%) than what historically has been seen with docetaxel therapy in CRPC (3%), as reported in TAX 327. In the STAMPEDE study, grade 3 or higher toxicities were enhanced by 20% in the docetaxel plus hormone therapy group, compared to the hormone therapy-only group (52% vs. 32%). Toxicity was the most common reason for premature discontinuation of the study before all docetaxel cycles were complete. Therefore, it is very important to administer docetaxel treatment only to properly selected and essential patients or prevent of neutropenia and neutropenic fever. During the GETUG-AFU 15 trial, four treatment-related deaths occurred in the ADP plus docetaxel group (two of which were neutropenia-related), after which the data monitoring committee recommended addition of prophylactic granulocyte colony-stimulating factor (5 μg/kg/day subcutaneously once a day) from day 5 to day 10 after each docetaxel treatment. After this amendment, the number of patients with grade 3–4 neutropenia fell from 51 (41%) of 123 to ten (15%) of 66 patients, and the number with grade 3–4 febrile neutropenia decreased from ten (8%) of 123 to four (6%) of 66. After this recommendation, no further treatment-related deaths occurred. Although many taxane-associated toxicities are transient and not life-threatening, febrile neutropenia is a relatively uncommon but potentially serious adverse event [8]. The American Society of Clinical Oncology (ASCO) recommends that primary prophylaxis with a CSF starts in the first cycle and continues through subsequent cycles of chemotherapy in patients who have an approximately 20% or higher risk for febrile neutropenia on the basis of patient, disease, and treatment-related factors. And secondary prophylaxis with CSFs is recommended for patients who experienced a neutropenic complication from a previous cycle of chemotherapy (for which primary prophylaxis was not received) [9].

20.7 Further Direction

It is unlikely that there will exist only one, unified, optimal approach to managing mHSPC. TAX 327 demonstrated a modest overall survival benefit of about 3 months with docetaxel chemotherapy in patients with mCRPC. However the overall survival benefits with docetaxel chemotherapy in hormone-sensitive setting of prostate cancer were 13.6 months in CHAARTED and 10 months in STAMPEDE. These show evidence that there are molecular alterations during hormone therapy that negatively affect the efficacy of docetaxel and presumably of other active drugs. This may give more validity to early docetaxel use in mHSPC. Indeed, numerous events altering signaling, gene expression, and cellular outcome were identified during hormone therapy [10]. In terms of finding proper patients group that can have benefits of maximal effectiveness and minimal side effects, further development of predictive biomarkers, such as molecular signatures derived from whole blood or circulating tumors cells should be continued.

20.8 Summary

It is unlikely that there will exist only one, unified, optimal approach to managing mHSPC. The GETUG-AFU 15 study concluded that there was no improvement in overall survival with the addition of docetaxel in mHSPC patients. However, the overall survival benefits with docetaxel chemotherapy in addition to standard ADT for patients with HSPC were found in CHAARTED and STAMPEDE studies. All of the three RCTs reported that docetaxel chemotherapy in HSPC setting had higher rates of febrile neutropenia than docetaxel therapy in CRPC setting. However, in the GETUG-AFU 15 study, the rates of neutropenia and febrile neutropenia were markedly decreased after addition of prophylactic granulocyte colony-stimulating factor. The overall survival benefits in two large studies suggest that early chemotherapy in hormone-sensitive setting of prostate cancer is effective and consistent. The data up to now show a definite usefulness of docetaxel in high-volume mHSPC disease, but it is expected that the indication will be extended to low-volume disease with high-risk features in the future. In addition to volume factor, other various molecular and clinical parameters should be supplemented. At the same time, maximal efforts to reduce toxicities and properly treat them should be made.

References

1. Tannock IF, de Wit R, Berry WR, Horti J, Pluzanska A, Chi KN, et al. Docetaxel plus prednisone or mitoxantrone plus prednisone for advanced prostate cancer. N Engl J Med. 2004;351(15):1502–12.
2. Petrylak DP, Tangen CM, Hussain MH, Lara PN Jr, Jones JA, Taplin ME, et al. Docetaxel and estramustine compared with mitoxantrone and prednisone for advanced refractory prostate cancer. N Engl J Med. 2004;351(15):1513–20.
3. Gravis G, Fizazi K, Joly F, Oudard S, Priou F, Esterni B, et al. Androgen-deprivation therapy alone or with docetaxel in non-castrate metastatic prostate cancer

(GETUG-AFU 15): a randomised, open-label, phase 3 trial. Lancet Oncol. 2013;14(2):149–58.
4. Gravis G, Boher JM, Joly F, Soulie M, Albiges L, Priou F, et al. Androgen deprivation therapy (ADT) plus docetaxel versus ADT alone in metastatic non castrate prostate cancer: impact of metastatic burden and long-term survival analysis of the randomized phase 3 GETUG-AFU15 trial. Eur Urol. 2016;70(2):256–62.
5. Sweeney CJ, Chen YH, Carducci M, Liu G, Jarrard DF, Eisenberger M, et al. Chemohormonal therapy in metastatic hormone-sensitive prostate cancer. N Engl J Med. 2015;373(8):737–46.
6. Liaw BC, Oh WK. Is docetaxel chemotherapy a new standard of care for metastatic hormone-sensitive prostate cancer? Am J Hematol/Oncol. 2015;11(9)
7. James ND, Sydes MR, Clarke NW, Mason MD, Dearnaley DP, Spears MR, et al. Addition of docetaxel, zoledronic acid, or both to first-line long-term hormone therapy in prostate cancer (STAMPEDE): survival results from an adaptive, multiarm, multistage, platform randomised controlled trial. Lancet. 2016;387(10024):1163–77.
8. Tsao CK, Galsky MD, Oh WK. Docetaxel for metastatic hormone-sensitive prostate cancer: urgent need to minimize the risk of neutropenic fever. Eur Urol. 2016;70(5):707–8.
9. Smith TJ, Bohlke K, Lyman GH, Carson KR, Crawford J, Cross SJ, et al. Recommendations for the use of WBC growth factors: American Society of clinical oncology clinical practice guideline update. J Clin Oncol Off J Am Soc Clin Oncol. 2015;33(28):3199–212.
10. Katzenwadel A, Wolf P. Androgen deprivation of prostate cancer: leading to a therapeutic dead end. Cancer Lett. 2015;367(1):12–7.

Systemic Chemotherapy in Metastatic Castration-Resistant Prostate Cancer

21

Dong Hoon Lee and Sung-Woo Park

21.1 Introduction

Most chemotherapeutic agents available for prostate cancer have been used by single agents or various combinations. Historically, cyclophosphamide, 5-fluorouracil, estramustine, cisplatin, carboplatin, doxorubicin, mitoxantrone, paclitaxel, and docetaxel have been used [1]. With the exception of docetaxel (and the related agent, cabazitaxel) and mitoxantrone, the other agents for cytotoxic chemotherapy are not being used anymore because these agents have not been proved with either symptomatic improvements or survival benefit. Clinical trials using chemotherapy regimens used since 2000 have shown that the survival benefit of metastatic castration-resistant prostate cancer (mCRPC) patients is between 16 and 20 months when used as a first-line chemotherapy [2, 3], but less than 6–12 months when using historical chemotherapy regimens before 2000s [1].

Cytotoxic chemotherapy using alkylating agent in prostate cancer patients started in the 1950s [1]. However, the rate of response to cytotoxic chemotherapy was low and no significant effect was achieved, suggesting that prostate cancer was a chemotherapy-resistant disease [1]. In 1996, mitoxantrone and prednisone for cytotoxic chemotherapy were first approved by the US FDA for mCRPC [4]. However, mitoxantrone was not effective in improving the survival rate and only palliation was effective [4]. Since 2004, a randomized control study using docetaxel by Tannok et al. [3] has been published and is recognized as a standard treatment for mCRPC. Currently, it has been developed to cabazitaxel and is recognized as a cytotoxic chemotherapy regimen following docetaxel.

D. H. Lee · S.-W. Park (✉)
Department of Urology, Pusan National University Yangsan Hospital,
Yangsan, Gyeongsangnam-do, South Korea
e-mail: psw@pusan.ac.kr

21.1.1 Mitoxantrone

Mitoxantrone was the first chemotherapy of mCRPC patients. This agent is a semisynthetic anthracycline, and it had previously shown modest symptomatic improvement for mCRPC patients but with minimal effect on the antitumor activity including overall survival. Furthermore, mitoxantrone had the maximal palliative effect with additional low-dose corticosteroids [4]. Based on the clinical data with its modest toxicity profile, mitoxantrone (12 mg/m^2 every 3 weeks) plus prednisone (5 mg daily) was investigated against prednisone alone in a phase III randomized clinical trial using the 161 patients with symptomatic mCRPC [4]. When the investigators evaluated the palliative response as the primary outcome of this study, they defined a 2-point decrease of pain evaluated on a

C. S. Kim (ed.), *Management of Advanced Prostate Cancer*,
https://doi.org/10.1007/978-981-10-6943-7_21

6-point pain scale without an increase in analgesic use. The palliative response rate was significantly higher among patients receiving mitoxantrone than those receiving prednisone alone (29% vs. 12%; $p < 0.001$). However, overall survival was not statistically improved between the two groups. Although mitoxantrone was well tolerated generally among patients receiving mitoxantrone, the most relevant toxicities included neutropenia and cardiotoxicity [4]. Two phase III randomized clinical trials (CALGB 9182 and the US Oncology trials) tried to demonstrate a survival benefit to giving mitoxantrone plus a steroid in comparison with a steroid alone. However, both studies failed to describe a statistically significant benefit of overall survival. They confirmed a benefit for these agents including prostate-specific antigen response rates, time to progression, and improvements in overall pain scores [5, 6]. According to these two studies, mitoxantrone plus prednisone was used as the standard of care in this disease in the pre-docetaxel era.

21.1.2 Docetaxel

Despite the relief of pain and prostate-specific antigen responses, mitoxantrone plus steroid failed to show the improvement of overall survival for mCRPC patients compared with steroid alone. The next significant advance in the chemotherapy for these patients came with docetaxel. This agent is a member of the taxane family and acts by stabilizing microtubules, the intracellular filaments that are part of the cell's cytoskeleton. Microtubules are involved in cell shape, vesicle transport, transcription factor trafficking, mitochondrial functioning, and cell signaling, as well as their best-known role in chromosome separation during cell division and mitosis. The binding of taxane molecules to microtubules prevents their disassembly, which leads to cell cycle arrest in metaphase–anaphase [7]. With cell cycle progression blocked, cells eventually die by apoptosis. Taxanes most likely promote apoptosis by inhibiting the anti-apoptotic function of the B-cell CLL/lymphoma 2 (BCL2) family and upregulating cyclin-dependent kinase inhibitor 1A (p21, Cip1) and tumor protein p53, which arrest the cell cycle. Recently, however, it has been proposed that the clinical efficacy of taxanes may actually be due to their inhibition of essential interphase cellular mechanisms involving microtubules rather than their effect on mitosis [8].

Early data with docetaxel chemotherapy demonstrated prostate-specific antigen responses in a significant proportion of patients studied [9]. Based on this result, the TAX-327 trial investigated docetaxel plus prednisone in mCPRC. The TAX-327 randomized 1006 men to 1 of 3 treatment arms: docetaxel 75 mg/m^2 given every 3 weeks; docetaxel 30 mg/m^2 given weekly for 5 of every 6 weeks; and mitoxantrone 12 mg/m^2 given every 3 weeks. Prednisone 5 mg was given orally twice daily to all patients of groups. The study designed to prove that docetaxel had survival benefit in comparison with mitoxantrone but was not sought to compare the 3 week versus weekly schedules. Patients in docetaxel group (given every 3 weeks) showed a 24% reduction in the risk of death compared with mitoxantrone group (HR 0.76; 95% CI 0.62–0.94; $p = 0.009$), and the median overall survival between the two groups was 18.9 and 16.5 months. Patients treated with docetaxel also had significant improvements in prostate-specific antigen response, pain response rates, and improvements in quality of life. However, there was no significant difference in overall survival among the weekly docetaxel group compared with mitoxantrone group. Docetaxel with prednisone was generally well tolerated, but patients group which received docetaxel in the every 3 week experienced more grade 3 and 4 toxicity including neutropenia, fatigue, alopecia, and gastrointestinal problem. The cardiac toxicity was more frequently observed in patients treated with mitoxantrone [3].

Another phase III clinical trial (the Southwest Oncology Group: SWOG-9916) demonstrated the survival benefit in comparison with docetaxel every 3 weeks (60 mg/m^2 which was escalated to 70 mg/m^2 if there was no severe toxicity during cycle 1) plus estramustine (280 mg three times daily on days 1 through 5 every 3 weeks) and mitoxantrone every 3 weeks plus prednisone. Patients with docetaxel did experience a 20% decrease in risk of death (HR 0.80; 95% CI 0.67–0.97; $p = 0.02$) with a median survival of 17.5 months vs. 15.6 months in comparison with mitoxantrone group. Patients receiving docetaxel plus estramustine had more grade 3 and 4 febrile neutropenia, nausea, and clinically significant cardiovascular events than mitoxantrone group [1]. However, estramustine had thromboembolic toxicities, so it is no longer generally used and remained as only a historic regimen currently.

So, with the result of these clinical trials, docetaxel plus prednisone was approved by the US FDA for use in patients with mCRPC based on the survival benefit. It is considered a category 1 recommendation for the first-line treatment of patients with symptomatic CRPC by the National Comprehensive Cancer Network (NCCN). Recent data suggest that docetaxel 50 mg/m^2 given every 2 weeks is effective and better tolerated than 3-week scheduled regimen [10].

Several experimental agents have been evaluated in combination with docetaxel to improve the efficacy over the single-agent docetaxel. However, most phase III trials of docetaxel-based combination therapy did not show the significant results. Some antiangiogenic agents (bevacizumab, aflibercept, and lenalidomide) combined with docetaxel have not improved overall survival even though serum vascular endothelial growth factor levels correlate inversely with survival. Also, combinations of bone-targeted agents including atrasentan, zibotentan, and dasatinib have produced similar results. High-dose vitamin D (calcitriol) with weekly docetaxel also showed no survival advantage over docetaxel alone. Investigators thought that potential reasons for the failure of combination therapies with docetaxel include marginal activity of the combined agents with docetaxel had lack of well-conducted randomized phase II trials before phase III studies, as well as dose reductions of docetaxel that were often required as a result of additional drug toxicities [11].

21.1.3 Cabazitaxel

Despite the significant effect of docetaxel in mCRPC, response rates are modest, and all the patients finally will experience disease progression. However, there were no other chemotherapy agent which was approved by the US FDA for these patients. And then, cabazitaxel changed it in 2010 for the treatment of mCRPC patients who showed progression after docetaxel based on the results of a phase III (TROPIC) trial [12]. Cabazitaxel is a novel taxane that binds to the same microtubule-binding site as docetaxel and was investigated in several clinical trials using the activity of docetaxel- and paclitaxel-resistant PC cell lines. In studies using cancer cell lines and mouse models, cabazitaxel was demonstrated to be effective in both docetaxel-sensitive tumors as well as in those with docetaxel resistance [13]. The TROPIC trial was an international, multicenter, phase III clinical trial of 755 men with mCRPC who had progressed after docetaxel. They were randomized to receive mitoxantrone plus prednisone (12 mg/m^2 every 3 weeks) or cabazitaxel plus prednisone (25 mg/m^2 every 3 weeks). Cabazitaxel group showed a 30% decrease in risk of death (HR 0.70; 95% CI 0.59–0.83; $p < 0.0001$), with a median survival of 15.1 months vs. 12.7 months in comparison with mitoxantrone group. Progression-free survival, prostate-specific antigen responses, and radiographic responses also were significantly higher in cabazitaxel group. Using the results of this study, it formed the basis for the US FDA's approval of cabazitaxel plus prednisone in 2010 as the second-line agent for docetaxel-refractory mCRPC patients.

According to TROPIC trial, which enrolled patients previously treated with docetaxel and had no significant residual neuropathy, cabazitaxel also did not lead to clinically significant peripheral neuropathy. However, cabazitaxel plus prednisone was associated with significant toxicity in this late-stage setting, about a 5% treatment-related mortality rate, primarily attributed to neutropenia and/or diarrhea. So, experts recommend prophylaxis with white blood cell colony-stimulating factors for the patients older than 65 years, with extensive prior radiation therapy, serious comorbidities, or poor performance status even though not meeting criteria for primary prophylaxis by some organizations [14]. The most common serious adverse events related to cabazitaxel were hematologic toxicity of grade 3 or 4 neutropenia in 82% of patients including febrile neutropenia in 8%. Older patients over 65 years reported a 6.6% higher rate of grade 3 neutropenia than younger. This incidence of hematologic suppression brought the trials of whether a lower dose of cabazitaxel may have been more appropriate; a phase III randomized trial (PROSELICA) comparing the safety and efficacy between two doses (25 mg/m^2 vs. 20 mg/m^2 every 3 weeks) is now being investigated. Other reported non-hematologic toxicities were greater than or equal to grade 3 diarrhea (6%) and fatigue (5%). Diarrhea was more common in old-aged patients and also in those with a previous radiation therapy history. In case of neuropathy, peripheral neuropathy (all grades) was observed in 14% of patients, and only 1% of men developed grade 3 neuropathy [12]. Although the patients receiving cabazitaxel had these toxicities, this novel agent demonstrated an overall survival benefit and is recommended as a category 1 cytotoxic agent by the NCCN for symptomatic mCRPC patients who have progressed after docetaxel chemotherapy [15]. Additionally, a randomized phase III trial (FIRSTANA) to compare docetaxel and cabazitaxel (20 mg or 25 mg/m^2) in chemotherapy naive mCRPC patients has been completed, and we wait the result of this trial. Also, a phase II study (TAXYNERGY) is randomizing patients to compare docetaxel versus cabazitaxel as first-line treatment. This trial is designed to allow the switching to the alternative taxane agent if the enrolled patients do not show more than a 30% prostate-specific antigen decline within the first four cycles of chemotherapy. This trial is also collecting circulating tumor cells to find the association between the androgen receptor and microtubules, and it will be helpful to investigate the mechanisms of response and resistance of taxane drugs in mCRPC patients.

21.1.4 Other Trials of Novel Agents

The continued evaluation of novel chemotherapy agents is warranted because of the significant effects of cabazitaxel following docetaxel and the potential overlapping cross-resistance between docetaxel and androgen-targeting agents. According to this effort, several agents of different classes have introduced with some promising results in several clinical studies. Eribulin mesylate, a non-taxane halichondrin B analogue microtubule inhibitor, resulted in ≥50% PSA responses in 22.4% of taxane-naive m CRPC patients and 8.5% of mCPRC patients who were treated with taxane ($n = 108$). The reported toxicity profile was excellent, and this agent does not require additional corticosteroid [16]. In case of satraplatin in the phase III SPARC (Satraplatin and Prednisone Against Refractory Cancer) study, an oral platinum analogue, it did not demonstrate overall survival benefit compared with placebo in mCRPC patients who had progression after one previous chemotherapy. It had the improvement in prostate-specific antigen levels and a decrease in the time to progression [17]. Other platinum-based chemotherapies, including carboplatin and cisplatin, combined with taxanes also investigated for docetaxel-refractory patients and several studies report that a subset of patients with mCRPC were effective when they received these combined chemotherpy agents. Ross et al. [18] combined docetaxel with carboplatin as second-line chemotherapy in mCRPC patients who showed the progression within 45 days of docetaxel-based chemotherapy ($n = 34$). This trial showed a ≥ 50% reduction in PSA level in 18% of patients. A retrospective analysis of patients with mCRPC who received docetaxel and carboplatin with ($n = 24$) or without estramustine ($n = 30$) as first-line and second-line chemotherapy, respectively, had excellent prostate-specific antigen response rates. This study reported a ≥50% reduction in prostate-specific antigen level in 88% and 20% of patients in docetaxel/carboplatin/estramustine group and docetaxel/carboplatin group, respectively [19]. With the development of new agents, patients have more survival gain and neuroendocrine transformation associated with N-Myc and aurora kinase. Gene alterations may occur more commonly [20]. Neuroendocrine transformation is not well investigated, and to date only one phase II study has evaluated to treat patients with tumors that have transformed. Four cycles of docetaxel/carboplatin chemotherapy followed by 4 cycles of etoposide plus cisplatin were administered to 120 patients with features of anaplastic disease. The study reported a median overall survival of 16 (13.6–19.0) months [21].

21.1.5 Chemotherapy for Neuroendocrine Prostate Cancer

Even though androgen deprivation therapy and cytotoxic chemotherapy using taxanes are highly effective in prostate cancer, it is well known that the effects of these drugs are less effective in neuroendocrine prostate cancer (NEPC). Although the characteristics of NEPC have yet to be cleared, NEPC shares histopathologic findings with small-cell carcinomas when examined, and it has different tumor characteristics from prostatic adenocarcinoma. This has little relationship with prostate-specific antigen and tumor burden and appears to more visceral and lytic bone metastases in comparison with bone and lymph node metastasis in prostatic adenocarcinoma. Platinum chemotherapy combinations are generally tried to use for the treatment of NEPC patients because of the clinical and histologic similarity to small carcinoma of the lung [22, 23]. However, we found that most of NEPC patients have mixed NEPC and prostatic adenocarcinomas not NEPC alone. So, patients treated with cisplatin and etoposide also have prostatic adenocarcinoma as the predominant histologic subtype present in sites of relapse [22, 23]. To avoid the relapse pattern of NEPC, taxane with platinum combination has been used to target both histologic subtypes. In a phase II trial, 120 men with metastatic NEPC were treated with carboplatin (day 1 every 3 weeks) plus docetaxel (75 mg/m^2, day 1 every 5 weeks) after etoposide (120 mg/m^2, days 1–3 every 3 weeks) plus cisplatin (25 mg/m^2, days 1–3 every 3 weeks). The median survival was 16 months (95% CI 12.6–19.0), and median time to progression was 5.1 months (95% CI 4.2–6.0) after first-line therapy and 3.1 months (95% CI 1.6–3.5) after the second-line regimen. About 50% of patients had clinical benefit from both therapies and 33.8% from carboplatin plus docetaxel alone. General toxicities were febrile neutropenia, thrombosis, thrombocytopenia, fatigue, and vomiting [21]. Nevertheless, most NEPC patients experienced the quick progression after treatment even though platinum regimens have modest tumor response. To find the novel agents for this prostate cancer variant including NEPC represents an unmet need and further molecular characterization to find chemotherapy alternatives, such as aurora-kinase inhibitors are currently investigated.

21.2 Evaluation of Treatment Efficacy

The measure of therapeutic results in the clinical trial for all prostate cancer patients including mCRPC might be confused by significant methodologic challenges. Bone is the most common metastatic site in these patients, and it contains the diffuse osteoblastic bone lesions that cannot be measured by current methods (termed "nonmeasurable" lesion). Generally, soft-tissue or visceral metastatic sites that we could measure serially ("measurable" lesion) are uncommon metastatic sites and represent a small proportion of metastatic site for prostate cancer patients. To choose the bidimensionally measurable lesion in metastatic site for the evaluation of therapeutic efficacy by serial measurements of tumor has been the subject of significant criticism, because many patients may only have bone metastases—"nonmeasurable" lesion. Furthermore, prostate cancer patients who had visceral metastasis are often considered a subgroup with little different biologic and clinical characteristics distinct from those with bone-only metastases. As a result of these potential limitations, it is discouraged to subject the tumor response rate as the primary end point of clinical trials for mCRPC patients, and the evaluation of progression-free survival of bone and/or soft-tissue lesions using radiographic finding has become a reliable end point [24].

Several predictors to evaluate baseline and posttreatment characteristics were developed for the dissection of the heterogeneity of mCRPC in the context of various cytotoxic and non-cytotoxic therapies. Among them, the patient's functional status (performance status), presence of pain, baseline hemoglobin level, baseline prostate-specific antigen level, baseline alkaline phosphatase, baseline LDH level, extent of bone involvement (number of lesions or pattern/distribution of bone lesions), and presence of visceral disease were introduced as clinical and laboratory parameters with prognostic significance. In the recent studies, quantitative methods to count the circulating tumor cell numbers and various prostate-specific antigen constructs including >30% prostate-specific antigen reduction are identified as the most significant posttreatment parameters [25, 26].

Preclinical experiments reported that some drugs could decrease prostate-specific antigen secretion without affecting tumor growth, whereas other drugs may affect tumor growth without reducing prostate-specific antigen levels. However, these findings required a careful validation by several clinical setting even though these laboratory observations are likely to be clinically effective to prostate cancer. A prostate-specific antigen consensus meeting developed by several leading investigators discussed initial guidelines about the role of the prostate-specific antigen test for clinical trials in mCRPC patients. These guidelines were updated and now also provide a consensus on the use of radiologic end points as well as other clinical end points including pain to evaluate mCRPC patients [24]. In the future, other novel biomarkers are investigated to identify the proper treatments for mCRPC, and the enumeration of circulating tumor cells may be one of such markers at baseline and after a period of treatment nowadays [26]. Furthermore, the evolution of non-cytotoxic and targeted agents for mCRPC might need a new biomarker to identify mechanism-specific biologic activity and new clinical end points.

21.3 Summary

- Docetaxel is the standard first-line cytotoxic chemotherapy for mCRPC. This cytotoxic agent has progression-free and overall survival benefit, pain relief, and improves quality of life.
- The standard treatment regimen of docetaxel is a 3-week regimen (docetaxel 75 mg/m^2 given every 3 weeks). And also, bi-weekly regimen (docetaxel 50 mg/m^2 given every 2 weeks) is available for mCRPC patients.
- Toxicity of docetaxel generally includes myelosuppression, fatigue, peripheral edema, neurotoxicity, hyperlacrimation, and nail dystrophy.
- Cabazitaxel has approved as a second-line chemotherapy option for mCRPC patients who have had progression during or after docetaxel chemotherapy.
- Toxicity of cabazitaxel includes neutropenia including febrile neutropenia and diarrhea.
- Mitoxantrone has been approved to palliate symptoms associated with metastasis even though it has no survival benefit, and it is often used in patients who have previously received docetaxel and/or cabazitaxel or in those who would not tolerate these agents.

References

1. Eisenberger MA. Chemotherapy for prostate carcinoma. NCI Monogr. 1988;7:151–63.
2. Petrylak DP, Tangen CM, Hussain MH, Lara PN Jr, Jones JA, Taplin ME, et al. Docetaxel and estramustine compared with mitoxantrone and prednisone for advanced refractory prostate cancer. N Engl J Med. 2004;351(15):1513–20.
3. Tannock I, DeWit R, Berry W, Horti J, Pluzanska A, Chi KN, et al. Docetaxel plus prednisone or mitoxantrone plus prednisone for advanced prostate cancer. N Engl J Med. 2004;351(15):1502–12.
4. Tannock IF, Osoba D, Stockler MR, Ernst DS, Neville AJ, Moore MJ, et al. Chemotherapy with

mitoxantrone plus prednisone or prednisone alone for symptomatic hormone-resistant prostate cancer: a Canadian randomized trial with palliative end points. J Clin Oncol. 1996;14(6):1756–64.
5. Berry W, Dakhil S, Modiano M, Gregurich M, Asmar L. Phase III study of mitoxantrone plus low dose prednisone versus low dose prednisone alone in patients with asymptomatic hormone refractory prostate cancer. J Urol. 2002;168(6):2439–43.
6. Kantoff PW, Halabi S, Conaway M, Picus J, Kirshner J, Hars V, et al. Hydrocortisone with or without mitoxantrone in men with hormone-refractory prostate cancer: results of the cancer and leukemia group B 9182 study. J Clin Oncol. 1999;17(8):2506–13.
7. Jordan MA, Wilson L. Microtubules as a target for anticancer drugs. Nat Rev Cancer. 2004;4(4):253–65.
8. Komlodi-Pasztor E, Sackett D, Wilkerson J, Fojo T. Mitosis is not a key target of microtubule agents in patient tumors. Nat Rev Clin Oncol. 2011;8(4):244–50.
9. Sun Y, Wang BE, Leong KG, Yue P, Li L, Jhunjhunwala S, et al. Androgen deprivation causes epithelial-mesenchymal transition in the prostate: implications for androgen-deprivation therapy. Cancer Res. 2012;72(2):527–36.
10. Kellokumpu-Lehtinen PL, Harmenberg U, Joensuu T, McDermott R, Hervonen P, Ginman C, et al. 2-weekly versus 3-weekly docetaxel to treat castration-resistant advanced prostate cancer: a randomised, phase 3 trial. Lancet Oncol. 2013;14(2):117–24.
11. Antonarakis ES, Eisenberger MA. Phase III trials with docetaxel-based combinations for metastatic castration-resistant prostate cancer: time to learn from past experiences. J Clin Oncol. 2013;31(14):1709–12.
12. de Bono JS, Oudard S, Ozguroglu M, Hansen S, Machiels JP, Kocak I, et al. Prednisone plus cabazitaxel or mitoxantrone for metastatic castration-resistant prostate cancer progressing after docetaxel treatment: a randomised open-label trial. Lancet. 2010;376(9747):1147–54.
13. Attard G, Greystoke A, Kaye S, De Bono J. Update on tubulin-binding agents. Pathol Biol. 2006;54(2):72–84.
14. Smith TJ, Khatcheressian J, Lyman GH, Ozer H, Armitage JO, Balducci L, et al. 2006 update of recommendations for the use of white blood cell growth factors: an evidence-based clinical practice guideline. J Clin Oncol. 2006;24(19):3187–205.
15. Mohler JL, Kantoff PW, Armstrong AJ, Bahnson RR, Cohen M, D'Amico AV, et al. Prostate cancer, version 2.2014. J Natl Compr Cancer Netw. 2014;12(5):686–718.
16. Fossa SD, Miller A. Treatment of advanced carcinoma of the prostate with estramustine phosphate. J Urol. 1976;115(4):406–8.
17. Sternberg CN, Petrylak DP, Sartor O, Witjes JA, Demkow T, Ferrero JM, et al. Multinational, double-blind, phase III study of prednisone and either satraplatin or placebo in patients with castrate-refractory prostate cancer progressing after prior chemotherapy: the SPARC trial. J Clin Oncol. 2009;27(32):5431–8.
18. Ross RW, Beer TM, Jacobus S, Bubley GJ, Taplin ME, Ryan CW, et al. A phase 2 study of carboplatin plus docetaxel in men with metastatic hormone-refractory prostate cancer who are refractory to docetaxel. Cancer. 2008;112(3):521–6.
19. Nakabayashi M, Sartor O, Jacobus S, Regan MM, McKearn D, Ross RW, et al. Response to docetaxel/carboplatin-based chemotherapy as first- and second-line therapy in patients with metastatic hormone-refractory prostate cancer. BJU Int. 2008;101(3):308–12.
20. Mosquera JM, Beltran H, Park K, MacDonald TY, Robinson BD, Tagawa ST, et al. Concurrent AURKA and MYCN gene amplifications are harbingers of lethal treatment-related neuroendocrine prostate cancer. Neoplasia. 2013;15(1):1–10.
21. Aparicio AM, Harzstark AL, Corn PG, Wen S, Araujo JC, Tu SM, et al. Platinum-based chemotherapy for variant castrate-resistant prostate cancer. Clin Cancer Res. 2013;19(13):3621–30.
22. Amato RJ, Logothetis CJ, Hallinan R, Ro JY, Sella A, Dexeus FH. Chemotherapy for small cell carcinoma of prostatic origin. J Urol. 1992;147(3):935–7.
23. Papandreou CN, Daliani DD, Thall PF, Tu SM, Wang X, Reyes A, et al. Results of a phase II study with doxorubicin, etoposide, and cisplatin in patients with fully characterized small-cell carcinoma of the prostate. J Clin Oncol. 2002;20(14):3072–80.
24. Scher HI, Halabi S, Tannock I, Morris M, Sternberg CN, Carducci MA, et al. Design and end points of clinical trials for patients with progressive prostate cancer and castrate levels of testosterone: recommendations of the prostate cancer clinical trials working group. J Clin Oncol. 2008;26(7):1148–59.
25. Scher HI, Eisenberger M, D'Amico AV, Halabi S, Small EJ, Morris M, et al. Eligibility and outcomes reporting for clinical trials for patients in the state of a rising PSA: recommendations from the prostate-specific antigen working group. J Clin Oncol. 2004;22(3):537–56.
26. de Bono JS, Scher HI, Montgomery RB, Parker C, Miller MC, Tissing H, et al. Circulating tumor cells predict survival benefit from treatment in metastatic castration-resistant prostate cancer. Clin Cancer Res. 2008;14(19):6302–9.

Radiopharmaceutical Therapy in Metastatic CRPC

22

Kwang Suk Lee and Byung Ha Chung

22.1 Introduction

The treatment options of metastatic castration-resistant prostate cancer (mCRPC) have changed due to the introduction of several new drugs. Docetaxel was the first drug to demonstrate an important survival benefit to mitoxantrone in prolonging the overall survival (OS) of patients with mCRPC [1]. Recently, cabazitaxel and new endocrine therapies such as abiraterone acetate and enzalutamide improved the survival rate of patients treated with docetaxel [2–6]. Finally, radium-223, an innovative radiopharmaceutical, is associated with an increased survival rate in patients with mCRPC, regardless of previous docetaxel administration [7]. However, there were no sequential guidelines for the purpose of achieving cumulative benefit in survival. Therefore, the cooperation of experienced medical professionals is the best way to provide comprehensive treatment that requires consideration of the patient's physical, psychological, and financial status [8].

K. S. Lee · B. H. Chung (✉)
Department of Urology, Yonsei University College of Medicine, Seoul, South Korea
e-mail: chung646@yuhs.ac

22.2 Overview of Bone-Targeted Radiopharmaceuticals

Bone is the most common site for metastasis in mCRPC patients [9]. The most common bone metastasis sites are the lumbar, spine, and pelvis and are often complicated by pain. Systemic treatment such as hormonal therapy, chemotherapy, and immunotherapy for metastatic prostate cancer can lead to pain reduction, prolongation of the first bone-related symptoms, and OS [10]. However, it is difficult to optimally alleviate malignant bone pain [11]. Analgesics such as opiates and nonsteroidal anti-inflammatory drugs are frequently used, but they may provoke several side effects.

Localized pain caused by a single metastasis can be controlled by external beam radiation therapy (EBRT) in about 80% of patients. In case of pain due to diffuse multifocal osteoblastic metastases, bone can be treated with radiopharmaceuticals [12]. The most commonly used bone-seeking radiopharmaceuticals are phosphorus-32 (^{32}P), strontium-89-chloride (^{89}Sr), samarium-153-EDTMP (^{153}Sm), rhenium-186-HEDP (^{186}Re), rhenium-188-HEDP (^{188}Re), and radium-223-chloride (^{223}Ra). These radionuclides bind to the ligands that bind to the bone matrix and accumulate in the increased bone turnover position. The radiation is then delivered at the osteoblastic sites. The most important side effect

C. S. Kim (ed.), *Management of Advanced Prostate Cancer*,
https://doi.org/10.1007/978-981-10-6943-7_22

of these radiopharmaceuticals is bone marrow suppression.

^{32}P was the first US Food and Drug Administration (FDA)-approved radiopharmaceuticals in 1952 [13]. ^{32}P, a β-emitter that can relieve cancer-related bone pain, localizes to remodeling areas in bone including those in osteoblastic lesions. ^{89}Sr was FDA approved for management of bone in patients with mCPRC in 1993 [14]. ^{89}Sr is a β-particle emitter with a half-life of 50.6 days. A phase III in bone metastatic CRPC demonstrated improvement in palliation of bone pain after one injection with no survival benefit. ^{153}Sm is a β- and γ-emitter that was FDA approved in 1997 as a chelate with ethylenediamine tetramethylene phosphonic acid (Sm-EDTMP or ^{153}Sm-lexidronam) [15]. The FDA approval was based on phase III studies demonstrating pain palliation, but not survival benefit after one injection in bone metastatic disease, with a second study focusing exclusively on prostate cancer [16].

Radium-223, like ^{89}Sr, is part of an alkaline earth metal that acts as a calcium mimetic when injected. The α-particle consists of two protons and two neutrons. These particles produce a short range of high-density ionizing high-linear energy transfer radiation. Bone-targeted radiopharmaceuticals under investigation include rhenium-186 (^{186}Re), ^{188}Re, tin-117 (^{117}Sn)-DTPA, strontium-85, and holmium-166-DOTMP. Each of these agents is β-emitters, except 117Sn, which emits a conversion electron [17].

22.3 Radium-223

22.3.1 Mechanism of Action

Radium-223 as the target radiopharmaceutical was an alpha particle-emitting radioactive material with a half-life of 11.4 days. It causes double-stranded DNA breaks with the release of two protons and two neutrons at short distances, which is more difficult to repair than single-strand breaks caused by beta-radioactive isotopes. The α-particles are enormously energetic and cause dense ionization in tissues. Radium-223 dichloride, which selectively affects the active site of bone remodeling, is associated with bone metastasis. It has an advantageous bio-distribution and shows a 15% lower concentration in the bloodstream at 15 minutes after intravenous administration; at 24 hits, 99% of the bone is concentrated. Disintegration of radium-223, a stable isotope of lead, is mainly through the internal organs, but only 5% is removed via urine [18].

22.3.2 Administration

Radium-223 is supplied in disposable vials and the concentration is 1100 kBq/mL. Each vial contains 6 mL of solution (total radioactivity is 6600 kBq/vial). Radium-223 must be received, used, and managed only by authorized personnel of a dedicated nuclear medical unit. Due to contamination due to radioactivity and bodily fluids, healthcare workers must use gloves and barriers to avoid contamination suitable for handling and management of radium-223 [19].

22.3.3 Clinical Efficacy

FDA approved radium-223 dichloride for metastatic CRPC in patients with symptomatic bone metastases and no visceral metastatic disease in 2013. Approval was based on clinical data from a multicenter, phase III, randomized trial (ALSYMPCA) which included 921 patients with CRPC and symptomatic bone metastases to receive 6 injections of radium-223 or placebo plus best standard of care [7]. Compared to placebo, radium-223 was significantly associated with improved OS (median 14.9 months vs. 11.3 months, HR 0.70 (0.0158–0.830), $p < 0.001$) and prolonged time to first skeletal-related events (median 15.6 months vs. 9.8 months). Of these cohorts, 57% received previous docetaxel. In the subset analysis, survival benefits were maintained regardless of previous docetaxel use [20]. Radium-223 improves or slows down the quality of life. In the ALSYMPCA trial, subset analysis showed a slow decline in the quality of life of EuroQol five-dimensional (EQ-5D) over time and a significant improvement in EQ-5D utility score and FACT-P total score [21]. Patients with less advanced disease and/or receiving radium-223 earlier in the treatment sequence for mCRPC are more likely to complete six cycles of treatment [22]. Good ECOG performance scores, no pain, and low alkaline phosphatase (ALP) levels are a significant prognostic factor for OS, and patients taking concomitant use of denosumab or abiraterone have a long OS.

22.3.4 Adverse Events

The adverse events of radium-223 occurred in both hematological and non-hematological toxicities at low frequency. Grade 3/4 hematological toxicity was low (3% neutropenia, 5% thrombocytopenia, and 13% anemia), likely due to the short range of radioactivity [20]. Fecal elimination of the agent led to generally mild non-hematologic side effects, which included nausea, diarrhea, and vomiting. Mild non-hematological adverse events occurred in at least 10% of patients in either treatment group, with no differences in patients with or without prior docetaxel exposure [20]. In sub-analysis according to prior docetaxel use, patients previously treated with docetaxel had a higher incidence of grade 3–4 thrombocytopenia with radium-223 than with placebo. Radium-223 did not adversely affect later cycles of chemotherapy [20].

22.3.5 Evaluation of Patients Treated with Radium-223

22.3.5.1 Imaging Modalities

CT is the most widely used imaging modality of CRPC's diagnostic imaging workup for evaluating node, visceral, and bone metastases. As far as nuclear medicine is concerned, bone scintigraphy, positron emission tomography/computed tomography (PET/CT), and radiology techniques have been performed in CRPC patients. Bone evaluation by CT is limited by osteoporosis. In addition, interpretation of the osteoclastic flare response may be difficult. Although MRI is considered the most accurate radiation technique for detecting axial skeletal metastases and assessing spinal cord compression, MRI and especially diffusion-weighted images are being studied as a way to evaluate the response of bone metastases to CRPC patients [23, 24]. Conventional bone radiographs can be used to give specificity to bone scintigraphic findings and to assess the risk of limb fractures.

22.3.5.2 Markers

A recent analysis from the ALSYMPCA study showed significant differences between the radium-223-treated group and placebo in ALP reduction, normalization, and median time to ALP increase [7]. Radium-223 has been shown to increase OS in both patients with baseline ALP <220 U/L and>220 U/L. However, there are indications of a correlation of pretreatment ALP levels ($\geq$146 U/L) and increased risk of death, progression time, skeletal-related events, and bone marrow failure, suggesting baseline prognostic value [25].

22.3.5.3 Clinical Evaluation and Management of the Patient during Treatment

Survival benefits were consistent regardless of baseline pain level in ALSYMPCA [26]. During the first–second cycle, the patient may experience pain as a "flare phenomenon." However, this pain is often reduced and daily activity has been improved, after injections of radium-223. Considering the safety and feasibility observed in the ALSYMPCA trial, a careful balance of risks and advantages should be made with previous or concomitant external beam radiotherapy on bone metastases being considered [7]. Clinical trials show the benefits of pain and extended time to SSE development with radium-223, allowing the use of simultaneous bisphosphonates. In addition, there is an efficacy benefit when co-administered with denosumab as indicated in the International Standardized Access Program (iEAP), and co-administration is permitted. It is recommended that vitamin D (25-hydroxycholecalciferol) > 1000 UI/die and calcium 500 mg/die be properly administered when both radium-223 and bisphosphonate or denosumab are administered simultaneously. Vitamin D and calcium supplementation is not recommended for radium-223 administration without bone turnover inhibitors. If the diameter of the short axis is less than 3 cm, patients with nodular disease can be treated. Careful evaluation of lymph node status should be made for expansion and localization. Combining Radium-223 with the node EBRT is safe and can be considered.

22.4 Summary

Radium-223 therapy changed the treatment landscapes of mCRPC patients. With the establishment of radium-223 as a treatment option for prostate cancer, an ongoing investigation will help optimize sequencing, understand the potential benefits of hormone-sensitive prostate cancer, and identify new molecular, serological, or biologic predictors and the potential synergy of radium-223.

References

1. Tannock IF, de Wit R, Berry WR, Horti J, Pluzanska A, Chi KN, et al. Docetaxel plus prednisone or mitoxantrone plus prednisone for advanced prostate cancer. N Engl J Med. 2004;351(15):1502–12.
2. de Bono JS, Oudard S, Ozguroglu M, Hansen S, Machiels JP, Kocak I, et al. Prednisone plus cabazitaxel or mitoxantrone for metastatic castration-resistant prostate cancer progressing after docetaxel treatment: a randomised open-label trial. Lancet. 2010;376(9747):1147–54.
3. Beer TM, Armstrong AJ, Rathkopf DE, Loriot Y, Sternberg CN, Higano CS, et al. Enzalutamide in metastatic prostate cancer before chemotherapy. N Engl J Med. 2014;371(5):424–33.
4. de Bono JS, Logothetis CJ, Molina A, Fizazi K, North S, Chu L, et al. Abiraterone and increased survival in metastatic prostate cancer. N Engl J Med. 2011;364(21):1995–2005.
5. Ryan CJ, Smith MR, de Bono JS, Molina A, Logothetis CJ, de Souza P, et al. Abiraterone in metastatic prostate cancer without previous chemotherapy. N Engl J Med. 2013;368(2):138–48.
6. Scher HI, Fizazi K, Saad F, Taplin ME, Sternberg CN, Miller K, et al. Increased survival with enzalutamide in prostate cancer after chemotherapy. N Engl J Med. 2012;367(13):1187–97.
7. Parker C, Nilsson S, Heinrich D, Helle SI, O'Sullivan JM, Fossa SD, et al. Alpha emitter radium-223 and survival in metastatic prostate cancer. N Engl J Med. 2013;369(3):213–23.
8. Baldari S, Boni G, Bortolus R, Caffo O, Conti G, De Vincentis G, et al. Management of metastatic castration-resistant prostate cancer: a focus on radium-223: opinions and suggestions from an expert multidisciplinary panel. Crit Rev Oncol Hematol. 2017;113:43–51.
9. Saad F, Clarke N, Colombel M. Natural history and treatment of bone complications in prostate cancer. Eur Urol. 2006;49(3):429–40.
10. van Dodewaard-de Jong JM, Verheul HM, Bloemendal HJ, de Klerk JM, Carducci MA, van den Eertwegh AJ. New treatment options for patients with metastatic prostate cancer: what is the optimal sequence? Clin Genitourin Cancer. 2015;13(4):271–9.
11. Mercadante S. Malignant bone pain: pathophysiology and treatment. Pain. 1997;69(1–2):1–18.
12. Lam MG, de Klerk JM, van Rijk PP, Zonnenberg BA. Bone seeking radiopharmaceuticals for palliation of pain in cancer patients with osseous metastases. Anti Cancer Agents Med Chem. 2007;7(4):381–97.
13. Smart JG. The use of P32 in the treatment of severe pain from bone metastases of carcinoma of the prostate. Br J Urol. 1965;37:139–47.
14. Porter AT, McEwan AJ, Powe JE, Reid R, McGowan DG, Lukka H, et al. Results of a randomized phase-III trial to evaluate the efficacy of strontium-89 adjuvant to local field external beam irradiation in the management of endocrine resistant metastatic prostate cancer. Int J Radiat Oncol Biol Phys. 1993;25(5):805–13.
15. Serafini AN, Houston SJ, Resche I, Quick DP, Grund FM, Ell PJ, et al. Palliation of pain associated with metastatic bone cancer using samarium-153 lexidronam: a double-blind placebo-controlled clinical trial. J Clin Oncol. 1998;16(4):1574–81.
16. Sartor O, Reid RH, Hoskin PJ, Quick DP, Ell PJ, Coleman RE, et al. Samarium-153-Lexidronam complex for treatment of painful bone metastases in hormone-refractory prostate cancer. Urology. 2004;63(5):940–5.
17. Sartor O, Hoskin P, Bruland OS. Targeted radionuclide therapy of skeletal metastases. Cancer Treat Rev. 2013;39(1):18–26.
18. Carrasquillo JA, O'Donoghue JA, Pandit-Taskar N, Humm JL, Rathkopf DE, Slovin SF, et al. Phase I pharmacokinetic and biodistribution study with escalating doses of (2)(2)(3)Ra-dichloride in men with castration-resistant metastatic prostate cancer. Eur J Nucl Med Mol Imaging. 2013;40(9):1384–93.
19. Dauer LT, Williamson MJ, Humm J, O'Donoghue J, Ghani R, Awadallah R, et al. Radiation safety considerations for the use of (2)(2)(3)RaCl(2) DE in men with castration-resistant prostate cancer. Health Phys. 2014;106(4):494–504.

20. Hoskin P, Sartor O, O'Sullivan JM, Johannessen DC, Helle SI, Logue J, et al. Efficacy and safety of radium-223 dichloride in patients with castration-resistant prostate cancer and symptomatic bone metastases, with or without previous docetaxel use: a prespecified subgroup analysis from the randomised, double-blind, phase 3 ALSYMPCA trial. Lancet Oncol. 2014;15(12):1397–406.
21. Nilsson S, Cislo P, Sartor O, Vogelzang NJ, Coleman RE, O'Sullivan JM, et al. Patient-reported quality-of-life analysis of radium-223 dichloride from the phase III ALSYMPCA study. Ann Oncol. 2016;27(5):868–74.
22. Sartor O, Hoskin P, Coleman RE, Nilsson S, Vogelzang NJ, Petrenciuc O, et al. Chemotherapy following radium-223 dichloride treatment in ALSYMPCA. Prostate. 2016;76(10):905–16.
23. Lecouvet FE, Geukens D, Stainier A, Jamar F, Jamart J, d'Othee BJ, et al. Magnetic resonance imaging of the axial skeleton for detecting bone metastases in patients with high-risk prostate cancer: diagnostic and cost-effectiveness and comparison with current detection strategies. J Clin Oncol. 2007;25(22):3281–7.
24. Padhani AR, Makris A, Gall P, Collins DJ, Tunariu N, de Bono JS. Therapy monitoring of skeletal metastases with whole-body diffusion MRI. J Magn Reson Imaging. 2014;39(5):1049–78.
25. Fizazi K, Massard C, Smith M, Rader M, Brown J, Milecki P, et al. Bone-related parameters are the main prognostic factors for overall survival in men with bone metastases from castration-resistant prostate cancer. Eur Urol. 2015;68(1):42–50.
26. Parker C, Finkelstein SE, Michalski JM, O'Sullivan JM, Bruland O, Vogelzang NJ, et al. Efficacy and safety of Radium-223 dichloride in symptomatic castration-resistant prostate cancer patients with or without baseline opioid use from the phase 3 ALSYMPCA trial. Eur Urol. 2016;70(5):875–83.

Immunotherapy for CRPC

23

Sang Hyeon Cheon

23.1 Introduction

CRPC had been considered to be chemoresistant until 2004 when docetaxel was approved by US Food and Drug Administration (FDA) as a first-line treatment for metastatic castration-resistant prostate cancer. Thereafter, docetaxel has become the standard treatment for patients with metastatic CRPC. Within the last decade, four new drugs, abiraterone, cabazitaxel, enzalutamide, and radium-223, have been approved for the treatment of various stages of CRPC. Despite the therapeutic options for CRPC has improved, immunotherapy is still an attractive approach since it can offer more sustainable disease control and long-term survival benefit. There are several features of prostate cancer that make it an ideal subject for immunotherapy, and in 2010, FDA approved sipuleucel-T based on improvement in overall survival (OS) in patients with CRPC.

There are compelling evidences that prostate cancer may react to immunotherapy. There are studies that have examined the cellular components of prostate cancers showing that certain populations of immune cell may infiltrate the prostate gland [1, 2] such as natural effector cells, killer cells, and regulatory T cells, indicating that both the adaptive and innate routes of the immune system may play a role in initiating an attack against prostate cancer cells [3]. Even though immunotherapy for prostate cancer has fell short in the past, this modality has reclaimed the spotlight due to the recent success of immune checkpoint inhibition in other tumor types such as melanoma.

Since prostate cancer is an immeasurable disease by radiologic modalities, the main end point for most studies assessing the new drugs targeting prostate cancer is overall survival (OS). Although PSA response has shown to correlate with symptomatic improvement or survival by several studies, it still has not been accepted as a surrogate end point of OS, so far [4–8].

Prostate cancer has several characteristics that make it attractive for immunotherapy. It is an indolent tumor that has slow growth kinetics, allowing sufficient window to generate immune responses, and recurrence can be diagnosed early since the advent of PSA. Various tumor-associated antigens (TAAs) have been identified and characterized such as prostate-specific antigen (PSA) and prostate-specific membrane antigen (PSMA), which can serve as targets for activated immune cells. Vaccines can be used with a good safety profile since the prostate is not a vital organ such as the liver and colon, and elimination of residual normal prostate tissue by immune response leaves no clinical sequelae.

This chapter reviews the recent development of clinical trials and discusses the future

S. H. Cheon
Department of Urology, Ulsan University Hospital, Ulsan, South Korea

C. S. Kim (ed.), *Management of Advanced Prostate Cancer*, https://doi.org/10.1007/978-981-10-6943-7_23

perspectives for immunotherapy regarding CRPC treatment paradigms.

23.2 Vaccine-Based Immunotherapy

Vaccine-based immunotherapy is to stimulate the immune system to target specific tumor-associated antigens (TAAs) overexpressed on cancer target cells with less collateral damage to normal tissues. For CRPC, there are four types of vaccine-based immunotherapies classified as autologous, cell-based, viral-based, and peptide-based vaccines.

23.2.1 Sipuleucel-T (Provenge, APC8015)

Sipuleucel-T is an autologous dendritic cell-based vaccine designed to target PAP. APCs are collected from the patient's own blood via leukapheresis and in vitro incubated with a recombinant fusion protein containing granulocyte-macrophage colony-stimulating factor (GM-CSF) and PAP protein [9, 10]. The primed, antigen-loaded APCs (vaccine) are then reinfused into the patient three times at biweekly intervals to stimulate antitumor immune response [11]. Phase I/II trials showed appreciable T-cell-medicated immune responses and antibodies against the fusion protein and a 50% decrease in the PSA levels with low toxicity [12–15]. Three phase III clinical trials have been conducted with promising results. In the first two studies (D9901, D9902A), men with asymptomatic or minimally symptomatic CRPC were randomized to placebo or sipuleucel-T [16, 17]. The integrated analysis of both studies (n = 225) showed no improvement in TTP, the primary end point, but a median benefit of 4.3 months in OS compared with placebo, the risk of death being 33% reduced. In both studies, the toxicity profile was acceptable, the most common side effects being flu-like symptoms. The approval of sipuleucel-T to be the first therapeutic cancer vaccine by the FDA in 2010 was based on the third larger phase III trial (IMPACT; n = 512). The primary end point was OS rather than TTP. Sipuleucel-T improved survival by 4.1 months compared with placebo, and no significant difference was shown between groups in PSA response or PFS. Sipuleucel-T was well tolerated with minimal toxicity. Common adverse events were chill, fever, and headache [18].

An exploratory analysis was conducted to evaluate the prognostic and predictive value using data from the IMPACT trial showing that the strongest prognostic value was PSA and treatment effect of sipuleucel-T appeared to have an inverse relation with baseline PSA. Patient with a lower baseline PSA had a median OS of 41.3 months which is 13 months improvement than placebo. On the contrary, those with a higher baseline PSA had a median OS of 18.4 moths with only 2.8 months improvements [19]. This implies that immunotherapy should be started as early as possible with a greater treatment benefit in disease with more favorable baseline prognostic factors in the earlier stage.

23.2.2 GVAX

GVAX (Cell Genesys, Inc., San Francisco, CA, USA) is a cell-based vaccine based on a platform of irradiated castrate-sensitive (LNCaP) and castrate-resistant (PC3) cell lines modified genetically to bear GM-CSF, an immunostimulatory cytokine. Using the whole cells not only induces APC recruitment on the injection site but also activates the immune response medicated by macrophage and T cells [20]. Phase I/II dose escalating study of patients with metastatic castration-resistant prostate cancer showed that GVAX was associated with PSA decrease and stabilization, tolerable toxicity profiles, and a median OS time of 35, 0.0, 20.0, and 23.1 months for the high-, medium-, and low-dose groups, respectively. In patients in the medium- and low-dose level groups, there was a lower benefit (medium dose, 20 vs. 20 months; low dose, 18 vs. 23.1 months). The most common adverse events were injection site reactions and fatigue [21].

These results led to two phase III studies (VITAL-1 and VITAL-2) which failed to show improved outcomes, and the trials were terminated early according to futility. However, the GVAX group showed a tendency to improved survival after 22 months, implying that GVAX may especially benefit patients with an expected survival of >18 months [22–24]. It is unclear whether the failure reflects a defect in clinical design or a true deficiency of vaccine efficacy. GVAX continues to be explored in different schedules in order to optimize the efficacy, in combined regimens, and in other cancer types [25].

23.2.3 PROSTVAC (PSA-TRICOM)

Prostvac (Bavarian Nordic, Kvistgaard, Denmark) is a PSA-directed poxviral vector-based vaccine consisting of vaccinia virus and a fowlpox virus encoding human PSA and three co-stimulatory molecules (TRICOM; B7.1, intercellular adhesion molecule 1 (ICAM-1); and lymphocyte function-associated antigen 3 (LFA-3)) which serve to increase PSA-specific immune response [26]. Several early trials demonstrated that the prime-and-boost regimen was well tolerated with tolerable toxicities consisting mainly of fever and injection-site reactions [27–30]. In a multicenter phase II study of patients (n = 125) with minimally symptomatic CRPC, PROSTVAC resulted in an 8.5 months survival advantage (25.1 s 16.6 months) without any differences in terms of time to tumor progression. At 3-year follow-up, 30% of PROSTVAC arm was alive compared to 17.5% of control arm [31]. It is not sure whether the survival benefit reported in the lack of a PFS improvement is due to the distinctive patterns of responses with immunotherapy or due to a confounding factor, as has been proposed as occurring in the IMPACT trial. A global, randomized, double-blind, placebo-controlled phase III study (PROSPECT, NCT01322490) is to test whether PROSTVAC alone or in combination with GM-CSF is effective in prolonging OS in men with asymptomatic or minimally symptomatic in mCRPC patients [32]. 1297 patients were enrolled by January 2015, and the final results are expected in the fourth quarter of 2017.

23.2.4 Personalized Peptide Vaccination

The complexity of immune responses against heterogeneous tumor cells leads to an idea that a more tailored selection of vaccine antigens appropriate for individual patients could be a reasonable approach for developing more effective cancer vaccines. Personalized peptide vaccination (PPV) is an immunotherapy that uses multiple cancer peptides that are selected to complement preexisting host immunity [33]. PPV screens patients for their immune response against a panel of epitopes from TAAs before vaccinating them with up to four peptides to which they had reacted most strongly. Several phase I trials of PPV for mCRPC showed acceptable toxicity profiles, injection-site reactions being the most common [34–36]. In a crossover, randomized phase II trial of PPV plus low-dose estramustine phosphate (EMP) comparing standard dose EMP in CRPC patients (n = 57), median PFS was significantly longer in the PPV plus EMP arm (8.5 vs. 2.8 months), and median OS also favored the PPV plus EMP arm (p = 0.033) [37]. In a recent randomized controlled phase II trial of PPV plus low-dose dexamethasone versus dexamethasone only (n = 72) with chemotherapy-naïve CRPC, 6–9 PFS was significantly longer in the PPV plus dexamethasone arm (22 vs. 7 months) and so was the median OS (73.9 vs. 34.9 months) [38]. In spite of the promising results of the phase II trials, the low number of enrolled patients and the lack of a placebo arm are the limitations. A phase III, randomized, placebo-controlled trial of PPV is underway in Japan, enrolling 333 docetaxel-refractory mCRPC patients (UMIN000011308).

23.3 Immune Checkpoint Inhibitors

These new agents typically interfere with the autoregulatory mechanisms of immune system, thus promoting T-cell activity and potentiating antitumor effects [39]. They are antibodies that target immunological checkpoint regulators such as cytotoxic T-lymphocyte-associated protein 4 (CTLA-4) and PD-1 and its ligand (PD-L1).

23.3.1 Ipilimumab (Anti-cytotoxic T-lymphocyte Antigen 4 [CTLA-4], MDX-010)

Ipilimumab is a human monoclonal antibody that blocks negative signals sent to T cells through the cell-surface molecule cytotoxic T-lymphocyte antigen-4 (CTLA-4), thus inhibiting a negative checkpoint, removing the physiologic brake, and augmenting the T-cell-mediated immune response [40]. This was the first FDA-approved immune checkpoint inhibitor for the treatment of relapsed metastatic melanoma, based on OS benefit seen in clinical trials [41]. This agent has also been evaluated in prostate cancer across a various range of disease setting. Several phase I/II trials have evaluated different schedules, doses, and combinations in mCRPC patients [42, 43]. CA184-107 (n = 50) is an open-label, multicenter phase I/II trial, evaluated ipilimumab with or without radiotherapy [42]. PSA level declined in 25% of patients treated with ipilimumab monotherapy and in 12% treated with ipilimumab plus radiotherapy. The most common immune-related side effects affected the gastrointestinal tract, skin, and liver, and ipilimumab did not appear to potentiate radiotherapy-associated toxicity. A phase III trial evaluated ipilimumab vs placebo after bone-directed therapy (n = 799) in patients who progressed on docetaxel chemotherapy [44]. No significant difference was noted in the primary end point of OS (11.2 vs. 10 months), but a modest benefit was observed in PFS favoring the ipilimumab arm (4.0 vs. 3.1 months). Patients in the ipilimumab arm more frequently had >50% reduction of PSA (13.1 vs. 5.3%). A post hoc analysis of predefined subgroups demonstrated a greater benefit in patients with more favorable prognostic factors, such as no visceral metastases, alkaline phosphatase concentration < 1.5 times ULN, and hemoglobin concentration > 110 g/L. [44] In this group, median OS was 22.7 months and 15.8 months with ipilimumab and placebo, respectively (p-0.0038). A recent phase III trial assessing ipilimumab in the chemotherapy-naïve mCRPC is setting randomized patients to ipilimumab or placebo (n = 400) [45]. Median OS was not significantly different between both arms (28.7 vs. 29.7 months). However, ipilimumab arm showed a modest PFS benefit of approximately 2 months (5.6 vs. 3.8 months) and a better PSA response (23 vs. 8%). Diarrhea was the only grade 3/4 adverse event reported in ≥10% of ipilimumab-treated patients. Interestingly, contrary to the former study, this trial did not show a greater benefit of ipilimumab in patients with favorable prognostic factors.

23.3.2 Anti-PD1/PDL-1

T-cell surface molecule interacts with its ligand PD-L1 resulting in T-cell inhibition, and blocking this process potentiates antitumor immune response. The PD-1 pathway-targeting agents such as nivolumab and pembrolizumab and PD-L1 inhibitors such as atezolizumab have more recently received regulatory approval in other tumor types such as melanoma, bladder, lung, and kidney cancers [46–49]. There are more studies ongoing currently with all of these drugs in different settings.

23.4 Conclusion

Immunotherapy is a promising field in the evolving landscape of CRPC treatment but still in its infancy state. Many clinical data have shown that immune modulation can prolong survival with tolerable toxicities. However, surrogate biomarkers that can reflect the immune response and the impact of the treatments on OS need to be explored. Immunotherapy is thought to be most effective when disease burden is minimal or throughout the course of disease or with a combination yet to be discovered and schedule of different, complimentary mechanism of action. Further studies in this field may bring more light to the treatment approaches for CRPC.

23.5 Summary

The treatment options for metastatic castration-resistant prostate cancer (mCRPC) have been widened during the last decade. Immunotherapy has emerged as an attractive strategy for its possibility to provide durable disease control and long-term benefit. Since the approval of sipuleucel-T by FDA in 2010, several strategies targeting the immune system such as cancer vaccines and immune checkpoint inhibitors have shown promising results in many clinical trials.

References

1. Gannon PO, Poisson AO, Delvoye N, et al. Characterization of the intra-prostatic immune cell infiltration in androgen-deprived prostate cancer patients. J Immunol Methods. 2009;348:9–17.
2. May KF Jr, Gulley JL, Drake CG, et al. Prostate cancer immunotherapy. Clin Cancer Res. 2011;17:5233–8.
3. Cha E, Small EJ. Is there a role for immune checkpoint blockade with ipilimumab in prostate cancer? Cancer Med. 2013;2:243–52.
4. Berthold DR, Pond GR, de Wit R, et al. Survival and PSA response of patients in the TAX 327 study who crossed over to receive docetaxel after mitoxantrone or vice versa. Ann Oncol. 2008;19:1749–53.
5. Petrylak DP, Ankerst DP, Jiang CS, et al. Evaluation of prostate-specific antigen declines for surrogacy in patients treated on SWOG 99-16. J Natl Cancer Inst. 2006;98:516–21.
6. Smith DC, Dunn RI, Strawderman MS, et al. Change in serum prostate-specific antigen as marker of response to cytotoxic therapy for hormone-refractory prostate cancer. J Clin Oncol. 1988;16:1835–43.
7. Scher HI, Halabi S, Tannock I, et al. Design and end points of clinical trials for patients with progressive prostate cancer and castrate levels of testosterone recommendations of the prostate cancer clinical trials working group. J Clin Oncol. 2008;26:1148–59.
8. Armstrong AJ, Garrett-Mayer E, Ou Yang YC, et al. Prostate-specific antigen and pain surrogacy analysis in metastatic hormone-refractory prostate cancer. J Clin Oncol. 2007;25:3965–70.
9. Rini BI. Technology evaluation: APC-8015, Dendrron. Curr Opin Mol Ther. 2002;4:76–9.
10. Patel PH, Kockler DR. Sipuleucel-T: a vaccine for metastatic, asymptomatic, androgen-independent prostate cancer. Ann Pharmacother. 2008;42:91–8.
11. Simons JW, Mikhak B, Chang JF, et al. Induction of immunity to prostate cancer antigens: results of a clinical trial of vaccination with irradiated autologous prostate tumor cells engineered to secrete granulocyte-macrophage colony-stimulating factor using ex vivo gene transfer. Cancer Res. 1999;59:5160–8.
12. Small EJ, Fraresi P, Reese DM, et al. Immunotherapy of hormone-refractory prostate cancer with antigen loaded dendritic cells. J Clin Oncol. 2000;18:3894–903.
13. Burch PA, Breen JK, Buckner JC, et al. Priming tissue-specific cellular immunity in a phase I trial of autologous dendritic cells for prostate cancer. Clin Cancer Res. 2000;6:2175–82.
14. Burch PA, Croghan CA, Gastineau DA, et al. Immunotherapy (APC8015, ProvengeVR) targeting prostatic acid phosphatase can induce durable remission of metastatic androgen-independent prostate cancer: a phase 2 trial. Prostate. 2004;60:197–204.
15. Beinart G, Rini BI, Weinberg V, Small EJ. Antigen-presenting cells 8015 (Provenge) in patients with androgen-dependent, biochemically relapsed prostate cancer. Clin Prostate Cancer. 2005;4:55–60.
16. Small EJ, Schellhammer PF, Higano CS, et al. Placebo-controlled phase III trial of immunologic therapy with sipuleucel-T (APC8015) in patients with metastatic, asymptomatic hormone refractory prostate cancer. J Clin Oncol. 2006;24:3089–94.
17. Higano CS, Schellhammer PF, Small EJ, et al. Integrated data from 2 randomized, double-blind, placebo-controlled phase 3 trials of active cellular immunotherapy with sipuleucel-T in advanced prostate cancer. Cancer. 2009;115:3670–9.
18. Kantoff PW, Higano CS, Shore ND, IMPACT Study Investigators, et al. Sipuleucel-T immunotherapy for castration-resistant prostate cancer. N Engl J Med. 2010 363:411–22.
19. Schellhammer PF, Chodak G, Whitmore JB, et al. Lower baseline prostate-specific antigen is associated with a greater overall survival benefit from sipuleucel-T in the immunotherapy for prostate adenocarcinoma (IMPACT) trial. Urology. 2013;81:1297–302.
20. Warren TL, Weiner GJ. Uses of granulocyte-macrophage colony-stimulating factor in vaccine development. Curr Opin Hematol. 2000;7:168–73.
21. Higano CS, Corman JM, Smith DC, et al. Phase 1/2 dose-escalation study of a GM-CSF-secreting, allogeneic, cellular immunotherapy for metastatic hormone-refractory prostate cancer. Cancer. 2008;113:975–84.
22. Gerritsen WR, Shama P. Current and emerging treatment options for castration-resistant prostate cancer: a focus on immunotherapy. J Clin Immunol. 2012 32:25–35.

23. Higano C, Saad F, Somer B, et al. A phase III trial of GVAX immunotherapy for prostate cancer vs. docetaxel plus prednisone in asymptomatic, castration-resistant prostate cancer (CRPC) Proc Am Soc Clin Oncol. Genitourinary Cancer Symposium 2009.
24. Small E, Demkov T, Gerritsen W, et al. A phase III trial of GVAX immunotherapy for prostate cancer in combination with docetaxel vs. docetaxel plus prednisone in symptomatic, castration resistant prostate cancer (CRPC). Proc Am Soc Clin Oncol. Genitourinary Cancer Symposium, 2009.
25. Van den Eerttwegh AJ, Versluis J, van den Berg HP, et al. Combined immunotherapy with granulocyte-macrophage colony-stimulating factor-transduced allogeneic prostate cancer cells and ipilimumab in patients with metastatic castration-resistant prostate cancer; a phase I dose escalating trial. Lancet Oncol. 2012;13:509–17.
26. Madan RA, Arlen PM, Mohebtash M, et al. Prostvac-VF; a vector-based vaccine targeting PSA in prostate cancer. Expert Opin Investig Drugs. 2009;18:1001–11.
27. Arden PM, Skarupa L, Paxdur M, et al. Clinical safety of a viral vector-based prostate cancer vaccine strategy. J Urol. 2007;178:1515–20.
28. Eder JP, Kantoff PW, Roper K, et al. A phase I trial of a recombinant vacciniavirus expressing prostate-specific antigen in advanced prostate cancer. Clin Cancer Res. 2000;6:1632–8.
29. Marchall JI, Hoyer RJ, Toomey MA, et al. Phase I study in advanced cancer patients of a diversified prime-and-boost vaccination protocol using recombinant vaccine virus and recombinant non-replicating avipox virus to elicit anti-carcinoembryonic antigen immune responses. J Clin Oncol. 2000;18:3964–73.
30. Gulley J, Chen AP, Dahut W, et al. Phase I study of a vaccine using recombinant vaccine virus expressing PSA (rV-PSA) in patients with metastatic androgen-independent prostate cancer. Prostate. 2002;53:109–17.
31. Kantoff PW, Schuctz TJ, Blumenstein BA, et al. Overall survival analysis of a phase II randomized controlled trial of a Poxviral-based PSA-targeted immunotherapy in metastatic castration-resistant prostate cancer. J Clin Oncol. 2010;28:1099–105.
32. Gulley JL, Giacchino JL, Breitmeyer JB, et al. A randomized double-blind phase 3 efficacy study of PROSTVAC-VF immunotherapy in men with asymptomatic/minimally symptomatic metastatic castration-resistant prostate cancer. J Clin Oncol. 2015;33
33. Sasada T, Noguchi M, Yamada A, et al. Personalized peptide vaccination; a novel immunotherapeutic approach for advanced cancer. Hum Vaccin Immunother. 2012;8:1309–13.
34. Noguchi M, Kobayashi K, Suetsugu N, et al. Induction of cellular and humoral immune responses to tumor cells and peptides in HLA-A2 positive patients with metastatic hormone refractory prostate cancer patients by peptide vaccination. Prostate. 2003;57:80–92.
35. Noguchi M, Itoh K, Suekane S, et al. Phase I trial of patient-oriented vaccination in HLA-A2 positive patients with metastatic hormone refractory prostate cancer. Ann Pharmacother. 2008;42:91–8.
36. Noguchi M, Uemura H, Naito S, et al. A phase I study of personalized peptide vaccination using 14 kinds of vaccine in combination with low-dose estramustine in HLA-A24-positive patients with castration-resistant prostate cancer. Prostate. 2011;71:470–9.
37. Noguchi M, Kakuma T, Uemura H, et al. A randomized phase II trial of personalized peptide vaccine plus low dose estramustine phosphate (EMP) versus standard dose EMP in patients with castration resistant prostate cancer. Cancer Immunol Immunother. 2010;59:1001–9.
38. Yoshimura K, Minami T, Nozawa M, et al. A phase 2 randomized controlled trial of personalized peptide vaccine immunotherapy with low-dose dexamethasone versus dexamethasone alone in chemotherapy-naïve castration-resistant prostate cancer. Eur Urol. 2016;70:25–41.
39. Noguchi M, Koga N, Moriya F, et al. Immunotherapy in prostate cancer: challenges and opportunities. Immunotherapy. 2016;8:69–77.
40. Pardoll D, Drake C. Immunotherapy earns its spot in the rank of cancer therapy. J Exp Med. 2012;209:201–9.
41. Hodi FS, O'Day SJ, McDermott DF, et al. Improved survival with ipilimumab in patients with metastatic melanoma. N Engl J Med. 2010;363:711–23.
42. Small EJ, Tchekmedyian NS, Rini BI, et al. A pilot trial of CTLA-4 blockade with human anti-CTLA-4 in patients with hormone-refractory prostate cancer. Clin Cancer Res. 2007;13:1810–5.
43. Harzstark AL, Fong L, Weinberg VK, et al. Final results of a phase I study of CTLA-4 blockade in combination with GM-CSF for metastatic castration resistant prostate cancer (mCRPC). J Clin Oncol. 2010;28(Suppl. 15.);[abstr 4689].
44. Kwon ED, Drake CG, Scher HI, CA184-043 Investigators, et al. Ipilimumab versus placebo after radiotherapy in patients with metastatic castration-resistant prostate cancer that had progressed after docetaxel chemotherapy: a multicenter, randomized, double-blind, phase 3 trial. Lancet Oncol. 2014;15:700–12.
45. Beer TM, Kwon ED, Drake CG, et al. Randomized, double-blind phase 3 trial of ipilimumab versus placebo in asymptomatic or minimally symptomatic patients with metastatic chemotherapy-naïve castration-resistant prostate cancer. J Clin Oncol. 2016;35(1):40–7.
46. Weber JS, D'Angelo SP, Minor D, et al. Nivolumab versus chemotherapy in patients with advanced melanoma who progressed after anti-CTLA-4 treatment (CheckMate 037): a randomized, controlled, open-label, phase 3 trial. Lancet Oncol. 2015;37:5–84.

47. Robert C, Schachter J, Long GV, et al. Pembrolizumab versus ipilimumab in advanced melanoma. N Engl J Med. 2015;372(26):1909–20.
48. Motzer RJ, Escudier B, McDermott DF, et al. Nivolumab versus everolimus in advanced renal cell carcinoma. N Engl J Med. 2015;180:3–13.
49. Rosenberg JE, Hoffman-Censits J, Powles T, et al. Atezolizumab in patients with locally advanced and metastatic urothelial carcinoma who have progressed following treatment with platinum-based chemotherapy: a single-arm, multicenter, phase 2 trial. Lancet. 2016;387:1909–20.

Clinical Trials in CRPC

24

Yoon Seok Suh and Jae Young Joung

24.1 Introduction

Prostate cancer (PC) is the second most common cause of cancer-related mortality in US men, and 180,890 of new PC cases occurred in 2016 [1]. At the time of diagnosis, approximately 12% of patients had locally advanced PC, and about 4% of patients had PC with metastasis [2]. Cure for localized PC that is newly diagnosed is available with definitive therapy. However, almost 30% of patients with PC experience recurrence of PC and castration-resistant PC (CRPC) [2]. Many new drugs have been approved by the US Food and Drug Administration (FDA) as a therapeutic option for CRPC. Various pathways and targets have demonstrated major advances in understanding the mechanisms of acquiring castration resistance and showing progression of PC. In this chapter, the clinical trials in CRPC will be elaborated. A large number of new agents for CRPC that is based on various mechanisms are currently being studied worldwide. Clinical trials of CRPC are summarized in Table 24.1.

Y. S. Suh · J. Y. Joung (✉)
Department of Urology, Center for Prostate Cancer, Research Institute and Hospital, National Cancer Center, Goyang, Korea

24.2 Therapeutic Strategies

24.2.1 Cytotoxic Chemotherapy

Docetaxel has gained acceptance as the standard treatment for CRPC patients. However, the requirement for new cytotoxic agents with effectiveness has been emphasized due to the inevitable progression of PC after treatment with chemotherapeutic agents. In previous study, induction of more than 50% reduction of PSA in patients who showed progression after docetaxel chemotherapy was reported with carboplatin [3]. The anticancer effect and overcoming the chemotherapy resistance were demonstrated with the everolimus, mTOR inhibitor, in addition to platinum-based chemotherapy [4]. The efficacy of combination therapy that uses everolimus and carboplatin for treatment of patients with metastatic PC was evaluated in Phase II trial [5]. The median survival time was 12.5 months in patients with metastatic PC who had experienced progression after treatment with docetaxel. No pharmacokinetic interactions were noted with the combination therapy.

24.2.2 Androgen Pathway Targeted Therapy

The 5α-androstenedione pathway is considered as a predominant pathway. Using this pathway, testosterone-mediated modulation can be

C. S. Kim (ed.), *Management of Advanced Prostate Cancer*,
https://doi.org/10.1007/978-981-10-6943-7_24

Table 24.1 Ongoing clinical trials in castration-resistant prostate cancer

Drug	Registry number	Phase	Enroll	Completion date[a]	Subject group	Status
TAS3681	NCT02566772	I	130	Jun 2018	TAS3681	Recruiting
IPH2201	NCT02671435	I	208	Oct 2019	IPH2201	Recruiting
AZD8186	NCT01884285	I	180	Sep 2019	AZD8186 monotherapy vs. combination with AZD2014 or abiraterone	Recruiting
EC1169	NCT02202447	I	40	Dec 2017	EC1169 vs EC0652	Recruiting
VBIR	NCT02616185	I	133	Apr 2019	VBIR	Recruiting
ADXS31–142	NCT02325557	I, II	51	Dec 2019	ADXS31–142 vs. ADXS31–142 + pembrolizumab (MK-3475)	Recruiting
VT-464	NCT02012920	I, II	141	Aug 2016	Treatment-naïve vs. previous abiraterone and enzalutamide	Recruiting
Alisertib	NCT01848067	I, II	9	May 2018	Alisertib + abiraterone	Not recruiting
Ipilimumab	NCT01688492	I, II	57	Sep 2018	Ipilimumab + abiraterone	Not recruiting
EPI-506	NCT02606123	I, II	166	Dec 2018	EPI-506	Recruiting
ARN-509	NCT01171898	I, II	12	Dec 2017	Previously abiraterone-treated chemotherapy-naive mCRPC	Not recruiting
Onapristone	NCT02049190	I, II	75	Dec 2017	Onapristone	Recruiting
ODM-204	NCT02344017	I, II	75	Dec 2017	ODM-204	Not recruiting
SHR3680	NCT02691975	I, II	140	Jun 2020	SHR3680	Recruiting
LEE011 (ribociclib)	NCT02494921	I, II	47	Dec 2019	Docetaxel + ribociclib	Recruiting
MK-3475 (pembrolizumab)	NCT02312557	II	58	Jan 2020	Pembrolizumab + enzalutamide	Recruiting
GX301	NCT02293707	II	120	Nov 2019	GX301	Recruiting
Sipuleucel-T with ipilimumab	NCT01804465	II	54	Dec 2018	Immediate vs. delayed sipuleucel-T + ipilimumab vs.	Recruiting
Carfilzomib	NCT02047253	II	28	Apr 2019	Carfilzomib	Not recruiting
Olaparib	NCT01682772	II	89	Dec 2016	Olaparib	Recruiting
CYT107	NCT01881867	II	54	Jan 2017	CYT107 vs. no therapy	Recruiting
Indoximod	NCT01560923	II	47	Nov 2017	Indoximod vs. placebo	Not recruiting
LY3023414	NCT02407054	II	Aug	May 2019	LY3023414 + enzalutamide vs. placebo + enzalutamide	Recruiting
MLN8237 (alisertib)	NCT01799278	II	60	Jun 2017	Neuroendocrine prostate cancer	Not recruiting
LY2157299	NCT02452008	II	60	Jul 2019	LY2157299 + enzalutamide vs. enzalutamide	Recruiting
Galeterone	NCT01709734	II	126	Aug 2017	Galeterone	Not recruiting
KPT-330 (selinexor)	NCT02215161	II	14	Jun 2018	KPT-330	Not recruiting
Everolimus	NCT00976755	II	37	Dec 2017	Everolimus	Not recruiting
PROSTVAC	NCT02649855	II	38	Jan 2020	Simultaneous vs. sequential docetaxel + PROSTVAC	Recruiting
AMG386	NCT01553188	II	23	Jan 2018	Abiraterone + AMG386 vs. abiraterone	Not recruiting
AZD5363	NCT02525068	II	136	Jun 2018	AZD5363 + enzalutamide	Recruiting
177Lu-J591	NCT00859781	II	140	Dec 2018	177Lu-J591 + Keto vs. 111ln-J591 + Keto	Recruiting
BAY1841788 (ODM-201)	NCT02200614	III	1500	Jun 2020	BAY1841788 vs. placebo	Recruiting
DCVAC	NCT02111577	III	1170	Jun 2019	DCVAC + chemotherapy vs. placebo + chemotherapy	Recruiting
Enz with abiraterone	NCT01949337	III	1311	Dec 2019	Enzalutamide vs. enzalutamide + abiraterone + prednisone	Not recruiting
Enz	NCT02003924	III	1396	Jun 2017	Enzalutamide vs. placebo	Not recruiting

[a]Final data collection date for primary outcome measure

bypassed by CRPC. The 17,20-lyase activity of cytochrome P450 17 (CYP17), 3β-hydroxysteroid dehydrogenase, and 5α-reductase activity are able to make an alternative pathway with cholesterol precursors. Cytochrome P450 17 is regarded as a potential treatment target for metastatic CRPC. Androgen receptor (AR) amplification is demonstrated in about 30% of CRPC. Increased expression of AR mRNA has been proposed as a process associated with decrease of hormone sensitivity as well as enhancement of intracellular converting of androgens and dihydrotestosterone. The AR antagonists that are second generation have been approved; however, more potent AR antagonists are still required.

24.2.2.1 AR Inhibitors

N-terminal domain is essential for AR transcriptional activity. EPI-001 (ESSA, Vancouver, Canada) is related with AR N-terminal domain covalently [6]. EPI-001 inhibits the activity of AR transcription as well as its variants. And in xenograft model, it reduced the growth of CRPC. EPI-001 is expected to demonstrate efficacy in the treatment of CRPC showing progression after enzalutamide treatment. EPI-506 is an N-terminal domain inhibitor as well, and it is a prodrug of EPI-002 [7].

BAY1841788 (ODM-201, Bayer, Leverkusen, Germany) is second-generation ligand-domain-binding AR antagonist. It makes binding with greater affinity to AR compared to enzalutamide. Not accumulating in the central nervous system is an advantage of BAY1841788. The ARAMIS which is the third clinical trial is undergoing. In Phase I and II clinical trials (ARADES), the median time to prostate-specific antigen (PSA) progression was 72.3 weeks and 20.3 weeks in chemo-naïve patients and post-chemotherapy patients, respectively [8].

Another second-generation AR antagonist is JNJ-56021927 (ARN-509, Apalutamide, Aragon, San Diego, California). It binds to AR with high affinity, inhibits AR nuclear translocation, and blocks recruiting of coactivators. In the study of JNJ-56021927, the PSA response that was defined as reduction of PSA > 50% at 3 months was 91%, 88%, and 24% in treatment-naïve cases without metastasis, treatment-naïve cases with metastasis, and mild disease of post-abiraterone case, respectively. SPARTAN (NCT01946204) and ATLAS (NCT01171898) that are Phase III studies have been evaluating JNJ-56021927 in patients with nonmetastatic CRPC. Clinical trial using abiraterone is planned (NCT01792687).

24.2.2.2 CYP17 Inhibitors

Galeterone (VN/124-1, TOK-001, Tokai, Boston, Massachusetts, United States) is a semisynthetic steroid compound available orally. It inhibits PC with CYP17 inhibition and AR modulation. Optimal therapy in the aspect of efficacy and safety using galeterone in patients with CRPC who were treatment-naïve regardless of metastasis was investigated in ARMOR2 clinical trial (NCT 01709734). In treatment-naïve metastatic CRPC patients who were treated with 2550 mg daily, PSA responses were reported with 81–90% of patients achieving a PSA decline of >50% and 30%, respectively. Stable disease was reported in patients refractory to abiraterone, and this suggests the possibility of various responses for galeterone compared to other second-generation drugs [9].

ASP9521 (Astellas, Tokyo, Japan) is an oral, 17β-hydroxysteroid dehydrogenase inhibitor. It seems to bypass the requirement of prednisone and does not show interference with the glucocorticoids synthesis. No biochemical or radiological response was observed with ASP9521 in 13 patients who underwent chemotherapy in Phase I and II trials [10].

VT-464 (Viamet) is a novel CYP17 inhibitor with greater affinity to 17,20-lyase compared to 17-hydroxylase. It does not need steroid administration. VT-464 is on underway in Phase I and II trials (NCT02012920). More selective inhibition of androgen synthesis and AR antagonism were found with VT-464 compared to abiraterone in preclinical studies [11].

24.2.3 Target Agents

Target agents have been widely used in a variety of malignant tumors. Since a well-defined drug target in PC was not identified, the role of the target drug in PC was thought to be limited.

However, efforts for developing targeted agents suitable for PC are increasing. Alisertib (Takeda Pharmaceutical Company, Osaka, Japan) is an Aurora A kinase inhibitor and it exhibits antitumor activity [12]. The incidence of expression in PC is only 5% of PC; however, in the case of neuroendocrine PC, 40% of expression of Aurora A kinase is found [13]. Complete inhibition of neuroendocrine marker expression has been noted following treatment with aurora kinase inhibitors. Phase II trials are currently undergoing (NCT01848067).

OGX-011 (OncoGenex, Bothell, Washington, United States) has been reported to restore the sensitivity of docetaxel in PC cells which is docetaxel-resistant as an antisense inhibitor to clusterin [14]. In clinical trials of Phase II study, the overall survival was 23.8 months and 16.9 months in the OGX-011 group and in the placebo group, respectively. Progression-free survival of 7.3 months was reported after combination therapy with docetaxel OGX-011, and progression-free survival of 6.1 months was reported without OGX-011 [15]. Phase III clinical trial that was designed to compare combination therapy with cabazitaxel and prednisolone with OGX-011 was performed (NCT01578655).

Everolimus (Novartis, Basel, Switzerland) is a mTOR inhibitor. Combination therapy with everolimus and bicalutamide was effective in patients with CRPC without prior bicalutamide treatment in a Phase II study [16]. In this study, 75% of patients (18/24) had PSA response. Currently, Phase II clinical trial is undergoing to investigate the everolimus monotherapy (NCT00976755).

Tasquinimod (Ipsen, Paris, France) is a quinolone-3-carboxamide derivative. The median progression-free survival after treatment with tasquinimod was 7.6 months that is significantly longer than placebo (3.3 months) in Phase II trial [17]. Stable disease and partial response were 52% and 7%, respectively, after treatment with tasquinimod. CRPC patients accompanying bone metastases had better progression-free survival than patients with lymph node or visceral metastases after treatment with tasquinimod. Accordingly, Phase III clinical trial regarding metastatic CRPC and bone metastases was performed with 1200 patients (NCT01234311). Although the results are currently not available, Active Biotech (Lund, Sweden) demonstrated that tasquinimod did not prolong survival (hazard ratio, 1.09; 95% confidence interval, 0.94–1.28). Concurrent trials with cabazitaxel (NCT01513733) and sipuleucel-T (NCT02159950) are undergoing.

AZD5363 (Ootsuka, Japan) is a novel Akt inhibitor. It is known to induce autophagy [18]. In combination with docetaxel chemotherapy (NCT02121639) and enzalutamide (NCT02525068), Phase II clinical trials were conducted. KPT-330 (selinexor; Karyopharm, Newton, Massachusetts, United States) is a selective exportin-1 inhibitor that has anticancer effects in the PC model [19]. Phase II clinical trial has been conducted. It was found that Exportin-1-1 is overexpressed in PC and related with adverse pathologic findings. AMG386 (Amgen, Thousand Oaks, California, United States) which is known as trebananib is a new agent that inhibits endothelial cell proliferation in tumors. Currently, Phase I and Phase II clinical trials are undergoing to evaluate the efficacy of combination therapy with AMG386 and abiraterone in metastatic CRPC (NCT01553188).

Cabozantinib (South San Francisco, California, United States), known as Exelixis, is a multi-kinase inhibitor for endothelial cell growth factor receptor 2 and MET. In the Phase II trial, CRPC patients treated with cabozantinib demonstrated a median progression-free survival of 23.9 weeks, compared with 5.9 weeks in controls treated with placebo [20]. However survival gain was not found in Phase III clinical trials that were conducted in 2014.

Arginine deaminase decreases plasma arginine levels and arouses damage to cancer cells which have arginine succinate synthase deficiency. Because of its high immunogenicity, arginine deaminase binds with polyethylene glycol to produce a therapeutic agent pegylated arginine deaminase (ADI-PEG 20, Polaris, San Diego, California, United States) that has a longer half-life. Autophagy and apoptosis were found in PC cells after treatment with ADI-PEG 20 in preclinical study [21]. The drug was proven to be tolerable in combination therapy with docetaxel in a Phase I study [22].

24.2.4 Vaccines

DCVAC is a vaccine that is based on autologous dendritic cell. Docetaxel and DCVAC combined chemotherapy showed longer survival than expected without significant adverse events in Phase I and II trials (19 months vs. 11.8 months) [23]. Currently, Phase III study is underway that evaluates the efficacy of combined therapy of DCVAC and standard chemotherapy (NCT02111577).

PROSTVAC (Bavarian Nordic, Martinsried, Germany) is a cancer vaccine that is based on vector. In Phase II trial, it has been shown to be well tolerated in patients with symptomatic CRPC which is minimal and improved overall survival compared to the control (25.1 months vs. 16.6 months) [24]. But, benefit in overall survival was not found in another Phase II study that investigated the effect of the combination therapy of PROSTVAC and docetaxel [25]. Phase II clinical trial investigating the efficacy of simultaneous or sequential therapy of docetaxel with PROSTVAC is underway (NCT02649855).

GX301 (Genovax, London, United Kingdom) is a vaccine targeting human telomerase, and its safety and highly immunogenic efficacy were reported in patients with CRPC [26]. A Phase II study has been conducting (NCT02293707).

24.2.5 Immunotherapy and Gene Therapy

The humanized monoclonal antibody, 177Lu-J591 (ATLAB, Nantes, France), was developed in the form of a PET radioactive label that binds primarily to prostate-specific membrane antigen (PSMA) extracellular domain. It was reported that 177Lu-J591 J591 is a potential carrier of a cytotoxic agent conjugate that facilitates treatment effect [27]. Accordingly, it is considered as a promising radioimmunotherapy drug. Phase II clinical trial is underway (NCT00859781).

Ipilimumab (Bristol-Myers Squibb, New York, United States), known as Yervoy, blocks the cytotoxic T-lymphocyte-related protein 4 (CTLA-4) activity. It is a monoclonal antibody that was approved by the FDA in 2011. Potential effect of radiotherapy for activating immune system in patient with PC had been suggested with prior studies [28, 29]. However, in Phase III study, it failed to show improvement of overall survival in patients treated with ipilimumab after radiotherapy, compared with patients treated with placebo treated after radiotherapy (11.2 months and 10.0 months, respectively) [30]. Combination trials with ADT (NCT01498978), abiraterone (NCT01688492), PROSTVAC (NCT02506114), and sipuleucel-T (NCT01804465) are in progress.

A poly-ADT-ribose polymerase inhibitor Olaparib (AstraZeneca, London, UK) was approved for ovarian cancer treatment with BRCA1/2 mutations. The DNA repair process includes poly-ADT-ribose polymerase, and genetic aberrations which are found in CRPC are considered to render sensitivity to poly-ADT-ribose polymerase inhibitors. Response rate of 33% in patients with post-docetaxel PC with defective DNA repair genes was reported with Olaparib treatment [31]. A Phase II clinical trial has been conducted (NCT01682772).

24.3 Summary

Docetaxel has gained acceptance as a standard treatment for CRPC patients. But for it is not sufficient in terms of prolonging survival, hence, the requirements for new drugs continues to exist. PC therapeutic strategies have recently been changed owing to emergence of novel agents. Research and development of new drugs based on several mechanisms are underway or awaiting approval. Recent developments in agents are expected to provide basis of optimal therapeutic option to patients with CRPC.

References

1. Siegel RL, Miller KD, Jemal A. Cancer statistics, 2016. CA Cancer J Clin. 2016;66(1):7–30.
2. Shore ND. Radium-223 dichloride for metastatic castration-resistant prostate cancer: the urologist's perspective. Urology. 2015;85(4):717–24.
3. Ross RW, Beer TM, Jacobus S, Bubley GJ, Taplin ME, Ryan CW, et al. A phase 2 study of carboplatin plus docetaxel in men with metastatic hormone-refractory prostate cancer who are refractory to docetaxel. Cancer. 2008;112(3):521–6.
4. Fury MG, Sherman E, Haque S, Korte S, Lisa D, Shen R, et al. A phase I study of daily everolimus plus low-dose weekly cisplatin for patients with advanced solid tumors. Cancer Chemother Pharmacol. 2012;69(3):591–8.
5. Vaishampayan U, Shevrin D, Stein M, Heilbrun L, Land S, Stark K, et al. Phase II trial of carboplatin, everolimus, and prednisone in metastatic castration-resistant prostate cancer pretreated with docetaxel chemotherapy: a prostate cancer clinical trial consortium study. Urology. 2015;86(6):1206–11.
6. Brand LJ, Olson ME, Ravindranathan P, Guo H, Kempema AM, Andrews TE, et al. EPI-001 is a selective peroxisome proliferator-activated receptor-gamma modulator with inhibitory effects on androgen receptor expression and activity in prostate cancer. Oncotarget. 2015;6(6):3811.
7. Maughan BL, Antonarakis ES. Clinical relevance of androgen receptor splice variants in castration-resistant prostate cancer. Curr Treat Options in Oncol. 2015;16(12):57.
8. Fizazi K, Massard C, Bono P, Jones R, Kataja V, James N, et al. Activity and safety of ODM-201 in patients with progressive metastatic castration-resistant prostate cancer (ARADES): an open-label phase 1 dose-escalation and randomised phase 2 dose expansion trial. Lancet Oncol. 2014;15(9):975–85.
9. Montgomery B, Eisenberger MA, Rettig MB, Chu F, Pili R, Stephenson JJ, et al. Androgen receptor modulation optimized for response (ARMOR) phase I and II studies: galeterone for the treatment of castration-resistant prostate cancer. Clin Cancer Res. 2016;22(6):1356–63.
10. Loriot Y, Fizazi K, Jones RJ, Van den Brande J, Molife RL, Omlin A, et al. Safety, tolerability and anti-tumour activity of the androgen biosynthesis inhibitor ASP9521 in patients with metastatic castration-resistant prostate cancer: multi-centre phase I/II study. Investig New Drugs. 2014;32(5):995–1004.
11. Toren PJ, Kim S, Pham S, Mangalji A, Adomat H, Guns EST, et al. Anticancer activity of a novel selective CYP17A1 inhibitor in preclinical models of castrate-resistant prostate cancer. Mol Cancer Ther. 2015;14(1):59–69.
12. Falchook GS, Zhou X, Venkatakrishnan K, Kurzrock R, Mahalingam D, Goldman JW, et al. Effect of food on the pharmacokinetics of the investigational Aurora A kinase inhibitor alisertib (MLN8237) in patients with advanced solid tumors. Drugs R&D. 2016;16(1):45–52.
13. Beltran H, Rickman DS, Park K, Chae SS, Sboner A, MacDonald TY, et al. Molecular characterization of neuroendocrine prostate cancer and identification of new drug targets. Cancer Discov. 2011;1(6):487–95.
14. Sowery RD, Hadaschik BA, So AI, Zoubeidi A, Fazli L, Hurtado-Coll A, et al. Clusterin knockdown using the antisense oligonucleotide OGX-011 re-sensitizes docetaxel-refractory prostate cancer PC-3 cells to chemotherapy. BJU Int. 2008;102(3):389–97.
15. Chi KN, Hotte SJ, Yu EY, Tu D, Eigl BJ, Tannock I, et al. Randomized phase II study of docetaxel and prednisone with or without OGX-011 in patients with metastatic castration-resistant prostate cancer. J Clin Oncol. 2010;28(27):4247–54.
16. Chow H, Ghosh PM, de Vere White R, Evans CP, Dall'Era MA, Yap SA, et al. A phase 2 clinical trial of everolimus plus bicalutamide for castration-resistant prostate cancer. Cancer. 2016;122(12):1897–904.
17. Pili R, Häggman M, Stadler WM, Gingrich JR, Assikis VJ, Björk A, et al. Phase II randomized, double-blind, placebo-controlled study of tasquinimod in men with minimally symptomatic metastatic castrate-resistant prostate cancer. J Clin Oncol. 2011;29(30):4022–8.
18. Lamoureux F, Zoubeidi A. Dual inhibition of autophagy and the AKT pathway in prostate cancer. Autophagy. 2013;9(7):1119–20.
19. Gravina GL, Mancini A, Sanita P, Vitale F, Marampon F, Ventura L, et al. KPT-330, a potent and selective exportin-1 (XPO-1) inhibitor, shows antitumor effects modulating the expression of cyclin D1 and survivin in prostate cancer models. BMC Cancer. 2015;15(1):941.
20. Smith DC, Smith MR, Sweeney C, Elfiky AA, Logothetis C, Corn PG, et al. Cabozantinib in patients with advanced prostate cancer: results of a phase II randomized discontinuation trial. J Clin Oncol. 2012;31(4):412–9.
21. Kim RH, Coates JM, Bowles TL, McNerney GP, Sutcliffe J, Jung JU, et al. Arginine deiminase as a novel therapy for prostate cancer induces autophagy and caspase-independent apoptosis. Cancer Res. 2009;69(2):700–8.
22. Tomlinson BK, Thomson JA, Bomalaski JS, Diaz M, Akande T, Mahaffey N, et al. Phase I trial of arginine deprivation therapy with ADI-PEG 20 plus docetaxel in patients with advanced malignant solid tumors. Clin Cancer Res. 2015;
23. Podrazil M, Horvath R, Becht E, Rozkova D, Bilkova P, Sochorova K, et al. Phase I/II clinical trial of dendritic-cell based immunotherapy (DCVAC/PCa) combined with chemotherapy in patients with metastatic, castration-resistant prostate cancer. Oncotarget. 2015;6(20):18192.
24. Kantoff PW, Schuetz TJ, Blumenstein BA, Glode LM, Bilhartz DL, Wyand M, et al. Overall survival analysis of a phase II randomized controlled trial of a Poxviral-based PSA-targeted immunotherapy in

metastatic castration-resistant prostate cancer. J Clin Oncol. 2010;28(7):1099–105.
25. McNeel DG, Chen Y-H, Gulley JL, Dwyer AJ, Madan RA, Carducci MA, et al. Randomized phase II trial of docetaxel with or without PSA-TRICOM vaccine in patients with castrate-resistant metastatic prostate cancer: A trial of the ECOG-ACRIN cancer research group (E1809). Hum Vaccin Immunother. 2015;11(10):2469–74.
26. Fenoglio D, Traverso P, Parodi A, Tomasello L, Negrini S, Kalli F, et al. A multi-peptide, dual-adjuvant telomerase vaccine (GX301) is highly immunogenic in patients with prostate and renal cancer. Cancer Immunol Immunother. 2013;62(6):1041–52.
27. DiPippo VA, Olson WC, Nguyen HM, Brown LG, Vessella RL, Corey E. Efficacy studies of an antibody-drug conjugate PSMA-ADC in patient-derived prostate cancer xenografts. Prostate. 2015;75(3):303–13.
28. Chakraborty M, Abrams SI, Camphausen K, Liu K, Scott T, Coleman CN, et al. Irradiation of tumor cells up-regulates Fas and enhances CTL lytic activity and CTL adoptive immunotherapy. J Immunol. 2003;170(12):6338–47.
29. Slovin S, Higano C, Hamid O, Tejwani S, Harzstark A, Alumkal J, et al. Ipilimumab alone or in combination with radiotherapy in metastatic castration-resistant prostate cancer: results from an open-label, multicenter phase I/II study. Ann Oncol. 2013;24(7):1813–21.
30. Kwon ED, Drake CG, Scher HI, Fizazi K, Bossi A, Van den Eertwegh AJ, et al. Ipilimumab versus placebo after radiotherapy in patients with metastatic castration-resistant prostate cancer that had progressed after docetaxel chemotherapy (CA184-043): a multicentre, randomised, double-blind, phase 3 trial. Lancet Oncol. 2014;15(7):700–12.
31. Mateo J, Carreira S, Sandhu S, Miranda S, Mossop H, Perez-Lopez R, et al. DNA-repair defects and olaparib in metastatic prostate cancer. N Engl J Med. 2015;2015(373):1697–708.

25 Palliative Care for Metastatic Symptomatic CRPC

Kyo Chul Koo

25.1 Introduction

Symptom development in advanced castration-resistant prostate cancer (CRPC) patients can be attributed to local invasion of the tumor, metastasis to the bone, or compression of the spinal cord. Along the course of disease progression, 50–70% of the patients will eventually develop complications. Bone metastasis and consequent skeletal complications are the most common manifestations which may increase the risk of death from prostate cancer and decrease life quality. The clinical manifestations of bone metastasis include pain, skeletal-related events, and additional medical cost. Advancements in the understanding of the disease have resulted in the development of new palliation strategies. In this chapter, we examine several interventional options for local and systemic disease manifestation, bone-targeted palliative agents, and bone-targeted agents which potentially improve survival and management strategies for spinal cord compression. These treatments include various agents, namely, bisphosphonates, human monoclonal antibodies, and alpha- and beta-emitting radiopharmaceuticals.

K. C. Koo
Department of Urology, Yonsei University College of Medicine, Seoul, South Korea
e-mail: gckoo@yuhs.ac

25.1.1 Pain Caused by Local Manifestation

Palliation of local symptoms and maintaining a good quality of life are major goals in the treatment landscape of symptomatic metastatic castration-resistant prostate cancer (mCRPC). Early diagnosis and intervention of local manifestations related to progression of the disease are important for maximizing quality of life.

25.1.1.1 Bladder Outlet and Ureteric Obstruction

Prostate enlargement or local bleeding may cause bladder outlet and/or ureteric obstruction. For the treatment of lower urinary tract symptoms (LUTS), transurethral resection of the prostate (TURP) with palliative purpose is a feasible option for symptoms intractable to medication [1]. Palliative radiotherapy is an alternative treatment for symptoms caused by bladder outlet obstruction with treatment efficacy reported in up to 63% of patients [1].

Ureteric obstruction can be caused by both tumor infiltration and compression [2, 3]. For symptomatic patients, urinary diversion should be considered to relieve the obstruction. For asymptomatic patients, urinary diversion can be considered for the less dilated and better functioning kidney. A nephrostomy catheter is superior to a JJ stent; however, ureteral stenting can be considered for patients desiring an internal

C. S. Kim (ed.), *Management of Advanced Prostate Cancer*,
https://doi.org/10.1007/978-981-10-6943-7_25

diversion. Palliative radiotherapy is another option to relieve the obstruction with a response rate reported in up to 62% of patients.

25.1.1.2 Lymphedema

Patients with metastatic lymph nodes may present with lymphedema of the lower extremities. Supportive treatments including compressive stockings or pressure pumps may improve functional deficit and alleviate pain and discomfort.

25.1.1.3 Ileus

Ileus can be caused by local compression and obstruction of the rectum. Surgery and rectal stenting are options to relieve the mechanical obstruction. Laxatives may improve motility and reduce pain for paralytic ileus caused by tumor involvement of the nerve plexus or secondary constipation caused by opioid analgesics.

25.1.1.4 Neuropathy

Nerve plexopathies can be caused by extensive skull metastasis with cranial nerve involvement, direct pelvic tumor invasion, or by extensive liver metastasis. Complete neurological evaluation should be performed, followed by pharmacological pain management including tricyclic antidepressants (amitriptyline), anticonvulsants (gabapentin, pregabalin), or corticosteroids for cranial nerve involvement. Neurolytic procedures (nerve block) can be considered for neuropathies caused by direct tumor invasion. Discontinuation of neurotoxic drugs such as docetaxel or cabazitaxel can be considered for intractable symptoms.

25.1.2 Pain Caused by Bone Metastasis

Bone metastasis associated with prostate cancer (PCa) is predominantly a blastic feature, reflecting a predominance of osteoblastic activity [4]. Bone metastasis is the most common etiology of chronic pain in patients diagnosed with mCRPC, while more than 20% of patients with bone metastases do not suffer from pain [2, 5]. Painful areas shown on bone scan should be evaluated with plain x-rays or computed tomography imaging to exclude osteolytic lesions or pathologic fractures. This is more important when the painful area is at weight-bearing sites. The choice and initiation of interventional therapy should depend on the metastatic site and on the patient's performance status. Therapeutic options should be tailored for each patient, preferably those with fewest side effects being the first-line option.

25.1.2.1 Single Lesion

Radiation Therapy

Palliation of focal bone pain, improvement in the quality of life, and the reduction of the risk of pain arising from sites to become symptomatic can be achieved with external beam localized radiation therapy [6]. There are various techniques, from higher doses given in less fractions to lower doses given over a longer period. The biological effect of radiotherapy depends on the total dose that is delivered, the number of treatment fractions, and the total period of the radiation. Stereotactic ablative radiation therapy is a novel radiation therapy which uses organ-limited approaches and has been reported with excellent outcomes. With radiation therapy, approximately 70% of the patients have been reported to achieve a complete relief of symptoms [7].

Orthopedic Surgery

Orthopedic surgery should be considered if more than half of the thickness of the bony cortex is involved in the metastasis [8, 9]. A sequential combination of radiofrequency and cementoplasty is a feasible option for painful osseous metastases [10].

25.1.2.2 Multiple Lesions

Systemic Analgesics

Nonsteroidal anti-inflammatory drugs alone can be used for chronic pain due to bone metastases. Dose escalation can be considered according to the response and side effects. Tramadol and dihydrocodeine extended-release tablets are commonly used agents. Morphine is the treatment of choice for moderate to severe degree pain. An alternative is hydromorphone; however, no clinically significant difference was shown when compared to morphine [11].

Bisphosphonates

Bisphosphonates, a class of drugs that is used to treat osteoporosis by preventing loss of bone mass, can be alternatively used as a supportive care for patients with pain caused by bone metastases. Bisphosphonates reduce bone resorption through the inhibition of osteoclastic activity and proliferation. Zoledronic acid is a potent bisphosphonate which reduces the frequency of skeleton-related events, delays the time to the first occurrence, and reduces pain compared with placebo [12, 13]. Moreover, zoledronic acid and pamidronate increase bone mineral density in men receiving long-term androgen deprivation therapy [14, 15]. Zoledronic acid is given at a dose of 4 mg intravenously every 4 weeks. Side effects include myalgia, fatigue, and anemia. Concomitant administration of oral calcium supplements and vitamin D is recommended owing to the possibility of hypocalcemia. A devastating complication of zoledronic acid is the osteonecrosis of the mandibular bone and consequent severe jaw pain. The benefit of other bisphosphonates, including etidronate, clodronate, ibandronate, and alendronate, has been studied in prospective randomized clinical trials; however, the efficacies of other bisphosphonates are inconclusive [16, 17].

Receptor Activator of Nuclear Factor-κB Ligand Inhibitors

Denosumab is a fully human monoclonal antibody against RANKL. Compared to zoledronic acid, denosumab has shown to improve the time to first skeletal-related events by 3.6 months and to prolong the time to first and subsequent skeletal-related events [18]. However, denosumab showed no benefits over other bone-targeted agents with regard to quality of life, pain management, progression-free survival, and overall survival. Toxicities of denosumab include nausea, fatigue, hypocalcemia, hypophosphatemia, and osteonecrosis of the jaw. Therefore, supplementary use of calcium and vitamin D is recommended. The recommended dose of denosumab is 120 mg administered subcutaneously every 4 weeks.

Radiopharmaceuticals

Beta Emitter

The beta emitters, strontium-89 (89Sr) and samarium-153 (153Sm), were historically the most commonly used radiopharmaceutical compounds [6, 19]. These agents were effective adjunctive therapies to local field radiotherapy, which improved progression-free survival and reduced the risks of future radiotherapy and analgesic support [19, 20]. With the improvement in the quality of life, 89Sr and 153Sm were both FDA approved for the palliative management of mCRPC; however, neither radiopharmaceutical demonstrated to improve overall survival.

Alpha Emitter

The alpha-emitting radiopharmaceutical, radium-223 (Ra-223), is a new concept radiopharmaceutical which delivers intense and highly localized radiation to the bone [21]. Alpha particles are approximately 7000 times heavier than beta particles, and one or two hits can induce cell death, in comparison with hundreds or thousands of hits required with beta particles. Moreover, alpha particles have a very short path length (<100 μm), by which surrounding the healthy bone can be maximally spared [22].

The ALSYMPCA trial was a randomized, double-blind, placebo-controlled phase III trial which compared Ra-223 versus placebo in men diagnosed with mCRPC without visceral or lymph node metastases [23]. Ra-223 was administered at a dose of 50 kBq/kg (intravenous) every 4 weeks for a total of six doses. Overall survival was improved by Ra-223 compared to placebo which resulted with a median survival improvement of 3.6 months. Moreover, Ra-223 showed benefit for secondary endpoints including time to first symptomatic skeletal event and quality of life. Based on the results of this trial, Ra-223 gained FDA approval for its use in patients with symptomatic bone metastatic CRPC.

25.1.3 Spinal Cord Compression

The collapse of a vertebral body or pressure exerted from a metastatic tumor within the spinal canal may cause spinal cord compression. The overall incidence of spinal cord compression in patients with prostate cancer is less than 10%, and the most common site is the thoracic cord. Early identification and intervention of spinal metastasis are important to preserve ambulatory ability and bladder and bowel function and to prevent and delay the onset of pain [24].

High-dose intravenous glucocorticoids should be the first therapeutic intervention in patients with suspected or documented spinal cord compression. The most commonly used agent is dexamethasone at daily doses from 16 to 100 mg. A loading dose of 10 mg followed by 4–10 mg every 6 h is administered. On improvement of symptoms, dose tapering may be performed throughout a 2–3-week period.

Definitive surgical intervention using spinal stabilization with anterior decompression or radiotherapy can be considered. Although radiotherapy is the mainstay of spinal cord compression, primary decompressive surgery could be considered for patients with compression at a single site, paraplegia of less than a 48-h period, tumors that are not radiosensitive, and patients' survival that is predicted to be longer than 3 months [25]. This is evident from a report suggesting that decompressive surgery after radiotherapy could result with better surgical outcome compared to performing radiotherapy alone [26]. Treatment selection should depend on the overall prognosis of the patient and status of the underlying comorbidities.

25.2 Summary

1. Early diagnosis and intervention of local symptoms in symptomatic mCRPC patients are essential in maintaining a good quality of life.
2. The choice of treatment for bone metastasis should depend on the site and number of the pathology and on the patient's physical condition. Therapeutic options include systemic analgesics, external beam radiation therapy, surgery, bisphosphonates, RANKL inhibitors, and radiopharmaceuticals, which should be tailored for each patient.
3. Initial treatment for spinal cord compression symptom should include high-dose intravenous glucocorticoid injection. Definitive treatment with surgery or radiotherapy should then be considered.

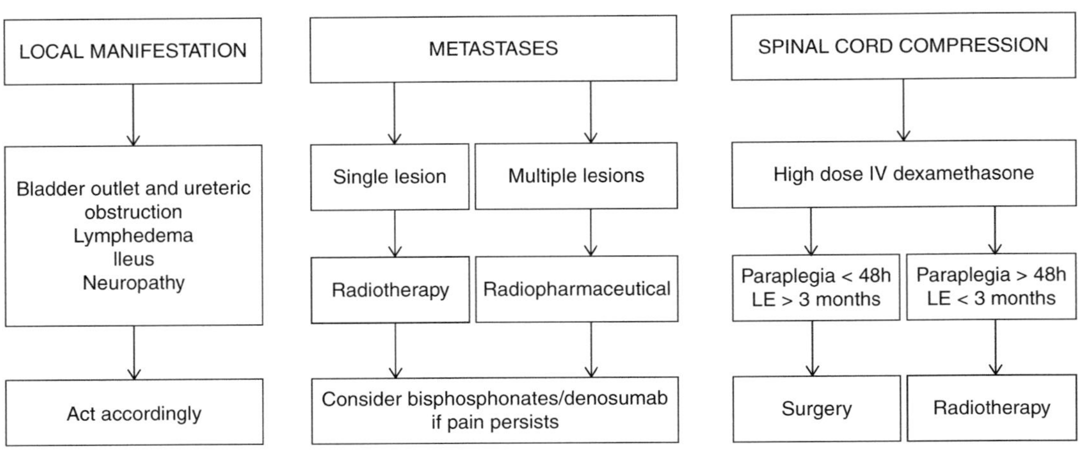

Modified from EAU Guidelines on Pain Management & Palliative Care, 2014

References

1. Cameron MG, Kersten C, Guren MG, Fosså SD, Vistad I. Palliative pelvic radiotherapy of symptomatic incurable prostate cancer—a systematic review. Radiother Oncol. 2014;110(1):55–60.
2. Banning A, Sjogren P, Henriksen H. Pain causes in 200 patients referred to a multidisciplinary cancer pain clinic. Pain. 1991;45(1):45–8.
3. Nielsen OS, Munro AJ, Tannock IF. Bone metastases: pathophysiology and management policy. J Clin Oncol. 1991;9(3):509–24.
4. Roodman GD. Mechanisms of bone metastasis. N Engl J Med. 2004;350(16):1655–64.
5. Wagner G. Frequency of pain in patients with cancer. Recent Results Cancer Res. 1984;89:64–71.
6. Porter AT, McEwan AJ, Powe JE, Reid R, McGowan DG, Lukka H, et al. Results of a randomized phase-III trial to evaluate the efficacy of strontium-89 adjuvant to local field external beam irradiation in the management of endocrine resistant metastatic prostate cancer. Int J Radiat Oncol Biol Phys. 1993;25(5):805–13.
7. Tiedje LB, Kingry MJ, Stommel M. Patient attitudes concerning health behaviors during pregnancy: initial development of a questionnaire. Health Educ Q. 1992;19(4):481–93.
8. Pathological fractures due to bone metastases. Br Med J (Clin Res Ed). 1981;283(6294):748.
9. Galasko CS. The management of skeletal metastases. J R Coll Surg Edinb. 1980;25(3):144–61.
10. Lane MD, Le HB, Lee S, Young C, Heran MK, Badii M, et al. Combination radiofrequency ablation and cementoplasty for palliative treatment of painful neoplastic bone metastasis: experience with 53 treated lesions in 36 patients. Skelet Radiol. 2011;40(1):25–32.
11. Miles CL, Fellowes D, Goodman ML, Wilkinson S. Laxatives for the management of constipation in palliative care patients. Cochrane Database Syst Rev. 2006;18(4):CD003448.
12. Smith MR. Zoledronic acid to prevent skeletal complications in cancer: corroborating the evidence. Cancer Treat Rev. 2005;31(Suppl 3):19–25.
13. Saad F, Gleason DM, Murray R, Tchekmedyian S, Venner P, Lacombe L. Long-term efficacy of zoledronic acid for the prevention of skeletal complications in patients with metastatic hormone-refractory prostate cancer. J Natl Cancer Inst. 2004;96(11):879–82.
14. Smith MR, McGovern FJ, Zietman AL, Fallon MA, Hayden DL, Schoenfeld DA, et al. Pamidronate to prevent bone loss during androgen-deprivation therapy for prostate cancer. N Engl J Med. 2001;345(13):948–55.
15. Smith MR, Eastham J, Gleason DM, Shasha D, Tchekmedyian S, Zinner N. Randomized controlled trial of zoledronic acid to prevent bone loss in men receiving androgen deprivation therapy for nonmetastatic prostate cancer. J Urol. 2003;169(6):2008–12.
16. Berry S, Waldron T, Winquist E, Lukka H. The use of bisphosphonates in men with hormone-refractory prostate cancer: a systematic review of randomized trials. Can J Urol. 2006;13(4):3180–8.
17. Van den Wyngaert T, Huizing MT, Fossion E, Vermorken JB. Bisphosphonates in oncology: rising stars or fallen heroes. Oncologist. 2009;14(2):181–91.
18. Fizazi K, Carducci M, Smith M, Damião R, Brown J, Karsh L, et al. Denosumab versus zoledronic acid for treatment of bone metastases in men with castration-resistant prostate cancer: a randomised, double-blind study. Lancet. 2011;377(9768):813–22.
19. Sartor O, Reid RH, Hoskin PJ, Quick DP, Ell PJ, Coleman RE, et al. Samarium-153-Lexidronam complex for treatment of painful bone metastases in hormone-refractory prostate cancer. Urology. 2004;63(5):940–5.
20. Roqué I, Figuls M, Martinez-Zapata MJ, Scott-Brown M, Alonso-Coello P. Radioisotopes for metastatic bone pain. Cochrane Database Syst Rev. 2011;(7):CD003347.
21. Tu SM, Millikan RE, Mengistu B, Delpassand ES, Amato RJ, Pagliaro LC, et al. Bone-targeted therapy for advanced androgen-independent carcinoma of the prostate: a randomised phase II trial. Lancet. 2001;357(9253):336–41.
22. Henriksen G, Fisher DR, Roeske JC, Bruland ØS, Larsen RH. Targeting of osseous sites with alpha-emitting 223Ra: comparison with the beta-emitter 89Sr in mice. J Nucl Med. 2003;44(2):252–9.
23. Parker C, Nilsson S, Heinrich D, Helle SI, O'Sullivan JM, Fosså SD, et al. Alpha emitter radium-223 and survival in metastatic prostate cancer. N Engl J Med. 2013;369(3):213–23.
24. Grossman SA, Lossignol D. Diagnosis and treatment of epidural metastases. Oncology (Williston Park). 1990;4(4):47–54; discussion 55,58.
25. George R, Jeba J, Ramkumar G, Chacko AG, Leng M, Tharyan P. Interventions for the treatment of metastatic extradural spinal cord compression in adults. Cochrane Database Syst Rev. 2015;9:CD006716.
26. Patchell RA, Tibbs PA, Regine WF, Payne R, Saris S, Kryscio RJ, et al. Direct decompressive surgical resection in the treatment of spinal cord compression caused by metastatic cancer: a randomised trial. Lancet. 2005;366(9486):643–8.

MIX
Papier aus verantwortungsvollen Quellen
Paper from responsible sources
FSC® C105338

If you have any concerns about our products,
you can contact us on
ProductSafety@springernature.com

In case Publisher is established outside the EU,
the EU authorized representative is:
Springer Nature Customer Service Center GmbH
Europaplatz 3, 69115 Heidelberg, Germany

Printed by Libri Plureos GmbH
in Hamburg, Germany

Berichte aus dem
Institut für Umformtechnik
der Universität Stuttgart
Herausgeber: Prof. Dr.-Ing. Dr. h.c. K. Lange

98

Wolfgang Schwab

Ermüdungsverhalten von massivumgeformten bauteilähnlichen Proben aus Stahl

Mit 81 Abbildungen und 3 Tabellen

Springer-Verlag Berlin
Heidelberg GmbH 1989

Dipl.-Ing. Wolfgang Schwab
Institut für Umformtechnik
Universität Stuttgart

Dr.-Ing. Dr. h. c. Kurt Lange
o. Professor em. an der Universität Stuttgart
Institut für Umformtechnik

D 93

ISBN 978-3-540-50805-2 ISBN 978-3-662-07112-0 (eBook)
DOI 10.1007/978-3-662-07112-0

Ursprünglich erschienen bei Springer-Verlag Berlin Heidelberg New York 1989.

Gesamtherstellung: Copydruck GmbH, Heimsheim
2362/3020—543210

GELEITWORT DES HERAUSGEBERS

Die Umformtechnik zeichnet sich durch sehr gute Werkstoffauswertung und hohe Mengenleistung in der Serienfertigung gegenüber anderen Fertigungsverfahren aus, wobei Beibehaltung der Masse, Änderung der Festigkeitseigenschaften während eines Vorgangs und elastische Rückfederung der Werkstücke nach einem Vorgang wesentliche Merkmale sind. Weiter sind die benötigten Kräfte, Arbeiten und Leistungen sehr viel größer als z.B. bei spanenden Verfahren. Die sichere Beherrschung eines Verfahrens in der industriellen Fertigung und die zunehmende Forderung nach Vermeidung bzw. Minimierung spanender Nacharbeit erzwingen die geschlossene Betrachtung des Systems 'Umformende Fertigung" unter zentraler Berücksichtigung plastizitätstheoretischer, werkstoffkundlicher und tribologischer Grundlagen.

Das Institut für Umformtechnik der Universität Stuttgart stellt entsprechend Forschung und Entwicklung zum einen auf die Erarbeitung von Grundlagenwissen in diesen Bereichen ab, zum anderen untersucht und entwickelt es Verfahren unter Anwendung spezieller Meßtechniken mit dem Ziel einer genauen quantitativen Ermittlung des Einflusses der Parameter von Vorgang, Werkstoff, Werkzeug und Maschine. Die Behandlung von Problemen des Maschinenverhaltens, der Maschinenkonstruktion sowie der Werkzeugauslegung und -beanspruchung, der Auswahl hochbeanspruchbarer, verschleißfester Werkzeugbaustoffe und schließlich der Tribologie gehört entsprechend ebenfalls zum Arbeitsgebiet, das durch die Erfassung organisatorischer und betriebswirtschaftlicher Fragen abgerundet wird.

Im Rahmen der "Berichte aus dem Institut für Umformtechnik" erscheinen in zwangloser Folge jährlich mehrere Bände, in denen über einzelne Themen ausführlich berichtet wird. Dabei handelt es sich vornehmlich um Abschlußberichte von Forschungsvorhaben, Dissertationen, aber gelegentlich auch um andere Texte. Diese Berichte sollen den in der Praxis stehenden Ingenieuren und Wissenschaftlern zur Weiterbildung dienen und eine Hilfe bei der Lösung umformtechnischer Aufgaben sein. Für die Studierenden bieten sie die Möglichkeit zur Vertiefung der Kenntnisse. Die seit zwei Jahrzehnten bewährte freundschaftliche Zusammenarbeit mit dem Springer-Verlag sehe ich als beste Voraussetzung für das Gelingen dieses Vorhabens an.

Kurt Lange

Vorwort

Die vorliegende Arbeit entstand während meiner Tätigkeit als wissenschaftlicher Mitarbeiter am Institut für Umformtechnik der Universität Stuttgart.

Herrn Professor Dr.-Ing. Dr. h. c. K. Lange danke ich für sein Vertrauen und seine wohlwollende Unterstützung bei der Durchführung der Arbeit.

Herrn Professor Dr.-Ing. K. H. Kloos bin ich für die eingehende Durchsicht dieser Arbeit und für wertvolle Anregungen zu Dank verpflichtet.

Mein Dank gilt ferner Herrn Dr.-Ing. habil. K. Pöhlandt für die Betreuung und kritische Durchsicht der Arbeit sowie allen Mitarbeiterinnen und Mitarbeitern des Instituts für Umformtechnik, die zum Gelingen der Arbeit beigetragen haben.

Die Mittel zur Durchführung der Untersuchung wurden von der Deutschen Forschungsgemeinschaft zur Verfügung gestellt. Für diese Förderung sei an dieser Stelle ebenfalls gedankt.

Leonberg-Eltingen, Juni 1988

Wolfgang Schwab

INHALTSVERZEICHNIS

Verzeichnis der wichtigsten Symbole

Allgemeine Zeichen

A	mm^2	Querschnittsfläche
A_g	%	Gleichmaßdehnung
A_V	J	Kerbschlagarbeit
A_5	%	Bruchdehnung
d	mm	Durchmesser
E	N/mm^2	Elastizitätsmodul
f	Hz	Frequenz
F	N	Kraft
F_a	N	Kraftamplitude
F_N	N	Nennkraft
F_{St}	N	Stempelkraft
h	mm	Höhe
k_f	N/mm^2	Fließspannung
L	mm	Länge
n	-	Verfestigungsexponent
N	-	Schwingspielzahl
N_B	-	Bruch-Schwingspielzahl
N_G	-	Grenz-Schwingspielzahl
r	mm	Radius
R	-	Spannungsverhältnis σ_u/σ_o
R_a	µm	Mittenrauhwert
R_m	N/mm^2	Zugfestigkeit
R_p	µm	Glättungstiefe
R_{pm}	µm	gemittelte Glättungstiefe
$R_{p0,2}$	N/mm^2	0,2-Dehngrenze
R_t	µm	Rauhtiefe
R_{ZDIN}	µm	gemittelte Rauhtiefe
t	mm	Kerbtiefe
T	°C	Temperatur
T_R	°C	Rohteiltemperatur
u_k	mm	Kerbaufweitung
u_{ka}	mm	Kerbaufweitungsamplitude
Z	%	Brucheinschnürung

α_k	-	Formzahl
ΔL	mm	Längenänderung
ΔN	-	Schwingspielzahländerung
$\Delta\varepsilon_m$	‰	Mitteldehnungsänderung
ε_a	‰	Dehnungsamplitude
ε_{ar}	‰	plastische Dehnungsamplitude
$\varepsilon_{ar}^{(ij)}$	‰	plastische Dehnungsamplitude von Meßebene i und DMS j (i = 1...3; j = 1...4)
ε_{at}	‰	Gesamtdehnungsamplitude
ε_{kt}	‰	Kerbgrundgesamtdehnung
ε_{kat}	‰	Kerbgrundgesamtdehnungsamplitude
ε_m	‰	Mitteldehnung
ε_t	%	Gesamtdehnung
ε_v	-	Vergleichsformänderung
ρ	mm	Kerbradius
σ	N/mm^2	Spannung
σ_a	N/mm^2	Spannungsamplitude
σ_{dF}	N/mm^2	Druckfließgrenze
σ_{dF}^K	N/mm^2	Druckfließgrenze im Kernbereich
σ_{dF}^R	N/mm^2	Druckfließgrenze im Randbereich
σ_E	N/mm^2	Eigenspannung
σ_{Ea}	N/mm^2	Axial-Eigenspannung
σ_{Et}	N/mm^2	Tangential-Eigenspannung
σ_{Er}	N/mm^2	Radial-Eigenspannung
σ_E^K	N/mm^2	Kerneigenspannung
σ_E^R	N/mm^2	Randeigenspannung
σ_{ka}	N/mm^2	Kerbspannungsamplitude
σ_m	N/mm^2	Mittelspannung
σ_n	N/mm^2	Nennspannung
σ_{na}	N/mm^2	Nennspannungsamplitude
σ_o	N/mm^2	Oberspannung
φ	-	Umformgrad
$\dot{\varphi}$	s^{-1}	Umformgeschwindigkeit
ψ	grd	Meßwinkel für die Probendrehung im Diffraktometer
2α	grd	Schulteröffnungswinkel

Abkürzungen

DMS	Dehnungsmeßstreifen
ES	Eigenspannung
FEM	Finite-Elemente-Methode
HRC	Rockwellhärte
HV	Vickershärte
IEC	International Electrotechnical Commission
REM	Rasterelektronenmikroskopie
RT	Raumtemperatur
SFE	Stapelfehlerenergie
Ssp	Schwingspiel
TEM	Transmissionselektronenmikroskopie
V	Vergrößerung
VVFP	Voll-Vorwärts-Fließpressen
Wz	Werkzeug

Indizes

min	Minimal...
max	Maximal...
0	Anfangs...
1	End...

0 EINLEITUNG

Der zunehmende Einsatz der Leichtbauweise erforderte im Rahmen der Betriebssicherheit und Wirtschaftlichkeit eine genaue Kenntnis der Belastung und Belastbarkeit der verwendeten Bauteile. Liegen hierüber - vornehmlich unter dem Aspekt der Schwingfestigkeit - gesicherte Informationen vor, so kann bei einer funktionsgerechten Gestaltung der Bauteile neben einer gezielten Werkstoffauswahl und besseren Werkstoffausnutzung eine effektivere Auswahl der Fertigungsverfahren vorgenommen werden. In diesem Zusammenhang liefern die Verfahren der Umformtechnik einen wichtigen Beitrag; sie sind energie- und werkstoffsparend, haben kurze Herstellzeiten und verbessern in vielen Fällen die Gebrauchseigenschaften. Das gilt insbesondere für solche Umformverfahren, bei denen sich eine fertigungsbedingte Werkstoffverfestigung neben einer hohen Maß- und Formgenauigkeit einstellt. Das führt oft unter Verwendung von Ausgangswerkstoffen niedriger Festigkeit und unter Einsparung etwaiger Fertigungsstufen (z. B. Wärmebehandlung) zu einbaufertigen oder nahezu einbaufertigen Werkstücken (neudeutsche Umschreibung mit "Near Net Shape Technology"). Hierbei erfordert eine Verbesserung der Bauteilendeigenschaften eine ganzheitliche Betrachtung und Optimierung von Werkstoff, Fertigung und konstruktiver Gestaltung.

Erfahrungsgemäß führen zeitlich veränderliche Beanspruchungen im Vergleich zu rein statischen aufgrund von Ermüdungsvorgängen im Werkstoff zu einer abnehmenden Bauteilfestigkeit. Zur Untersuchung der strukturmechanischen Änderungen im Werkstoff bei schwingender Beanspruchung eignen sich Hysteresismessungen. Dabei ist für die Bewertung des Ermüdungsverhaltens von fundamentaler Bedeutung, daß das Versagen durch plastische Verformungen über hinreichend viele Schwingspiele verursacht wird. Der Betrag der irreversiblen plastischen Dehnungsamplitude - die halbe Breite der Hysteresisschleife - kann bei aufgeprägten Belastungen unterhalb der makroskopischen Streckgrenze im Bereich der Mikroverformung liegen und dennoch zum Ermüdungsbruch führen /1/.

1 STAND DER KENNTNISSE

Nach DIN 8582 bzw. 8583 werden die Fertigungsverfahren der Umformtechnik "Voll-Vorwärts-Fließpressen" und "Verjüngen von Vollkörpern" in die Untergruppe der Durchdrückverfahren eingeordnet; in der industriellen Praxis gehören sie zu den Verfahren der Massivumformung. In den meisten Veröffentlichungen werden die Werkstückeigenschaften nach der Umformung durch statische Festigkeitskennwerte beschrieben /2-4/; über das dynamische Werkstoff- bzw. Bauteilverhalten sind im Schrifttum noch wenig Arbeiten zu finden. Da es sich zudem bei diesen Untersuchungen vorwiegend um kleinere Umformgrade beim Längen ($\varphi \leq 0{,}2$) handelt, erscheint es schwierig, Schlußfolgerungen für Umformgrade beim Fließpressen für $\varphi > 0{,}5$ zu ziehen. Außerdem sind die vorliegenden Ergebnisse oft unheitlich, was größtenteils auf die Oberflächenbeschaffenheit der Proben zurückzuführen ist. Weiterhin wird oft nur die Lebensdauer bis zum Bruch bzw. bis zum Anriß registriert und auf die Erfassung wichtiger Informationen während der Schwingbeanspruchung verzichtet. Zur Beurteilung des Ermüdungsverhaltens eignen sich z. B. die Deformation und die Temperatur als Indikator für strukturmechanische Abläufe im Werkstoff.

In der vorliegenden Arbeit interessiert vornehmlich eine Kaltumformung, die den ganzen Querschnitt des Werkstücks erfaßt. Im Gegensatz dazu steht die örtliche Kaltumformung beispielsweise durch Kugelstrahlen oder Glatt- und Festwalzen einer dünnen Schicht an der Werkstückoberfläche: dabei wird die Randzone verfestigt und es werden Druckeigenspannungen I. Art an der Oberfläche induziert, was sich dauerfestigkeitssteigernd auswirkt /5-10/.

Nach Hempel /11/ erhöht Kaltumformen durch Strecken, Fließpressen, Stauchen, Ziehen und Walzen zwar die Dauerfestigkeit, aber in weit geringerem Maße als die Streckgrenze und die Zugfestigkeit. Das Verhältnis der Wechselfestigkeit zur Zugfestigkeit nimmt mit wachsendem Umformgrad ab (Versuchswerte für unlegierte Stähle aus /12/). Neben dem Umformgrad beeinflußt die Umformgeschwindigkeit die Wechselfestigkeit. Bei unlegierten Stählen nimmt die Wechselfestigkeit infolge der Erhöhung der dynamischen Streckgrenze zu, während die instabilen austenitischen Stähle an Wechselfestigkeit verlieren, da sich bei hohen Umformgeschwindigkeiten weniger Austenit in Martensit umwandelt.

In /13/ wird vom Einfluß einer durch Längsdehnen aufgebrachten Kaltverformung auf das Anreiß- bzw. Zeitfestigkeitsverhalten von glatten Proben (mechanisch poliert in Längsrichtung auf $R_t \approx 1$ µm) aus Ck15N im Biegewechselversuch berichtet. Maier kommt dabei zu dem Schluß, daß es einen optimalen Verformungsgrad (Brucheinschnürung $Z = (A_0 - A)/A_0$ mit dem Bruchquerschnitt A) zwischen 25 und 40 % gibt, bei welchem zunehmende Verfestigung und abnehmendes Verformungsvermögen eine maximale Lebensdauer ergeben.

Durch eine vorangegangene Zugumformung an normalisierten Stahlblechen (zentrale Kerbe in Form einer Bohrung mit 2 mm Durchmesser) wird bei schwingender Beanspruchung (R = 0 und 0,125) die Rißeinleitungsphase verzögert und bei einer Kaltumformung von 6 und 9 % die Rißfortschrittsrate um den Faktor 2,4 und 3,7 verringert /14/. An ähnlichen Proben aus StE47 und STE70 (DIN 17006; auf bleibende Dehnungen von 1 und 5 % dehnungsgesteuert gelängt und anschließend gelocht, $\alpha_k = 2,5$) stellen Sonsino und Hagedorn /15/ aufgrund der Festigkeitssteigerung eine Lebensdauererhöhung im Zeitfestigkeitsgebiet ($\geq 5 \cdot 10^4$ Schwingspiele) fest. Im Bereich der Kurzzeitfestigkeit ($< 5 \cdot 10^4$ Schwingspiele) ist beim StE47 mit zunehmender Kaltverformung eine deutliche Minderung der Anrißlebensdauer zu erkennen. Parker und Montgomery /16/ beobachten an 40 % gleichmäßig biaxial gedehnten unlegierten Stahlproben (SAE 1008) ebenfalls eine geringere Lebensdauer im Bereich der Kurzzeitermüdung infolge reduzierter Werkstoffzähigkeit. Im dehnungskontrollierten Versuch zeigt der Werkstoff eine schnelle zyklische Entfestigung in der Anfangsphase und geht dann in einen Beharrungszustand über.

Um den Einfluß der Kaltverformung auf die Werkstoffeigenschaften der Stähle Ck15, Ck35 und 34Cr4 möglichst eindeutig nachweisen zu können, wählt Flemming /17/ als Modellversuche den einachsigen Zug- und Stauchversuch. Die Art der Probenherstellung und die Probenform sind darauf ausgerichtet, daß die Proben möglichst homogen umgeformt und frei von Eigenspannungen I. Art (einschließlich Bearbeitungsspannungen; Proben elektrolytisch poliert auf $R_t \approx 0{,}14$ µm, $R_p \approx 0{,}04$ µm und $R_a \approx 0{,}06$ µm) sind. Kleine Umformgrade ($\varphi \leq 0{,}05$) führen zu einem 10 bis 20 %-igen Abfall der Dauerfestigkeit, mittlere und hohe Umformgrade ($\varphi \leq 0{,}25$ beim Längen und $\varphi \leq 0{,}85$ beim Stauchen) dagegen verbessern die Wechselfestigkeit. Der Abfall beruht auf Eigenspannungen und ist von der Gefügehomogenität sowie der Fließgrenze des nicht umgeformten Werkstoffes abhängig. Der Anstieg der Dauerfestigkeit entspricht der Werkstoffverfestigung im statischen Versuch. Die Grenze zwischen beiden Bereichen ist werkstoffabhängig und liegt etwa bei $\varphi \approx 0{,}1$. Von diesem Umformgrad an überwiegt der Einfluß der Verfestigung den Einfluß der entfestigenden Eigenspannungen. Bilý /18/ führt Untersuchungen von Černjak /19/ an, welche die Ergebnisse von Flemming bestätigen.

Die Dauerfestigkeit eines Werkstoffs nimmt ab, wenn beim Herstellen, Weiterverarbeiten, Wärmebehandeln oder unter Betriebsbeanspruchung Oberflächenverletzungen auftreten, wie Narben, Kratzer oder Ziehriefen, Warmrisse, Zunderschichten oder Randentkohlung /11/. In diesem Zusammenhang untersuchte Woodward /20/ die Dauerfestigkeit von Proben aus verschiedenen Aluminiumlegierungen im stranggepreßten und gewalzten Zustand ohne spanende Nachbearbeitung. Bei 10^7 Schwingspielen liegt das Verhältnis Dauerfestigkeit unbearbeiteter Proben aus stranggepreßten Rundstangen zu bearbeiteten Proben aus der Legierung HE15-WP (entsprechend AlCuSiMnwa nach DIN 1725) zwischen 0,4 und 0,75. Die Entfernung einer 0,63 mm dicken Oberflächenschicht von stranggepreßten Rundstäben der obengenannten Legierung bewirkt eine Zunahme der Dauerfestigkeit bis zu einem Wert, der nur geringfügig unterhalb dem von kleinen Proben mit polierter Oberfläche liegt. Gewalzte Stäbe ähnlicher Legierungszusammensetzung zeigen ebenfalls eine verminderte Dauerfestigkeit, wenn sie im Walzzustand geprüft werden.

Ein wesentlicher Vorteil fließgepreßter Werkstücke ist der formgerechte Faserverlauf auch bei komplizierten Werkstücken. Wegen des Einflusses der Faserorientierung auf das statische und dynamische Bauteilverhalten ist darauf zu achten, daß die Faserrichtung mit der Richtung der höchsten Zugbelastung übereinstimmt /21/. Nach Hertel /5/ haben Versuche mit Rundstäben aus AlCuMg1 gezeigt, daß sich bei gleicher Lebensdauer für Längsfaserproben um 25 % höhere Spannungsamplituden einstellen.

Ein typisches Beispiel, bei dem die beiden Durchdrückverfahren Fließpressen und Verjüngen in Kombination mit dem Umformverfahren Stauchen angewendet werden, ist die Schraubenherstellung. An fließgepreßten und konventionell gefertigten (vergüteten) Schrauben überprüfte Flemming /17/, inwieweit seine - an den Modellversuchen Längen und Stauchen - gewonnenen Erkenntnisse auf reale Bauteile zu übertragen sind. Außerdem wurden zum Vergleich mit den gelängten und gestauchten Proben aus den über dem Querschnitt inhomogen umgeformten Schrauben Proben herausgearbeitet. Die Versuche an fließgepreßten Proben und Schrauben zeigen weitgehend das gleiche Werkstoffverhalten wie die gestauchten Proben. Die Festigkeitswerte der fließgepreßten Proben liegen trotz vergleichbarer Werkstoffe und Umformgrade deutlich über den gestauchten Proben. Dies dürfte durch die unterschiedliche Gefügeorientierung bedingt sein: während die Textur beim Stauchen quer zur Belastungsrichtung verläuft, liegt sie beim fließgepreßten Werkstoff in Belastungsrichtung. Die Eigenspannungen entsprechen allerdings denen des gestauchten Werkstoffes. Wegen der geringen Verfestigungsfähigkeit des kaltumgeformten Werkstoffes beim Gewindewalzen liegt die Dauerfestigkeit fließgepreßter Schrauben unter der vergüteter Schrauben. Erfolgt das Gewindewalzen vor dem Vergüten, ist die Dauerfestigkeit fließgepreßter Schrauben höher. Bei der Fertigung von Verbindungselementen aus austenitischen Werkstoffen mit gezielter Beeinflußung der Bauteilendeigenschaften kommt der Kaltumformung eine dominierende Bedeutung zu. Denn nur durch Kaltumformen läßt sich unter Beibehaltung der Korrosionsbeständigkeit - im Gegensatz zu thermischen Verfahren - die Bauteilfestigkeit steigern. Dabei weisen solche Schrauben der Güten A2 und A3 (DIN 276, Bl. 11) trotz niedrigerer Festigkeitswerte gegenüber Schrauben der Güte 8.8 (unlegierte oder niedriglegierte Stähle; DIN 276, Bl. 3 und 4) mindestens gleiche Dauerhaltbarkeit auf /22, 23/. Ergebnisse von einer umfassenden Untersuchung zur Dauerhaltbarkeit von Schraubenverbindungen sind in /24/ zusammengefaßt.

Während das Fließpressen üblicherweise mit starren Werkzeugen bei Raumtemperatur bzw. auch nach Anwärmen der Rohteile auf eine Temperatur im Bereich der Erholung und Rekristallisation durchgeführt wird, benutzt man beim hydrostatischen Fließpressen ein Wirkmedium (Hydraulikflüssigkeit) zur Kraftübertragung auf das Werkstück (siehe DIN 8583). Im Bereich der Preßschulter herrschen dadurch sehr günstige Reibungsbedingungen, was in Verbindung mit dem Wegfall der Reibung zwischen Rohteil und Aufnehmer zu einem verminderten Kraftbedarf führt /25/. Kerspe /26/ hat die Wöhlerlinien für hydrostatisch und konventionell fließgepreßte Werkstücke (φ = 1,3 u. 2α = 40°; σ_m = 240 N/mm^2 = konst.) gegenübergestellt. Hydrostatisch fließgepreßte Proben zeigen eine höhere Dauerfestigkeit, da beim Preßvorgang die starke Schubbelastung durch verringerte Reibung wesentlich herabgesetzt ist und somit in der Randzone eine etwas homogenere Umformung erreicht wird. Hydrostatisches Fließpressen mit einem Schulteröffnungswinkel der Matrize 2α = 40° und einem Umformgrad φ = 1,3 bewirkt im Vergleich zu φ = 1,0 höhere Lebensdauerwerte der Werkstücke bei gleicher Oberspannung σ_o (σ_m = 240 N/mm^2). Durch die Vergrößerung des Schulteröffnungswinkels von 40 auf 60° bei konstantem Umformgrad (φ = 1,3) stellen sich höhere Schwingfestigkeitswerte bei gleicher Schwingspielzahl ein, bei 2α = 90° hingegen fällt die Dauerfestigkeit ab, was der Autor durch den scharfkantigen Übergang zwischen Schulter und Fließpreßschaft erklärt (Kerbeffekt).

Beim Halbwarmumformen verfolgt man das Ziel, die Vorzüge des Warmumformens - geringere Kräfte, besseres Formänderungsvermögen - mit jenen des Kaltumformens - erhöhte Genauigkeit, gute

Oberflächenqualität - zu verbinden. Die Fließspannung wird beträchtlich herabgesetzt; bei Stahl ist sie z. B. für den Bereich $500 \leq T_R \leq 750$ °C um 30 bis 70 % geringer als bei Raumtemperatur /27/. Soweit bekannt, wird im Schrifttum nur für halbwarmfließgepreßte Sinterstähle über die Gebrauchseigenschaften unter dynamischer Beanspruchung berichtet. Schaub /28/ zeigt im Umlaufbiegeversuch (DIN 50113), daß der eingesetzte Sinterwerkstoff WPL 200 + 1 % MCM nach dem Halbwarmfließpressen (Proben aus den Werkstücken entnommen) im Vergleich zu äquivalenten Werkstoffen nach dem Sinterschmieden /29/ höhere Schwingfestigkeitswerte aufweist ($\Delta\sigma_a \approx 40$ N/mm^2).

Auf das Schmieden (Warmumformung) soll in diesem Zusammenhang nicht näher eingegangen werden; die Auswirkung der Einflußgrößen - Werkstoffgrundfestigkeit, Umformgrad, Schmiedetemperatur, Randentkohlung, Gratbildung etc. - auf die Schwingfestigkeit ist in /30-32/ beschrieben.

2 AUFGABENSTELLUNG

Die Schrifttumsrecherche zeigte, daß wenig fundierte Grundlagen über den Einfluß von Verfahrensparametern beim Fließpressen auf das Ermüdungsverhalten umgeformter Bauteile vorliegen.

Das Ziel der vorliegenden Arbeit ist es daher, einen Beitrag zu der angesprochenen Thematik zu leisten. Auf der Basis dieser Grundlagenuntersuchung werden Aussagen über diejenigen Verfahrensparameter gemacht, bei denen sich günstige Werkstückeigenschaften einstellen. Außerdem wird nach Möglichkeit versucht, einige Hinweise für die Konstruktion und Fertigung von schwingend beanspruchten Bauteilen zu geben.

Der Einfluß von Verfahrensparametern bei der Kalt- und Halbwarmmassivumformung auf das Ermüdungsverhalten der Werkstücke soll am Beispiel des Voll-Vorwärts-Fließpressens und Verjüngens untersucht werden. Zu diesem Zweck werden der Umformgrad, die Temperatur der Rohteile, der Schulteröffnungswinkel der Matrize und die Schmierungsbedingungen bei der Umformung variiert.

Für die Schwingprüfung sollen bauteilähnliche Proben hergestellt werden, die durch ihre gebunden umgeformte Oberfläche Bauteilendeigenschaften aufweisen. In diesem Zusammenhang wird eine numerische Simulation der kompletten Stufenfolge mit Hilfe der Finite-Elemente-Methode zur Berechnung des lokalen Umformgrades durchgeführt. Zur weiteren Charakterisierung der Schwingproben ist neben einer Ermittlung der Verformungseigenspannungen und mechanischen Kennwerte die Gefügeausbildung und Oberflächenstruktur nach der Umformung zu betrachten.

Die Untersuchung der makroskopischen Änderungen im Werkstoff macht den Aufbau eines Schwingprüfstandes mit der notwendigen Meß- und Datenverarbeitungstechnik erforderlich. Ein Rechnerprogramm zur Steuerung des Meßablaufs, der Meßwerterfassung, der Datenreduktion und Datenverarbeitung ist dafür zu erstellen. Die Ergebnisse sind in Form von Wechselverformungskurven, Wöhlerkurven (S/N-Kurven) und zyklischen Spannungs-Dehnungskurven darzustellen.

Die Werkstücke sollen ohne nachträgliche Bearbeitung der Oberfläche in Einstufenversuchen bei reiner Wechselbeanspruchung geprüft werden. Zu Vergleichszwecken werden Versuche mit unterschiedlichen Mittelspannungen gefahren, und die Wechselverformungskurven nicht umgeformter sowie weitgehend homogen umgeformter Proben (Entnahme aus dem Kernbereich umgeformter Werkstücke) aufgenommen. Weiterhin ist auch auf den Einfluß verschiedener Versuchsführungen, auf die Versuchsfrequenz und auf Kerbeffekte einzugehen.

Zur Deutung des Wechselverformungsverhaltens fließgepreßter Werkstücke sollen elektronenmikroskopische Untersuchungen durchgeführt werden. Diese beziehen sich einerseits auf die Ermüdungsfeinstruktur (Versetzungsanordnung) und andererseits auf das Bruchverhalten (Rißinitiierung, Rißfortschritt und Gewaltbruch).

3 VERSUCHSVORBEREITUNG

3.1 VERSUCHSPLAN

Der Einfluß von Verfahrensparametern beim Massivumformen auf das Ermüdungsverhalten der Werkstücke wird anhand der in Bild 2 aufgeführten Untersuchungen ermittelt. Dazu werden die Umformverfahren Voll-Vorwärts-Fließpressen (VVFP) und Verjüngen (Bild 1) gewählt und die folgenden Verfahrensparameter variiert:

- Umformgrad φ: $0{,}5 \le \varphi \le 1{,}6$ (VVFP) und $0{,}1 \le \varphi \le 0{,}3$ (Verjüngen);
- Schulteröffnungswinkel 2α: $30^{o} \le 2\alpha \le 150^{o}$ (VVFP) und $15^{o} \le 2\alpha \le 30^{o}$ (Verjüngen);
- Rohteiltemperatur T_R: RT, $500 \le T_R \le 700$ °C (VVFP);
- Schmierung: Alkaliseife in Lösung (Bonderlube 234) und wässrige MoS_2-Suspension (Molydag 15) für das Kaltfließpressen und im Halbwarmbereich wässrige Graphitdispersion für Rohteil (Delta 144) und Werkzeug (Stempel und Matrize; Stuart M1905);
- Geometrie: Glatte und gekerbte bauteilähnliche Proben mit kreisförmigem Prüfquerschnitt.

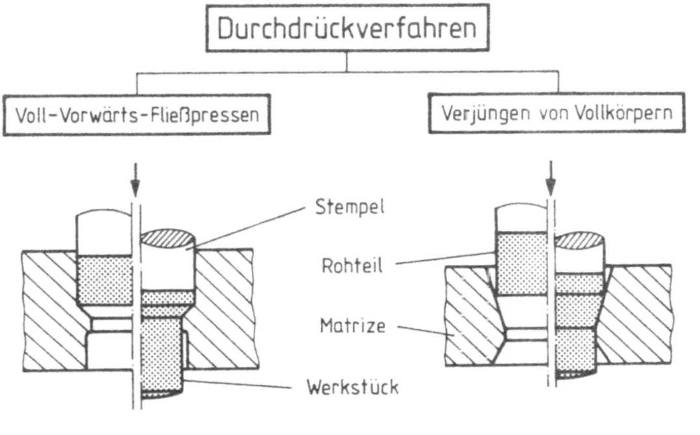

Bild 1: Prinzipdarstellung der eingesetzten Durchdrückverfahren.

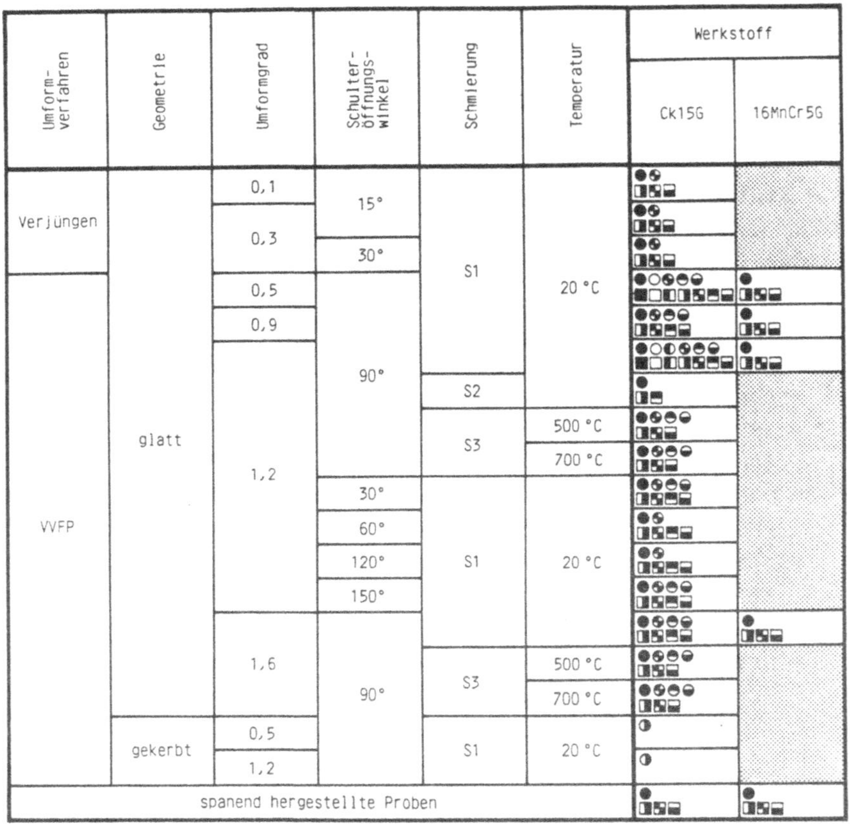

- Ermittlung der Wechselverformungskurven (Hysteresisaufnahmen; σ_a = konst. bzw. ε_{at} = konst.)
- Wechselverformungsverhalten von Proben aus dem Kern massivumgeformter Werkstücke
- Mitteldehnungskurven ($\sigma_m \neq 0$)
- Kerbgrundtotaldehnungskurven
- Wöhlerlinie / Zyklische Spannungs-Dehnungskurve
- Fraktographie (REM)
- Ermüdungsfeinstruktur (TEM)
- Werkstofffluß (Visioplasticity)
- Lokale Verfestigung (FEM)
- Eigenspannungsanalyse
- Mechanische Kennwerte
- Härteprofil
- Oberflächenbeschaffenheit
- Gefügeausbildung

S1 Phosphatschicht + Zinkseife (Bonderlube 234)

S2 Phosphatschicht + wässrige MoS_2-Suspension (Molydag 15)

S3 Rohteil: Wasserige Graphitdispersion (Delta 144)
Werkzeug: Wasserloslicher Öl-Graphit (Stuart M1905)

Bild 2: Untersuchungsprogramm.

Die Untersuchungen werden hauptsächlich mit dem unlegierten Fließpreßstahl Ck15G durchgeführt; in einigen Stichversuchen wird als weiterer Werkstoff 16MnCr5G geprüft.

Das Versuchsprogramm besteht aus drei Abschnitten:

- Erfassung der Eigenschaften der Werkstoffe vor der Umformung (Mechanische Kennwerte aus Zug- und Stauchversuch, Härte, Gefüge);
- Charakterisierung der bauteilähnlichen Proben (Werkstoff nach der Umformung). Außer den mechanischen Kennwerten aus Zug-, Stauch- und Kerbschlagbiegeversuch, dem Härteprofil, der Gefügeausbildung und Oberflächenbeschaffenheit, wird der örtliche Umformgrad berechnet und der Eigenspannungszustand experimentell ermittelt;
- Untersuchung der makroskopischen Auswirkung einzelner Versuchsparameter (Verfahrensparameter, Frequenz, Versuchsführung, etc.) auf das Ermüdungsverhalten. Dabei wird das Reaktionsverhalten des verfestigten Werkstoffs unter schwingender Beanspruchung aufgrund von Hysteresismessungen in Form von Wechselverformungskurven und zyklischen Spannungs-Dehnungskurven aufgezeigt sowie begleitende elektronenmikroskopische Untersuchungen (REM und TEM) durchgeführt. Zur lebensdauerorientierten Bewertung werden in Einstufenversuchen Wöhlerkurven aufgenommen.

Bei den Schwingproben handelt es sich vornehmlich um Fließpreßteile, deren Oberfläche keiner nachträglichen Behandlung unterzogen werden. Der Randzoneneinfluß wird untersucht, indem Proben aus dem Innern der Werkstücke (nahezu homogener Kernbereich mit quasistationärem Werkstofffluß) entnommen werden.

3.2 WERKSTOFF

Die Werkstoffe (Tabelle 1) lagen im Anlieferungszustand in Form warmgewalzter Stäbe vor.

Werkstoff-Bezeichnung (Werkstoff-Nr.)	C %	Si %	Mn %	P %	S %	Cr %
Ck15 (1.1141)	0,16	0,24	0,57	0,013	0,029	-
16MnCr5 (1.7131)	0,15	0,29	1,17	0,012	0,028	0,87

Tabelle 1: Chemische Analyse der Versuchswerkstoffe.

3.2.1 Gefügeausbildung

Zum Fließpressen wurde ein Werkstoffausgangszustand mit möglichst günstigem Dehnungsverhalten (niedrige Fließspannung und geringe Verfestigung) durch eine entsprechende Wärmebehandlung erreicht. Zu diesem Zweck wurden die beiden Stähle bei Temperaturen knapp unterhalb A_1 (720 °C) weichgeglüht mit anschließender Ofenabkühlung. Die Glühdauer wurde dabei für Ck15 auf 5 h und für 16MnCr5 auf 10 h angesetzt. Zur Beurteilung des Gefüges im Anlieferungszustand sowie nach dem Glühen wurden mikroskopische Schliffbilder angefertigt. Bild 3 zeigt die Gefügestruktur für die aus Ferrit und Perlit bestehenden Versuchswerkstoffe. Aus der Darstellung der beiden Zustände geht hervor, daß das Einformen des lamellaren Perlits zu körnigem Perlit durch das Weichglühen weitgehend erreicht wurde. Im Temperaturbereich nahe A_{c1} geht die Festigkeit des Zementits soweit zurück, daß die Lamellenstruktur aufreißt. Der kugelförmige Zementit im körnigen Perlit bietet der weichen, zähen, ferritischen Grundmasse einen verminderten Fließwiderstand bzw. verbessertes Formänderungsvermögen /33/. Dabei kann die Korngröße für den vorliegenden Ausgangszustand nach ASTM mit 7 ÷ 8 angegeben werden.

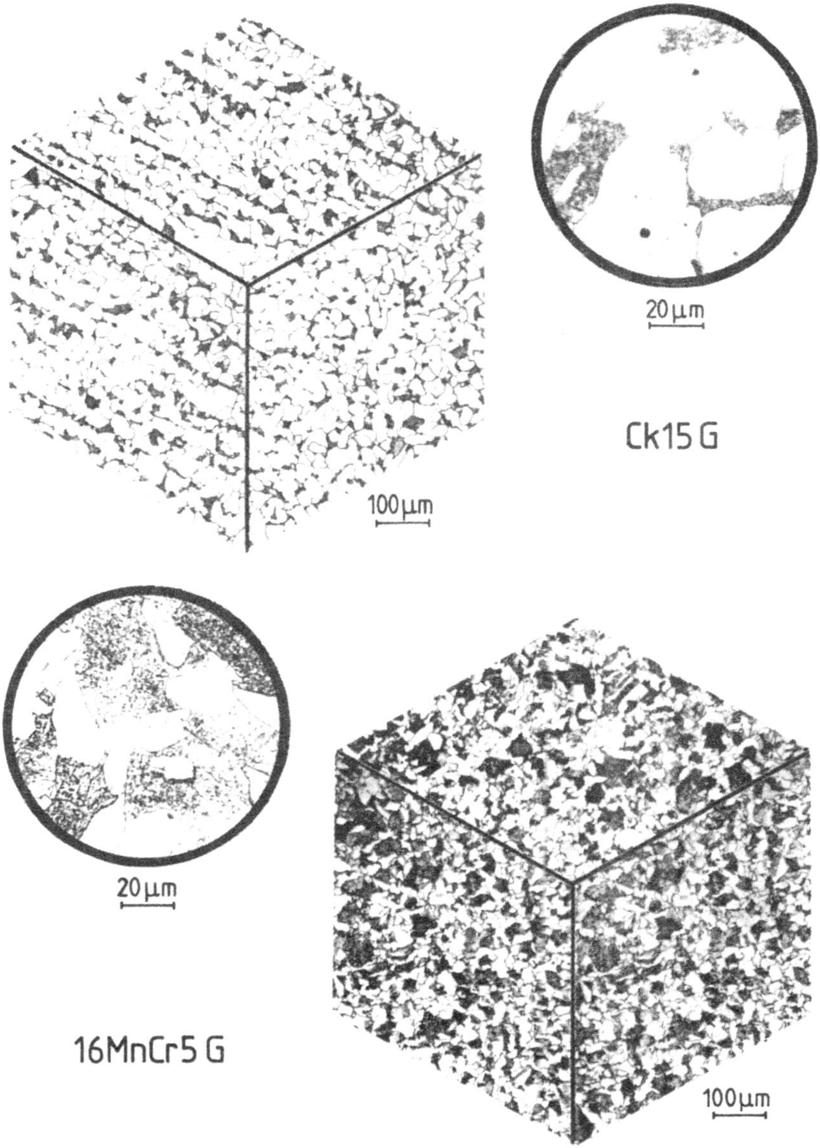

Bild 3: Gefügeaufnahmen der Versuchswerkstoffe Ck15 und 16MnCr5 im weichgeglühten Ausgangszustand.

3.2.2 Mechanische Kennwerte

Für die Ermittlung der mechanischen Eigenschaften der Werkstoffe im Ausgangszustand wurden an Proben aus der Stabmitte Härtemessungen und Zugversuche durchgeführt sowie die Fließkurven im Stauchversuch aufgenommen. Die mechanischen Kennwerte sind in Tabelle 2 zusammengefaßt.

Mechanische Kennwerte \ Werkstoff	Ck15		16MnCr5	
	ungeglüht	weichgeglüht	ungeglüht	weichgeglüht
Zugfestigkeit R_m N/mm²	472	414	622	490
0,2-Dehngrenze $R_{p0,2}$ N/mm²	354	304	372	293
Streckgrenzenverhältnis $R_{p0,2}/R_m$	0,75	0,73	0,60	0,60
Verfestigungsexponent n	0,20	0,23	0,16	0,20
Gleichmaßdehnung A_g %	23	25	17	22
Bruchdehnung A_5 %	37	42	29	36
Brucheinschnürung Z %	65	73	63	71
Härte HV5	155	112	179	150

Tabelle 2: Mechanische Eigenschaften der Versuchswerkstoffe im ungeglühten und weichgeglühten Zustand.

Die Fließkurven wurden im Stauchversuch mit mindestens drei zylindrischen Probekörpern (d_0 = 10 mm, h_0 = 16 mm) zwischen ebenen parallelen Stauchbahnen aufgenommen. Die Fließkurven bei Raumtemperatur wurden mit einer Umformgeschwindigkeit im Bereich $0{,}02 \leq \dot{\varphi} \leq 0{,}03$ auf einer hydraulischen Universalprüfmaschine (Hersteller Losenhausen, F_N = 400 kN) ermittelt. Dagegen wurden die Fließkurven bei 500 und 700 °C auf einer Exzenterpresse (Hersteller Schuler, F_N = 1000 kN) mit $\dot{\varphi} \approx 38\ s^{-1}$ erfaßt (dies entspricht in etwa der Umformgeschwindigkeit beim Halbwarmumformen). Die Fließkurven für die beiden Versuchswerkstoffe sind in Bild 4 zusammengestellt.

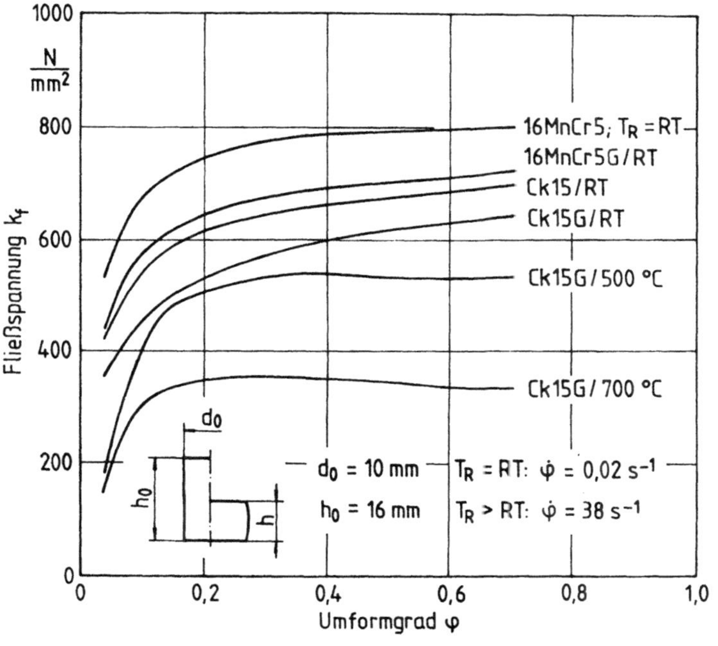

Bild 4: Fließkurven der Versuchswerkstoffe Ck15G und 16MnCr5G bei RT und $500 \leq T_R \leq 700$ °C.

3.3 HERSTELLUNG BAUTEILÄHNLICHER PROBEN

Im Hinblick auf die Schwingprüfung der Fließpreßteile, ohne nachträgliche Bearbeitung der gebunden umgeformten Schaftoberfläche, ist das Einspannen der Werkstücke problematisch. Normalerweise läßt sich das fließgepreßte Werkstück in drei Bereiche - Kopf-, Schulter- und Schaftteil - einteilen und zeigt unterschiedliche Verfestigung bzw. mechanische Eigenschaften durch unterschiedlichen Werkstofffluß. Die gewählte Vorgehensweise bei der Herstellung der Werkstücke wird im nächsten Abschnitt behandelt.

3.3.1 Stadienplan

Zur Fertigung der verwendeten Schwingproben (Bild 5) wurden, ausgehend von einem Schaftdurchmesser d_1 = 15 mm beim Voll-Vorwärts-Fließpressen und Verjüngen, die Umformbedingungen durch eine entsprechend gewählte Rohteilgeometrie (d_0, h_0) variiert. Dabei wurde ein Schaft mit quasistationärem Werkstofffluß und einer Ausgangslänge von 105 mm für das anschließende Kopfanstauchen benötigt. Die Rohteile wurden gesägt, vorgedreht, weichgeglüht (siehe Abschnitt 3.2.1) und fertiggedreht (Entfernen der randentkohlten Schicht). Die entfetteten Rohteile wurden für die Kaltmassivumformung durch Zink-Phosphatieren mit einer Schmierstoffträgerschicht (10 ÷ 15 µm Schichtdicke) versehen und dann entweder beseift (Bonderlube 234) oder in wässrige MoS_2-Suspension (Molydag 15) getaucht und getrommelt. Für die Halbwarmumformung wurden die

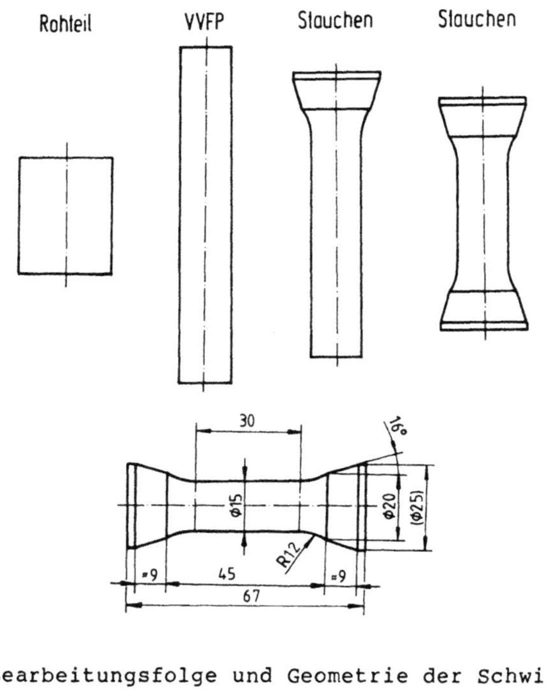

Bild 5: Bearbeitungsfolge und Geometrie der Schwingproben.

Rohteile zur besseren Haftung des Schmierstoffs auf rd. 100 °C vorgewärmt und mit wässriger Graphitdispersion Delta 144 beschichtet und im elektrisch beheizten Kammerofen auf die jeweilige Umformtemperatur gebracht. Die Rohteile wurden auf einer weggebundenen Exzenterpresse (Hersteller Schuler, F_N = 2000 kN) bis ca. 2 mm Kopfhöhe fließgepreßt; mit dem nächsten Rohteil wurde das Werkstück vollständig durch die Matrize hindurchgedrückt, so daß ein zylindrischer Schaft entstand. Hierbei verhinderte der Stützbund der Preßbüchse (siehe Bild 6) ein Durchbiegen der Schäfte beim Austritt. Die instationären Anfangs- und Endstücke wurden abgetrennt, und der quasistationär fließgepreßte Schaft auf definierte Länge gebracht. Danach wurde auf einer hydraulischen Presse (Hersteller Müller, F_N = 2000 kN) an beiden Schaftenden sukzessive ein kegliger Einspannkopf angestaucht.

3.3.2 Umformwerkzeuge

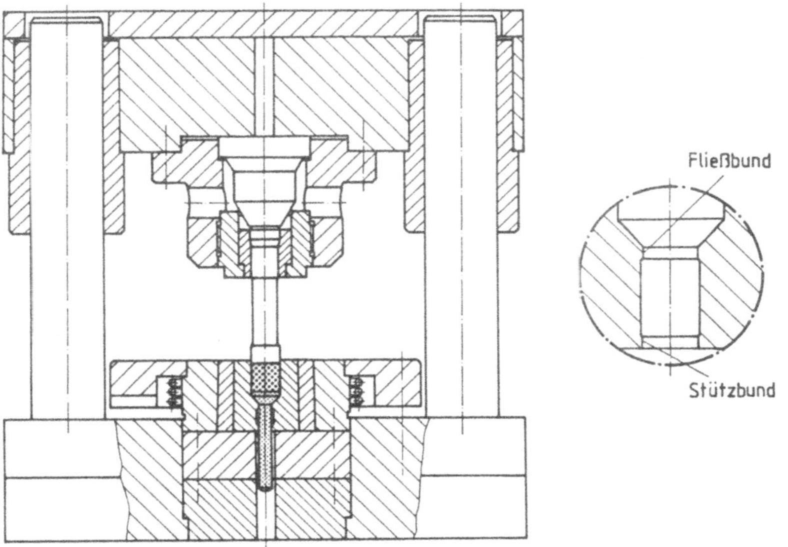

Bild 6: Werkzeug für das Voll-Vorwärts-Fließpressen.

Bild 6 zeigt das Fließpreßwerkzeug im Grundgestell. Für das Voll-Vorwärts-Fließpressen wurden ungeteilte und doppelt armierte Fließpreßmatrizen verwendet, deren Aufnehmer entsprechend der jeweiligen $\varphi/2\alpha$-Kombination für eine Zwischenform mit rd. 115 mm Schaftlänge (incl. der instationären An- und Auslaufteile) und 15 mm Schaftdurchmesser ausgelegt wurde. Bei der Halbwarmumformung wurde das Werkzeug mit einer um den äußeren Schrumpfring gelegten Heizwendel elektrisch beheizt (Temperatur an der Preßbüchse ca. 160 ^{o}C), um Temperaturschocks zu vermeiden. Der Stempel wurde zu Beginn ebenfalls vorgewärmt (ca. 130 ^{o}C).

Bild 7 zeigt die verwendeten Stauchwerkzeuge. Es handelt sich hierbei um eine einfach armierte (Auslegung nach /34/) und eine geteilte Matrize für das Anstauchen der Einspannenden im kalten Zustand.

Für die einzelnen Werkzeugkomponenten wurden folgende Werkzeugwerkstoffe eingesetzt:

Voll-Vorwärts-Fließpressen

Stempel:	Schnellarbeitsstahl S10-4-3-10 (63÷65 HRC)
Preßbüchse:	Schnellarbeitsstahl S6-5-2 (61÷63 HRC)
Armierungsring:	Warmarbeitsstahl X20CrW12 (50÷52 HRC)

Stauchen

Stempel:	Kaltarbeitsstahl X155CrMoV121 (60÷62 HRC)
Stauchmatrize: (geschlossen)	Kaltarbeitsstahl X155CrMoV121 (60÷62 HRC)
Armierungsring:	Warmarbeitsstahl X40CrMoV51 (50÷52 HRC)
Stauchmatrize: (geteilt)	Kaltarbeitsstahl X155CrMoV121 (60÷62 HRC)

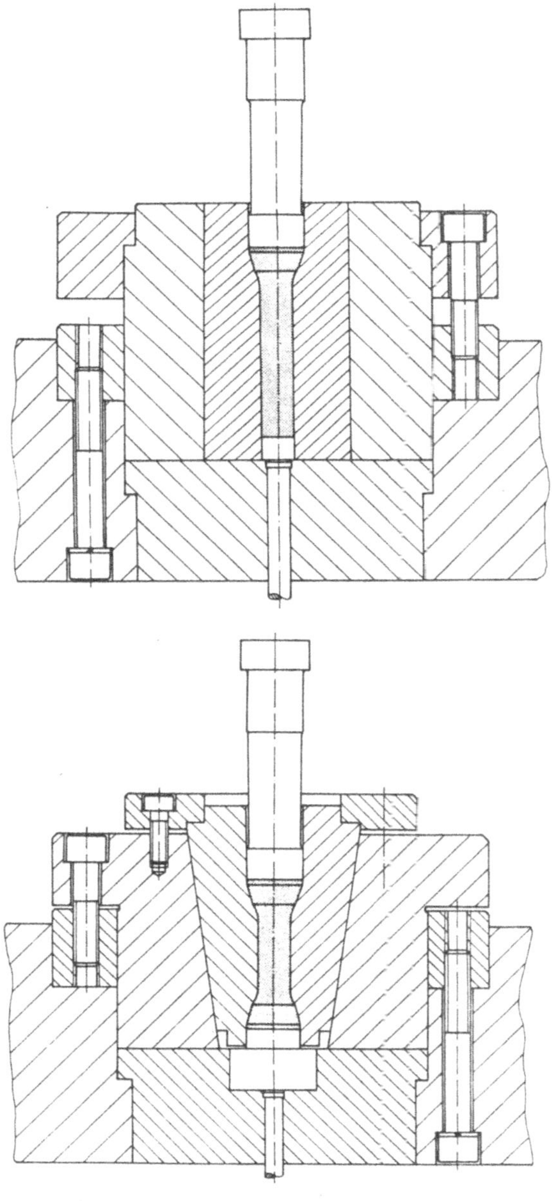

Bild 7: Stauchwerkzeuge für das Kopfanstauchen (geschlossene und geteilte Matrize).

4 EIGENSCHAFTEN DER UMGEFORMTEN WERKSTÜCKE

4.1 BERECHNUNG DES LOKALEN UMFORMGRADES MIT HILFE DER FINITE-ELEMENTE-METHODE

Zur Charakterisierung der verwendeten Schwingproben wurde für die komplette Umformfolge eine numerische Prozeßsimulation mit Hilfe von am Institut für Umformtechnik entwickelten Finite-Element-Programmen durchgeführt. Beide Programme - VVFPFEM (quasistationäres Fließpressen) und AXSTFEM (axialsymmetrisches Stauchen) /35/ - beruhen auf dem starrplastischen Werkstoffmodell nach von Mises. Die elastischen Dehnungen können gegenüber den plastischen Formänderungen bei den hier eingesetzten Verfahren der Kaltmassivumformung vernachlässigt werden. Die Grundlagen der Verfahren unter Verwendung der Methode der oberen Schranke sind in /35/ dargelegt. Wie aus der Stufenfolge in Abschnitt 3.3.1 zu ersehen, interessiert ausschließlich der quasistationär fließgepreßte Schaft. Bei der Berechnung des Fließpressens wurde daher ein FE-Modell zugrundegelegt, bei dem der Werkstoff durch ein raumfestes Gitter fließt. Dagegen ist beim instationären Stauchen das FE-Modell mit dem Werkstück gekoppelt und wird bei jedem Zeitschritt mitverformt.

Eingegeben wurden die Daten zur geometrischen Beschreibung des Problems unter Verwendung von isoparametrischen Viereckelementen mit vier Knoten für die Netzidealisierung. Durch die Anwendung von Pre-Prozessoren konnten für die vorliegenden Strukturen die Koordinaten und die Zuordnung der Knoten zu den jeweiligen Elementen generiert werden. Aufgrund der beschränkten Speicherkapazität der Rechenanlage (Cyber 170-835) wurde die Diskretisierung für das Fließpressen und Stauchen mit jeweils 144 Elementen und 175 Knoten durchgeführt. Die Übergänge beim Ein- und Auslauf aus der Fließpreßschulter wurden allerdings feiner idealisiert (siehe Bild 8), da an den Umlenkungspunkten große Formänderungsgeschwindigkeitsgradienten zu erwarten sind. Zusätzlich wird programmintern bei größeren Schulteröffnungswinkeln durch stufenweises Beschreiben dieses Winkels (entspricht einem sehr kleinen Radius) ein sanfterer Werkstofffluß erreicht /35/. Zur vollständigen Geometriebeschreibung

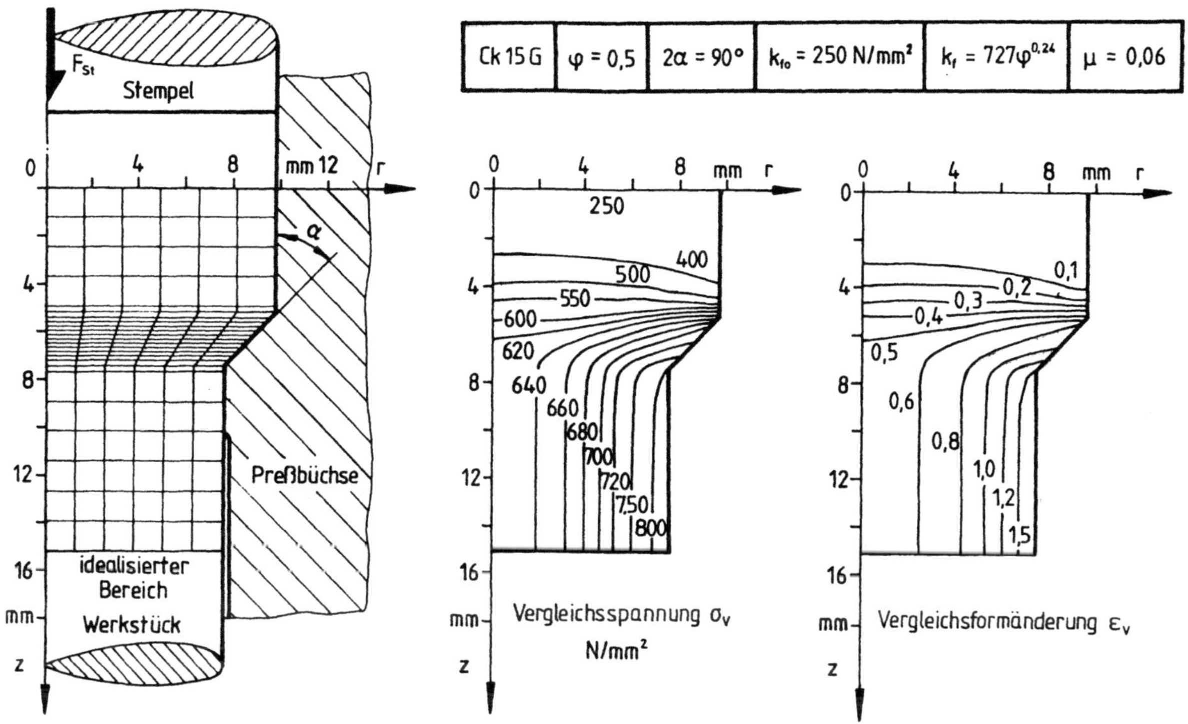

Bild 8: FE-Simulation des Voll-Vorwärts-Fließpressens (φ = 0,5 und 2α = 90°); Netzidealisierung, Vergleichsspannung σ_v und Vergleichsformänderung ε_v.

werden noch die Symmetrie- und Randbedingungen eingearbeitet, unter Verwendung einer Werkstückhälfte beim Fließpressen und eines -viertels beim Kopfanstauchen. Das Werkstoffverhalten wurde durch die Anfangsfließspannung $k_{f0} = 250\ N/mm^2$, und die Fließkurve durch den Ludwik-Ansatz $k_f = 727 \cdot \varphi^{0,24}$ auf der Basis der mechanischen Kennwerte aus dem Zugversuch für Ck15G beschrieben. Die Reibzahl wurde mit $\mu = 0,06$ beim Fließpressen und mit 0,1 beim Stauchen angenommen /36/.

Die Elementzahl in radialer Richtung, der Elementtyp und die Elementgröße für den Schaft beim Fließpressen entsprechen der Anordnung beim nachfolgenden Kopfanstauchen. Das Voll-Vorwärts-Fließpressen zeigt eine inhomogene Verfestigung über dem Querschnitt mit zunehmendem lokalem Umformgrad zum Rand hin. Im Kernbereich besteht annähernd homogene Umformung. Die Vergleichsformänderung ε_v nimmt für $\varphi = 0,5$ in radialer Richtung des Schaftes von ungefähr 0,6 bis 1,5 und für $\varphi = 1,2$ von 1,2 bis 2,2 zu (Bild 8 und linkes Teilbild in Bild 10). Analog dazu verhält sich auch die Vergleichsspannung σ_v ($k_f = f(\varphi)$ mit einem Gradienten zum Rand hin. Im Kopfbereich - vor der eigentlichen Umformzone stellt sich schon eine Verfestigung über dem Querschnitt ein mit ε_v-Werten von 0,1 bis annähernd 0,4 bei $\varphi = 1,2$. In Vorversuchen mit verschiedenen Diskretisierungen in den Bereichen Kopf/Schulter/Schaft zeigte sich ein gewisser Einfluß der Elementeinteilung im Kopfbereich auf den fließgepreßten Schaft.

Für das anschließende Kopfanstauchen wurde das Programm AXSTFEM dahingehend modifiziert, daß die inhomogene Verfestigung bzw. Verteilung der Vergleichsformänderung des fließgepreßten Schaftes als Ausgangszustand eingelesen werden konnte. Außerdem wurden das Einlegespiel und die elastische Aufweitung der Matrize durch eine Durchmesserdifferenz zwischen dem eigentlichen Fließpreßteil und dem mit Einspannköpfen versehenen Fertigteil berücksichtigt (Erweiterung des Werkzeugdurchmessers im Schaftbereich auf ca. 15,16 mm). Dadurch konnte ein geringes Aufstauchen des fließgepreßten Schaftes - das sich bei der Herstellung der Schwingproben gezeigt hatte - in den Berechnungsgang einbe-

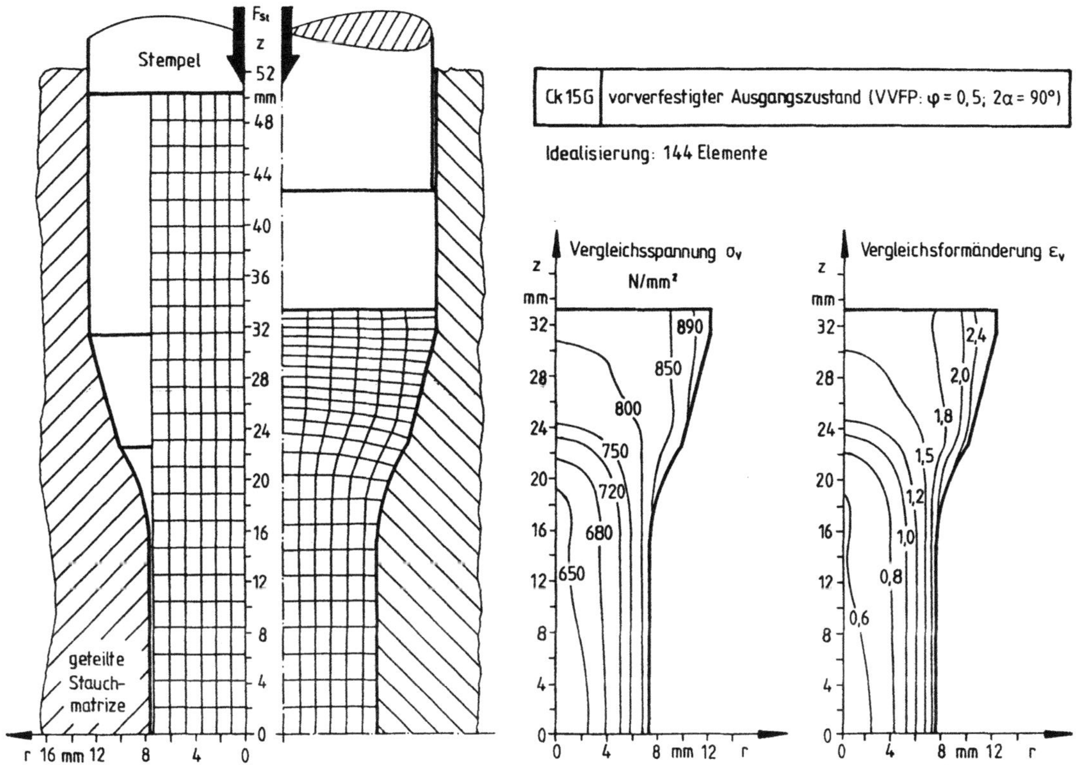

Bild 9: Kopfanstauchen an einem fließgepreßten Schaft ($\varphi = 0{,}5$ und $2\alpha = 90^{\circ}$); Netzidealisierung, umgeformter Endzustand, Vergleichsspannung σ_v und Vergleichsformänderung ε_v.

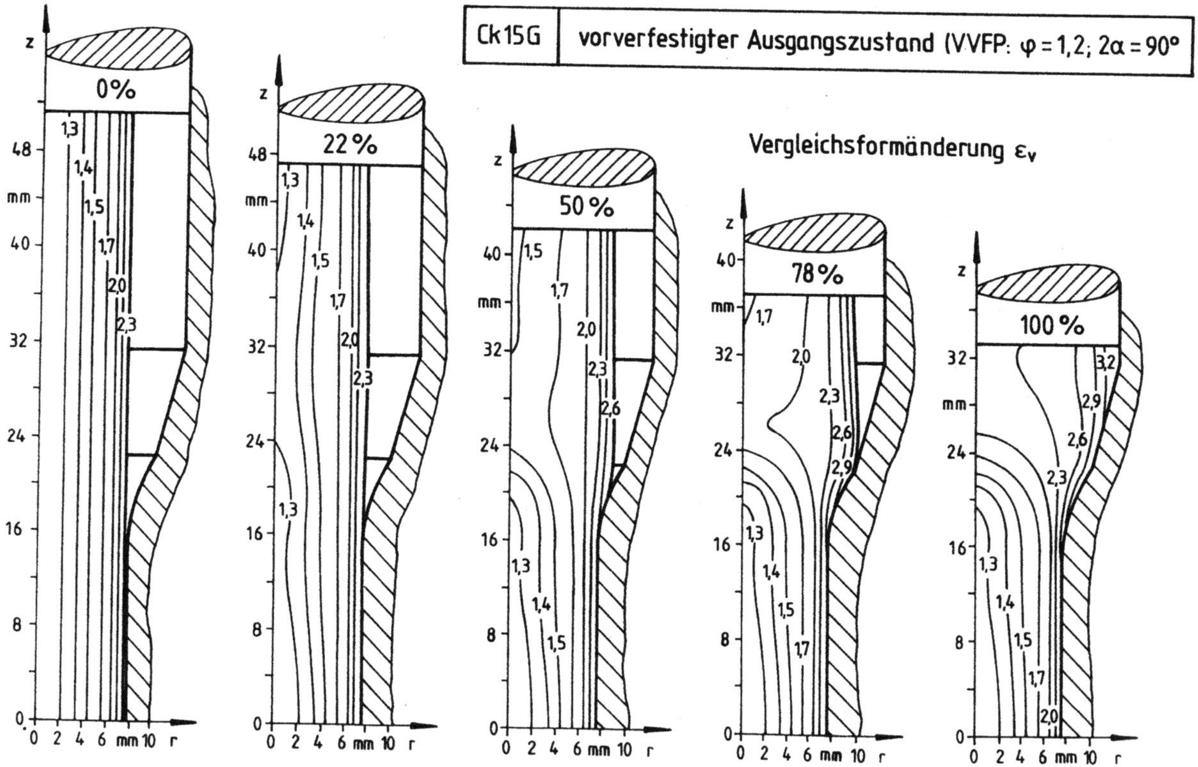

Bild 10: Axialsymmetrisches Kopfanstauchen; Vergleichsformänderung ε_v bei verschiedenen Stadien der Umformung (Höhenabnahme des Stauchkörpers in %).

zogen werden. Den Verlauf der Vergleichsformänderung ε_v für die mit $\varphi = 0{,}5$ und 1,2 vorverfestigten Werkstücke zeigt Bild 9 und Bild 10. Vor allem im Kernbereich des Schaftes (d. h. in der Zone, wo noch das größte Formänderungsvermögen vorhanden ist) ändert sich die ε_v-Verteilung geringfügig. Dies tritt in der Anfangsphase des Kopfanstauchens ein: nach ca. 22 %-iger Umformung ändert sich der Verlauf der Vergleichsformänderungen nicht mehr. Das bedeutet, daß die vom Fließpressen vorhandenen Linien gleicher Vergleichsformänderung parallel zur Längsachse der Probe in der Randzone praktisch unverändert bleiben. Eine zusätzliche Verfestigung ist bei beiden Umformgraden im Randbereich des Kopfes feststellbar.

Die Berechnungen wurden mit Ergebnissen aus visioplastischen Stoffflußuntersuchungen - auf die hier nicht weiter eingegangen werden soll - verglichen und stimmten beim Fließpressen gut überein. Auf eine Untersuchung des Anstauchens der Einspannköpfe nach der Methode der Visioplasticity mußte verzichtet werden, da für die halbierten Visioproben die Knickgrenze überschritten wurde und dementsprechend bei einem durchgeführten Versuch Faltenbildung am Probenkopf auftrat.

4.2 HÄRTEVERTEILUNG

Die Härteverteilung wurde für sämtliche Verfahrensparameterkombinationen (siehe Versuchsplan) ermittelt. Die Ergebnisse werden vornehmlich im Kapitel 6 im Zusammenhang mit den Wechselverformungskurven erörtert. Da ein Zusammenhang zwischen Vikkershärte und Vergleichsformänderung besteht /37/, läßt sich das Härteprofil bei der Charakterisierung kaltmassivumgeformter Schwingproben als Maß für die örtliche Umformung verwenden. Beim Halbwarmfließpressen hingegen ist eine eindeutige Beziehung zwischen Eindringhärte und örtlicher Formänderung nicht gegeben. Hierbei wird die Härte des Werkstückwerkstoffs außer von der Umformtemperatur und dem Umformgrad auch von Entfestigungs- und Ausscheidungsvorgängen im Gefüge während des Umformens und danach im Verlauf des Abkühlens bestimmt /38/.

Die Härteprüfung nach Vickers (DIN 50133) wurde mit der Prüflast 50 N (HV5) auf einem Kleinlast-Härteprüfgerät (Bauart Zwick Z 323) durchgeführt. Dazu wurden die fließgepreßten Schäfte (exemplarisch für die Umformgrade φ = 0,5 und 1,2) und bauteilähnlichen Proben in Längsrichtung bis zur Mitte abgefräst, geschliffen und poliert. Von der anderen Seite erhielten die Proben eine zur Prüffläche parallele Auflagefläche. Beim Ausmessen betrug der Abstand der Meßpunkte senkrecht zur Probenachse 1 mm und in Achsrichtung 2 mm.

Es wurden keine meßbaren Unterschiede im quasistationären Fließpreßschaft festgestellt, gleichgültig ob der Einspannkopf in der oder gegen die Fließpreßrichtung angestaucht wurde. Um einen Vergleich zur FE-Berechnung (Abschnitt 4.1) zu ermöglichen, ist in Bild 11 für die mit φ = 0,5 und 1,2 vorverfestigten Werkstücke der Verlauf konstanter Härtewerte darstellt.

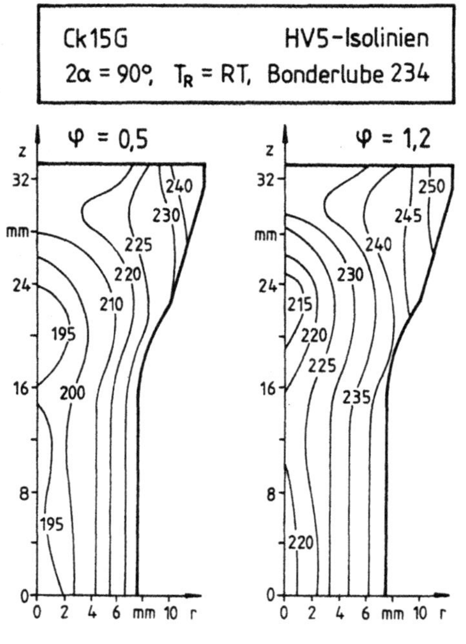

Bild 11: Härteverteilung der bauteilähnlichen Proben.

Die höchsten Härtewerte treten in der Randzone der Einspannköpfe auf. Dies wirkt sich bei der vorhandenen vollständigen Anschmiegung der Oberflächen der gebunden umgeformten Einspannköpfe und der nitrierten Spannelemente hinsichtlich der hohen Flächenpressung günstig aus. Die ursprünglich zur Längsachse der fließgepreßten Schäfte parallelen Linien gleicher Vickershärte wurden durch das Anstauchen der Einspannköpfe im Bereich des Übergangsradius zum Spannkopf quer zur Stauchrichtung umgelenkt. Die geringste Härte ergibt sich jeweils entlang der Mittelachse des Werkstücks, im für die Ermüdungsversuche interessanten Fließpreßschaft. In Längsrichtung des Prüfschaftes stellt sich ein weitgehend homogener Härteverlauf ein; beim Umformgrad φ = 0,5 macht sich der Einfluß des Kopfanstauchens durch leicht gekrümmte Isolinien im Kernbereich bemerkbar. Über dem Querschnitt stellt sich ein inhomogener Härteverlauf mit einem Härteanstieg zum Rand hin ein. Dieser Anstieg ist begründet in den vermehrt auftretenden Schiebungen in der Randzone; der Werkstofffluß zeigt einen gleichmäßigen Verzerrungszustand, der durch eine gleichmäßige Elementumformung - Voreilung der inneren gegen die weiter außen liegenden Elemente - gekennzeichnet ist. Im Randbereich stellten sich keine meßbaren Veränderungen der Vickershärte gegenüber dem fließgepreßten Schaft vor dem Kopfanstauchen ein; die HV-Linien bleiben achsparallel.

4.3 GEFÜGEAUSBILDUNG

Die Proben für die Gefügeuntersuchungen wurden jeweils nach dem Voll-Vorwärts-Fließpressen sowie nach dem Anstauchen der Einspannköpfe aus dem quasistationären Schaft der Werkstücke an verschiedenen Stellen entnommen: aus dem Kernbereich mit 0,5 mm Abstand von der Probenlängsachse und aus der Randzone mit 0,5 mm Abstand von der Oberfläche. Die Längsschliffe wurden mit 1 %-iger alkoholischer Salpetersäure geätzt. Die Gefüge wurden bei 100- und 500-facher Vergrößerung aufgenommen.

Bild 12 zeigt Gefügeaufnahmen aus dem quasistationären Fließpreßschaft der Schwingproben aus Ck15G. Als Parameter dient der

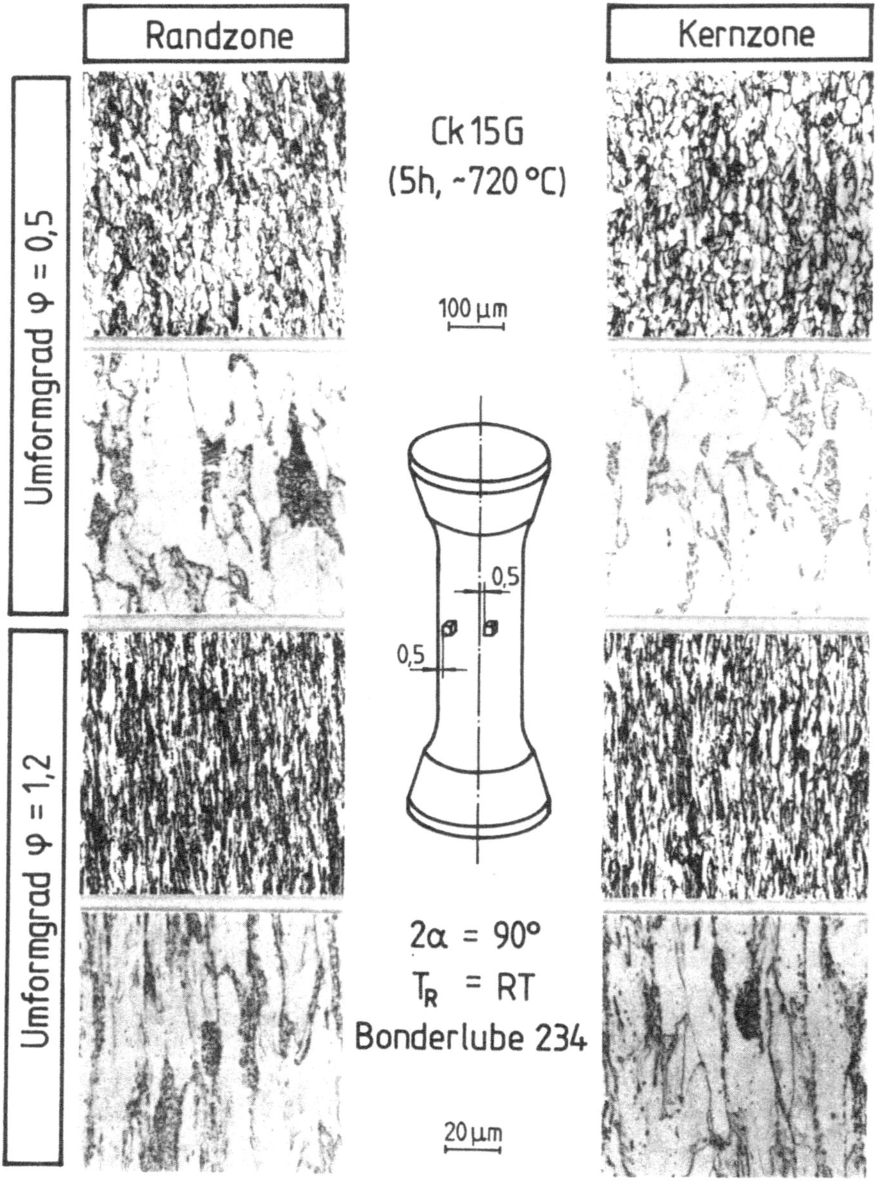

Bild 12: Werkstoffgefüge von Ck15G nach der Umformung bei verschiedenen Umformgraden.

Umformgrad φ. Die durch die Behandlungsvorgeschichte des Stahles (Warmwalzen) hervorgerufene Zeiligkeit der Körner wird - wie aus Abschnitt 3.2.1 bekannt - auch nach einer Weichglühung teilweise beibehalten. Durch das Durchdrücken entsteht eine Streckung der Körner mit Gefügeorientierung in Umformrichtung. Der spröde Zementit (Fe_3C-Karbid) ist durch das vorangegangene Weichglühen der Rohteile - wie auch nach der Umformung ersichtlich - innerhalb der von α-Mischkristallen umgebenen zeilenförmig ausgerichteten Perlitbereiche globular eingebettet bzw. koaguliert. Die Aufnahmen mit $\varphi = 0{,}5$ und V = 500 deuten auf eine Ablenkung des noch nicht vollständig eingeformten lamellaren Zementits quer zur Stauchrichtung hin. Beim größeren Umformgrad ist zwischen den Gefügeaufnahmen des quasistationären Schaftes vor bzw. nach dem Anstauchen der Einspannköpfe visuell kein Unterschied zu erkennen. Durch das Fließpressen mit $\varphi = 1{,}2$ ist die Streckung der Perlitkörner verfahrensbedingt stärker fortgeschritten und zeigt in der Randzone des Schaftes eine kompaktere Anordnung. Diese Gefügestruktur stimmt qualitativ mit der inhomogenen Verfestigung über dem Querschnitt (ε_V- bzw. Härteverlauf) überein.

4.4 MECHANISCHE KENNWERTE

Zur Kennzeichnung des Werkstoffzustandes nach der Umformung bzw. des Ausgangszustandes vor der schwingenden Beanspruchung wurden aus dem Innern der Werkstücke Zug- und Kerbschlagbiegeproben entnommen. Die Festigkeits- und Zähigkeitskennwerte aus dem Zugversuch (DIN 50125) bzw. dem Kerbschlagbiegeversuch (DIN 50115) für die jeweiligen Bedingungen beim Fließpressen sind in Tabelle 2 zusammengestellt. Daraus wird deutlich, daß mit steigendem Umformgrad bzw. Schulteröffnungswinkel zwar die Festigkeitswerte R_m und $R_{p0,2}$ zunehmen, aber die Zähigkeitswerte A_g, A_5, Z und A_V abnehmen; umgekehrtes Verhalten ist mit steigender Rohteiltemperatur zu beobachten. Die Stauchproben ($h_0/d_0 = 1{,}5$) wurden aus dem quasistationären Fließpreßschaft (ohne angestauchte Einspannköpfe) entnommen und auf $h_0/2$ gestaucht (entspricht $\varphi \approx 0{,}7$). Bei den kaltvorverfestigten Proben stellt

Umformverfahren	Werkstoff	Umformgrad φ	Schulteröffnungswinkel 2α	Rohteiltemperatur T_R °C	Zugfestigkeit R_m N/mm²	0,2-Dehngrenze $R_{p0,2}$ N/mm²	Streckgrenzenverhältnis $R_{p0,2}/R_m$	Gleichmaßdehnung A_g %	Bruchdehnung A_5 %	Brucheinschnürung Z %	Kerbschlagarbeit A_v J
		0,5			603	505	0,84	4,2	14,2	57	62
		0,9		20	691	536	0,78	3,8	12,3	51	53
			90		744	539	0,72	3,7	10,9	49	52
				500	742	524	0,71	7,7	15,1	52	72
				700	546	461	0,84	8,8	15,8	63	117
Voll-Vorwärts-Fließpressen	CK15G	1,2	30		720	536	0,74	4,2	13,1	52	56
			60		730	537	0,74	4,1	12,9	50	54
			120	20	744	543	0,73	4,2	12,8	49	49
			150		743	545	0,73	4,4	12,9	49	51
					804	556	0,69	4,2	13,0	49	64
		1,6		500	662	478	0,72	9,1	16,8	58	107
				700	489	383	0,78	13,0	23,2	68	121
		0,5	90		692	540	0,78	4,5	14,6	56	–
	16MnCr5G	0,9			775	559	0,72	4,9	14,4	56	–
		1,2		20	829	562	0,68	4,9	13,5	53	–
		1,6			912	585	0,64	5,5	13,4	53	–

Tabelle 3: Mechanische Eigenschaften nach der Umformung.

sich anfänglich noch eine Fließspannungszunahme ein ($\Delta\varphi \approx 0{,}1$). Im weiteren k_f-Verlauf wird im allgemeinen - bedingt durch den Bauschinger Effekt /39/ - eine meist leicht fallende Tendenz beobachtet. Ursachen hierfür sind nach /40/ einerseits Versetzungsanhäufungen, die bei Umkehr der Formänderungsrichtung (Fließpressen ≡ Querstauchen; Stauchen ≡ Längsstauchen) die Gleitung der Versetzungen erleichtern, anderseits Eigenspannungen zwischen zwei heterogenen Phasen. Durch die unterschiedlichen elastischen und plastischen Eigenschaften des Ferrits und Zementits der verwendeten Stähle steht nach dem Voll-Vorwärts-Fließpressen der weiche Ferrit unter Druck- und das harte Fe_3C-Karbid unter Zugeigenspannungen. Beim Stauchversuch addieren sich die äußeren Druckspannungen zu den Druckeigenspannungen des Ferrits (Superposition von Last- und Eigenspannungen), so daß plastisches Fließen im Gegensatz zum nicht vorverfestigten, eigenspannungsfreien Zustand bei einer niedrigeren Lastspannung einsetzt. Die im Halbwarmbereich fließgepreßten Proben verfestigen allerdings kontinuierlich (siehe Bild 13).

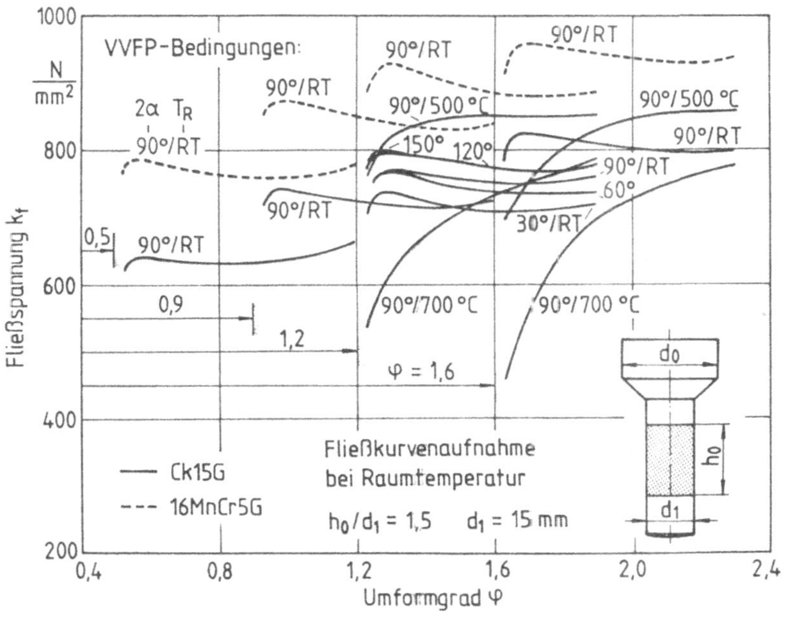

Bild 13: Fließverhalten der vorverfestigten Versuchswerkstoffe.

4.5 OBERFLÄCHENBESCHAFFENHEIT

Von besonderer Bedeutung ist der Einfluß der Oberflächenbeschaffenheit auf die Ermüdung, da - von speziellen Ausnahmen abgesehen - an der Oberfläche kurze Risse unter Schwingbeanspruchung entstehen, die sich bei zeitlich veränderlicher Belastung ausbreiten und zu einer wesentlichen Schädigung des Bauteils führen.

Die Oberflächenschicht des voll-vorwärts-fließgepreßten Schaftes der Schwingproben ergibt sich aus der ursprünglichen Rohteiloberfläche und Oberflächenwandlung durch den Umformvorgang. Nach /41/ wird die Feingestalt der Schaftoberfläche beim Voll-Vorwärts-Fließpressen durch die Auswirkungen zweier Vorgänge bestimmt. Der erste Vorgang ist die dem Umformgrad nahezu proportionale Aufrauhung in der Schulter. Der anschließende Glättungsgang im Fließbund wandelt die frei gerauhte Schulteroberfläche zur gebunden umgeformten Schaftoberfläche.

Die Oberflächenfeingestalt des Schaftes wurde nach dem Fließpressen und dem Anstauchen der Einspannköpfe untersucht. Es wurde ein mikroprozessorgesteuertes Meß- und Auswertegerät (Hommel T20) verwendet, das nach dem Tastschnittverfahren arbeitet. Der Tastweg betrug 4 mm. Um den statistischen Eigenschaften der Oberfläche wenigstens teilweise gerecht zu werden, wurden mindestens 10 Einzelmessungen in Längs- und Umfangsrichtung durchgeführt (1 Meßpunkt im Schaubild entspricht dem Mittelwert aus 10 Messungen). Die Oberflächenmaßzahlen "Mittlere Rauhtiefe" R_{ZDIN} und "Mittlere Glättungstiefe" R_{pm} geben eine quantitative Beschreibung der Oberflächenfeingestalt. Die Kennzeichnung der gedrehten Rohlteil-Mantelfläche kann wie folgt angegeben werden: R_{ZDIN} = 12,6 µm und R_{pm} = 5,8 µm. Die Werkstücke wurden nach der Umformung gereinigt, um einen Einfluß von Schmierstoffresten weitgehend auszuschließen.

Bild 14 zeigt die Oberflächenbeschaffenheit der Schwingproben mit dem Umformgrad als Parameter. Tendenziell stellt sich ein ähnlicher Verlauf wie nach dem Fließpressen ein; die Senkrecht-maße liegen bis auf den R_{ZDIN}-Wert am mit $\varphi = 1{,}2$ umgeformten Schaft (gemessen in Umfangsrichtung) unter den Ausgangswerten des gedrehten Rohteils und lassen auf einen Glättungsvorgang schließen. Bei kleinem Umformgrad bleibt die Aufrauhung gering, während sich bei großem Umformgrad ein hoher Glätteffekt einstellt; die "Mittlere Rauhtiefe" erreicht demzufolge bei mittleren Umformgraden ein Maximum. Die auf den fließgepreßten Schaft bezogene Stauchung ist gering. Daher reicht die Durchmesserzunahme im Schaftbereich nicht aus, um die Werkstückoberfläche mit einer zur deutlichen Veränderung der Oberfläche ausreichenden Flächenpressung an die Stauchwerkzeugoberfläche anzulegen.

Um einen qualitativen Eindruck von den umgeformten Oberflächen zu vermitteln, sind in Bild 14 die REM-Aufnahmen der Schwingprobenoberfläche bei verschiedenen Umformgraden gegenübergestellt. Bei einem höher verfestigten Werkstück sind größere Plateaus festzustellen, die auf eine Einebnung der Rauhbergspitzen durch Mikroprägevorgänge zurückzuführen sind. Bei-

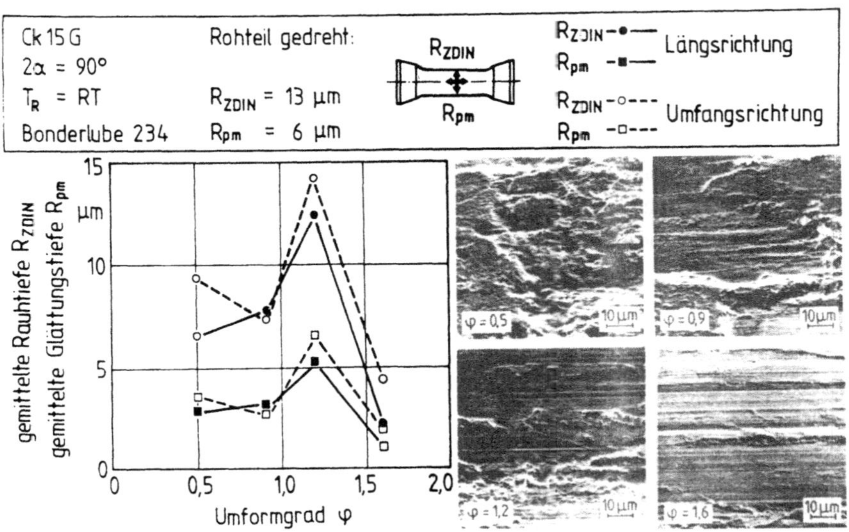

Bild 14: Oberflächenstruktur der Schwingproben.

spielsweise zeigt die Oberfläche des mit φ = 0,5 umgeformten Werkstücks gegenüber dem mit φ = 1,6 umgeformten keine ausgesprochenen Umformspuren in Form von Durchdrückriefen. Auf eine mögliche Rißinitiierung an der Oberfläche wird in Abschnitt 7.2 detailliert eingegangen.

4.6 EIGENSPANNUNGSANALYSE

4.6.1 Definitionen

Eigenspannungen (ES) werden nach /42/ je nach der räumlichen Erstreckung wie folgt eingeteilt:

- Eigenspannungen I. Art sind über größere Werkstoffbereiche (mehrere Körner) nahezu homogen. Die mit den Eigenspannungen verbundenen inneren Kräfte und Momente befinden sich im mechanischen Gleichgewicht. Jeder Eingriff in dieses Gleichgewicht bewirkt makroskopische Maßänderungen.
- Eigenspannungen II. Art sind über kleine Werkstoffbereiche (ein Korn oder Kornbereiche) nahezu homogen. Die mit den Eigenspannungen verbundenen inneren Kräfte und Momente sind über hinreichend viele Körner im Gleichgewicht. Bei Eingriffen in dieses Gleichgewicht können makroskopische Maßänderungen auftreten.
- Eigenspannungen III. Art sind über kleinste Werkstoffbereiche (mehrere Atomabstände) inhomogen. Ursache dieser Eigenspannungsart sind alle Gitterbaufehler (Leerstellen, Fremdatome, Versetzungen, Ausscheidungen usw.).

Nachfolgend werden unter Eigenspannungen bzw. Makroeigenspannungen ausschließlich solche I. Art verstanden.

4.6.2 Mechanische und röntgenographische Ermittlung

Die Bestimmung der Umformeigenspannungen im fließgepreßten Schaft vor und nach dem Anstauchen der Einspannköpfe wurde - bedingt durch den Prüfdurchmesser der Werkstücke (d_1 = 15 mm) -

mechanisch und röntgenographisch durchgeführt /43/.

Um den Eigenspannnungszustand im Kernbereich zu erfassen, wurde das Sachssche Ausbohrverfahren /44/ mit der Auswertung nach Bühler und Schreiber /45/ angewandt. Zur Aufnahme der axialen, radialen und tangentialen Eigenspannungen wurde je ein Dehnungsmeßstreifen (DMS; Typ 06/120 LY11, Hottinger Baldwin Meßtechnik) um 180° versetzt im Abstand von 45 mm ($3 \cdot d_1$) von der Probenstirnfläche appliziert. Das sukzessive Abtragen der Querschnittsfläche bei dem relativ kleinen Durchmesser erfolgte durch 9 Bohrungen. Die Messung der Dehnungsänderungen wurde bei einer Restwanddicke von etwa 2 mm abgebrochen, um zu vermeiden, daß beim Ausbohrvorgang des rotationssymmetrischen Restkörpers plastische Deformationen zu falschen Eigenspannungen führen. Da es nicht möglich war, in der größten Bohrung von 11,6 mm an die gewünschte Stelle Dehnungsmeßstreifen zu kleben, um so durch Abdrehen des Außendurchmessers weitere Dehnungsänderungen zu bestimmen, wurden die oberflächennahen Eigenspannungen röntgenographisch ermittelt.

Die Messungen wurden auf einem automatisierten ψ-Diffraktometer mit CrK_{α}-Strahlung am Institut für Werkstoffkunde I der Universität Karlsruhe durchgeführt. Es wurden die Gitterdehnungsmessungen in 11 verschiedenen ψ-Richtungen im Bereich $-45^{o} \leq \psi \leq +45^{o}$ an den $\{211\}$-Netzebenen oberflächennaher Ferritkristallite vorgenommen. Der vom Röntgenstrahl erfaßte Werkstoffbereich war kreisförmig mit einem Durchmesser von etwa 1 mm. Die Proben rotierten während der Messung um ihre Längsachse, so daß die in den Bildern 15 und 16 angegebenen Spannungen Mittelwerte über dem Schaftumfang darstellen. Der Tiefenverlauf an allen Werkstücken wurde durch elektrolytischen Oberflächenabtrag gewonnen und nach /46/ korrigiert, so daß es sich bei den eingetragenen Versuchspunkten um die wirklich vorliegenden Eigenspannungen in der jeweiligen Tiefe vor dem Abtrag handelt. Die Spannungsberechnung erfolgte nach dem $\sin^2\psi$-Verfahren unter Zugrundelegung des Elastizitätsmoduls E = 210000 N/mm^2 und der Querkontraktionszahl $\nu = 0{,}3$. Effekte der elastischen Anisotropie blieben unberücksichtigt.

Die Eigenspannungsverläufe im quasistationär fließgepreßten Schaft zeigt Bild 15. Für die beiden Umformgrade (φ = 0,5 und 1,2) stellen sich im Kernbereich in axialer, tangentialer und radialer Richtung Druckeigenspannungen ein. An der Oberfläche sind für φ = 0,5 geringe tangentiale und axiale Zugeigenspannungen vorhanden (σ_{Et} = 24 N/mm^2, σ_{Ea} = 31 N/mm^2). Für den Umformgrad φ = 1,2 wurde zwar ebenfalls eine tangentiale Zugei-

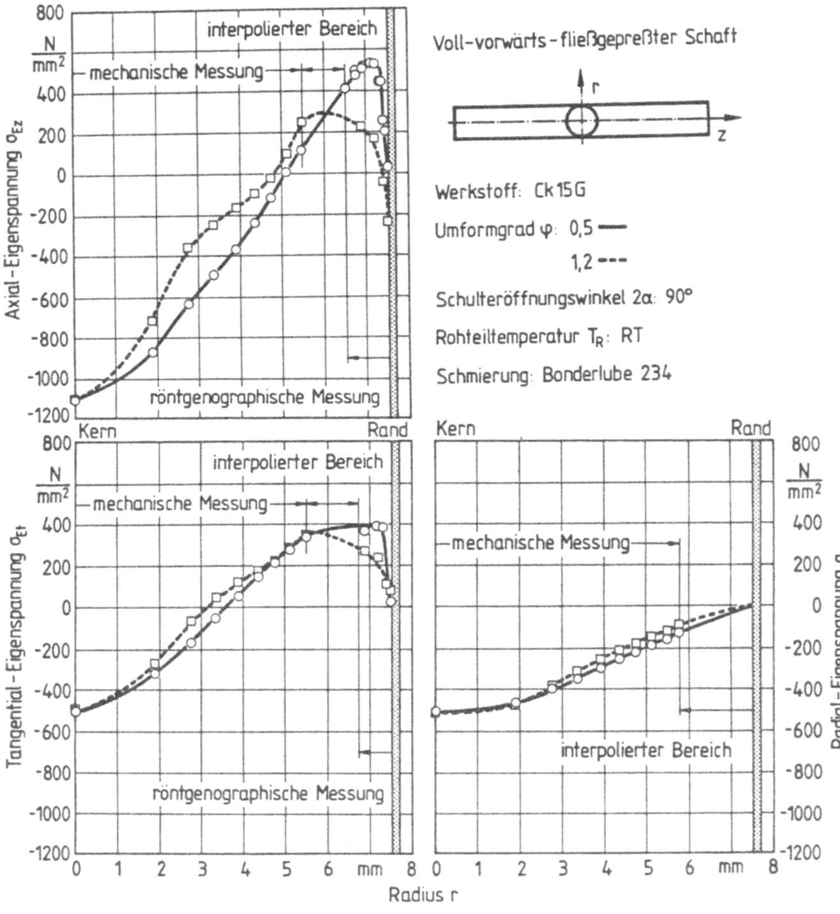

Bild 15: Eigenspannungsverläufe im fließgepreßten Schaft (φ = 0,5 und 1,2; 2α = 90°).

genspannung (σ_{Et} = 55 N/mm^2) an der Oberfläche ermittelt, aber zugleich auch eine hohe Druckeigenspannung σ_{Ea} = -250 N/mm^2. Für beide Umformgrade zeigen sich mit zunehmender Tiefe unter der Schaftoberfläche ansteigende Spannungswerte; die höchsten wurden für φ = 0,5 erfaßt (kompatible Ergebnisse in /47, 48/). Tekkaya /49/ interpretiert den Einfluß des Umformgrades anhand eines gedanklichen Modells und erklärt eine Abnahme der Eigenspannungen beim Fließpressen mit zunehmendem Umformgrad durch die Existenz eines "Eigenspannungsextremums" im Bereich des Umformgrades $\varphi \approx 0,3$.

Im Bild 16 sind die Eigenspannungsverläufe im fließgepreßten Schaft nach dem Anstauchen der Einspannköpfe zusammengefaßt. Für beide Umformgrade stellt sich ein ähnlicher Eigenspannungsverlauf ein. Die beim Fließpressen gebildeten Eigenspannungen werden durch das Kopfanstauchen offenbar vollständig geändert, so daß niedrige Eigenspannungswerte zurückbleiben. Im randnahen

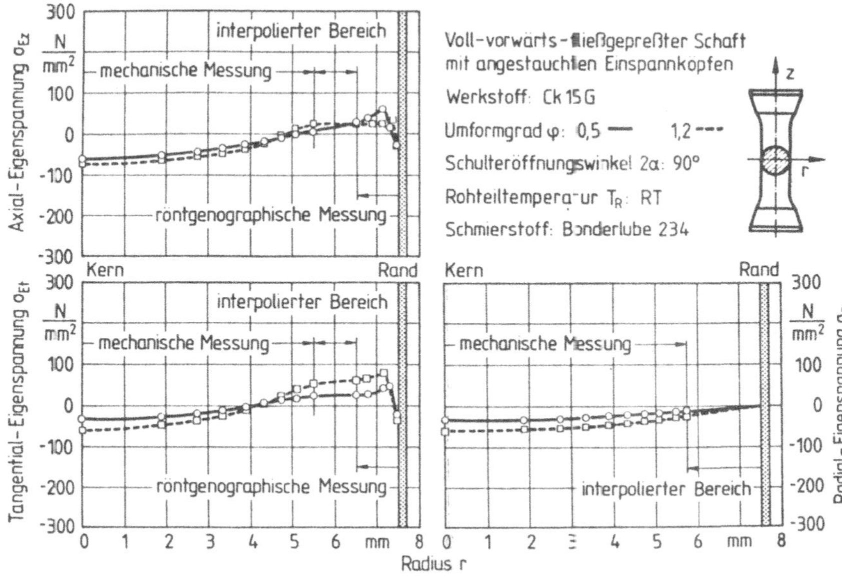

Bild 16: Eigenspannungsverläufe im fließgepreßten Schaft nach dem Kopfanstauchen (φ = 0,5 und 1,2; 2α = 90°).

Bereich stellten sich durchweg Druckeigenspannungen ein. Das instationäre Stauchen - bezogen auf den Schaftquerschnitt - von geringfügigem Ausmaß ruft einen ähnlichen Effekt hervor wie das Auswerfen der Werkstücke nach einer Stempelentlastung. In beiden Fällen tritt durch einsinniges Umformen ein ES-Abbau ein /50/. In einer theoretischen Untersuchung mit Hilfe der Finite-Elemente-Methode (φ = 0,7 und 2α = 60°; Ck15) weist Tekkaya /49/ nach, daß die gefährlichen Eigenspannungen während des Auswerfens der Werkstücke weitgehend abgebaut werden. Die Zugeigenspannungen gehen dabei fast auf Null zurück. Anhand des in Bild 17 wiedergegebenen Spannungs-Dehnungs-Diagramms läßt sich in stark vereinfachter Weise das Abbauverhalten im Schaft durch eine geringe Plastifizierung beim Kopfanstauchen betrachten. Aufgrund der inhomogenen Verfestigung über dem Querschnitt wird angenommen, daß die Druckfließgrenze σ^R_{dF} im Randbereich größer ist als die Druckfließgrenze σ^K_{dF} im homogen umgeformten Kernbe-

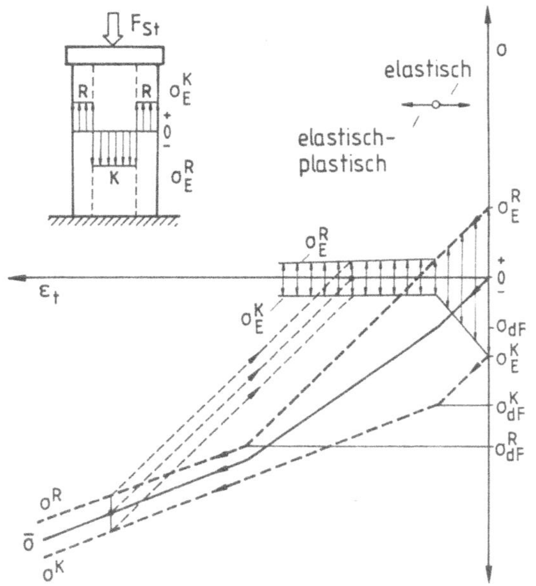

Bild 17: Vereinfachtes Modell zum Eigenspannungsabbau durch Kopfanstauchen.

reich. Weiterhin soll Verfestigung mit konstantem Anstieg auftreten; im Rand jedoch mit kleinerer Steigung bedingt durch ein geringeres Formänderungsvermögen. Bei einem Stauchvorgang erreicht eher der Kern bei einem kleineren ε_t-Wert die Druckfließgrenze σ_{dF} als der unter Zugspannungen stehende Probenrand. Im Kern setzt somit zuerst plastisches Fließen ein. Wird nun der Schaft durch Stempelrückzug entlastet, bleiben selbst bei vorangegangenen sehr geringen Formänderungen im Kern- und Randbereich nur noch stark reduzierte Eigenspannungen zurück.

5 SCHWINGPRÜFEINRICHTUNG

5.1 VERSUCHSANLAGE

Der Prüfstand für die Ermüdungsversuche mit der in Bild 18 aufgegliederten Anordnung enthält eine servo-hydraulische Zug-Druck-Schwingprüfmaschine (Bauart Instron 1343; F_a = 250 kN) mit Kraft-, Weg- und Längenänderungsregeleinheit in Verbindung mit einem Spitzenwertregler. Letzterer gewährleistet eine annähernde Konstanz der Beanspruchungsamplitude, die sonst von der Prüfmaschine oft nicht zufriedenstellend nachgeregelt werden kann. Derartige Schwierigkeiten treten z. B. bei der Untersuchung duktiler Werkstoffzustände mit hohen Spannungsamplituden auf, die folglich große Dehnungsamplituden bedingen /1/, oder allgemein bei schnellen strukturmechanischen Änderungen meist kurz vor dem Probenbruch.

Die Prüfmaschine wurde mit hydraulischen Spannköpfen zur Aufnahme der bauteilähnlichen Proben bestückt, vgl. Bild 19. Die Werkstücke werden mit Hilfe von zwei halbschalenförmigen Spannelementen in der Aufnahmeplatte fixiert. Die Druckflüssigkeit beaufschlagt jeweils nur eine Kolbenseite mit dem notwendigen Spanndruck (Druckbereich 220 ÷ 330 bar); die hydraulische Kraft bewirkt die Bewegung in einer Richtung und die Rückstellung erfolgt durch Federkraft. Bei einem eventuellen Setzvorgang tritt kein Spiel auf, da der Spanndruck konstant gehalten wird, indem der Hydrospeicher der Einspanneinrichtung seine gespeicherte Energie zur Verfügung stellt. Außerdem enthalten die Spannköpfe integrierte Kühlflansche. In einem geschlossenen Kühlkreislauf mit Umwälzpumpe und hintereinandergeschalteten Kühlflanschen wird ein vom Arbeitskolben der Maschine vornehmlich auf die untere Einspannung übertragener Wärmestrom abgeführt, und so für einen Temperaturausgleich gesorgt.

Die Steuer- und Regelelektronik /51/ liefert die analogen Sollwertsignale für die Kraft F und die Längenänderung ΔL (Extensometer 2620-603, Hersteller Instron; L_0 = 15 mm). Die Kraft dient bei spannungskontrollierter Versuchsführung, und die Längenänderung bei totaldehnungskontrollierter zur externen

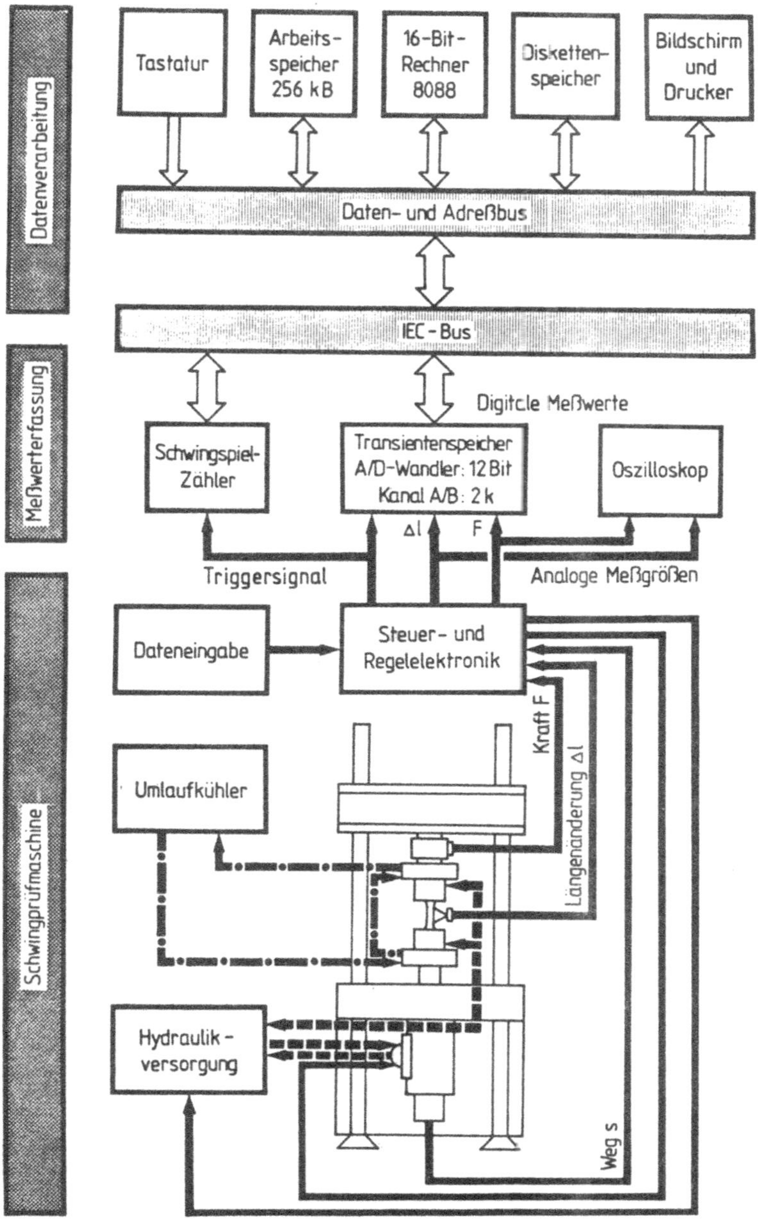

Bild 18: Versuchsaufbau.

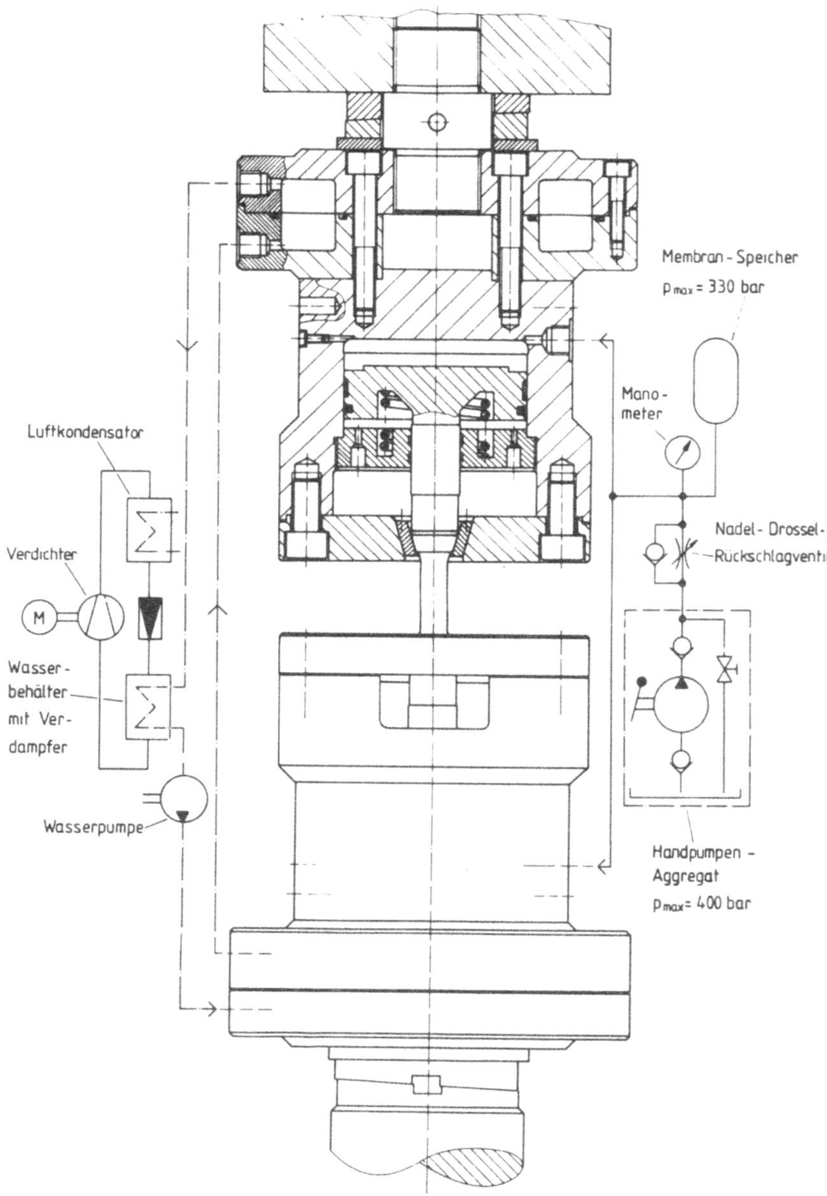

Bild 19: Hydraulische Werkstück-Spanneinrichtung.

Zählung der Schwingspiele. Außerdem wird dieses Signal - Vollausschlag der Amplitudensteuerung des dynamischen Funktionsgenerators (100 %-Peak) - am Transientenspeicher zum externen Triggern verwendet. Anfangs wurde das am ersten Kanal des Transientenspeichers (Bauart Krenz TRC 4010) anliegende geregelte Istwertmeßsignal als externe Triggerquelle benutzt; dabei kam es aber zu Problemen bei kleinen Schwingbeanspruchungen. Zur Triggerung wird die positiv ansteigende Signalflanke gewählt. Die beiden analogen Signale werden im Transientenspeicher digitalisiert (A/D-Wandler mit 12 Bit Auflösung) und zwischengespeichert (Speichertiefe pro Kanal 2k). Es können etwa 2000 Meßwerte pro Kanal, d. h. beispielsweise 16 Hysteresen mit 125 Meßpunkten (F/ΔL-Wertepaare) aufgenommen werden. Zur Erfassung der Meßdaten wurde folgende IEC-Bus-Konfiguration realisiert (Bild 20):

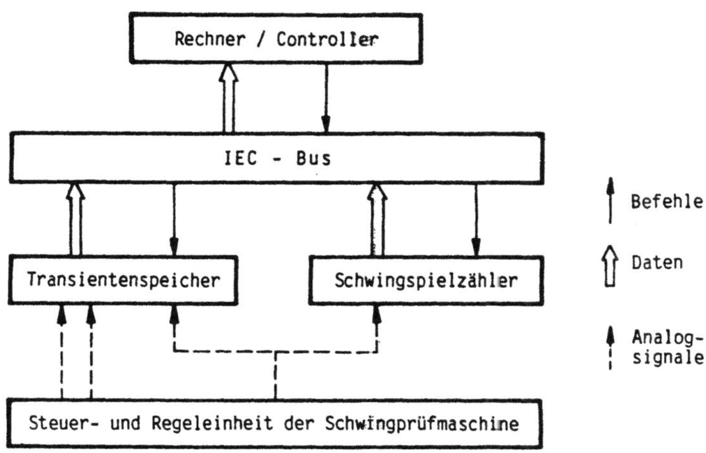

Bild 20: IEC-Bus-Anordnung.

Die Steuerung der Meßabläufe und die Auswertung der Meßergebnisse übernimmt ein Rechner der Bauart Sirius I.

Das Programm zur Meßdatenerfassung führt unter anderem auch die Controllerfunktion gemäß dem IEC-Bus-Standard /52/ aus:

- Adressierung der Meßgeräte
- Datenaustausch von den Meßgeräten zum Rechner (Meßdaten)
- Datenaustausch vom Rechner zu den Meßgeräten (Setzen von Funktionstasten)

Der Ablauf der Meßdatenerfassung erfolgt nach folgendem Schema:

1. Einlesen der Schwingspielzahl vom Ereigniszähler;
2. Anstoßen der Aufnahmephase am Transientenspeicher (TRC);
3. Lesen und Konvertieren der Meßdaten vom TRC (TRC-Meßdaten in INTEGER-Werte) sowie Zwischenspeichern im Rechner;
4. Auswertung der Meßwerte;
5. Speicherung der Kenngrößen der Hysteresisschleifen; und 1 - 5 Wiederholen bis zum Probenbruch bzw. Erreichen der Grenz-Schwingspielzahl;
6. Ausgabe der Kenngrößen in Tabellenform und im Schaubild.

5.2 PROGRAMM ZUR STEUERUNG DES MESSABLAUFS, DER DATENERFASSUNG UND DATENVERARBEITUNG

Das erstellte Programmsystem SWING setzt sich aus dem Hauptprogramm STRECON für spannungskontrollierte und STRACON für totaldehnungskontrollierte Versuchsführung sowie den Programmen PRINT und PLOT zur Ausgabe der Ergebnisse zusammen. Sämtliche Quellprogramme sind in der Programmiersprache FORTRAN geschrieben.

5.2.1 Hauptprogramm

Die Hauptprogramme STRECON und STRACON mit ihren Unterprogrammen dienen bei Einstufenversuchen zur kontinuierlichen Aufnahme und Auswertung von mechanischen Hysteresen. Eine Versuchsunter-

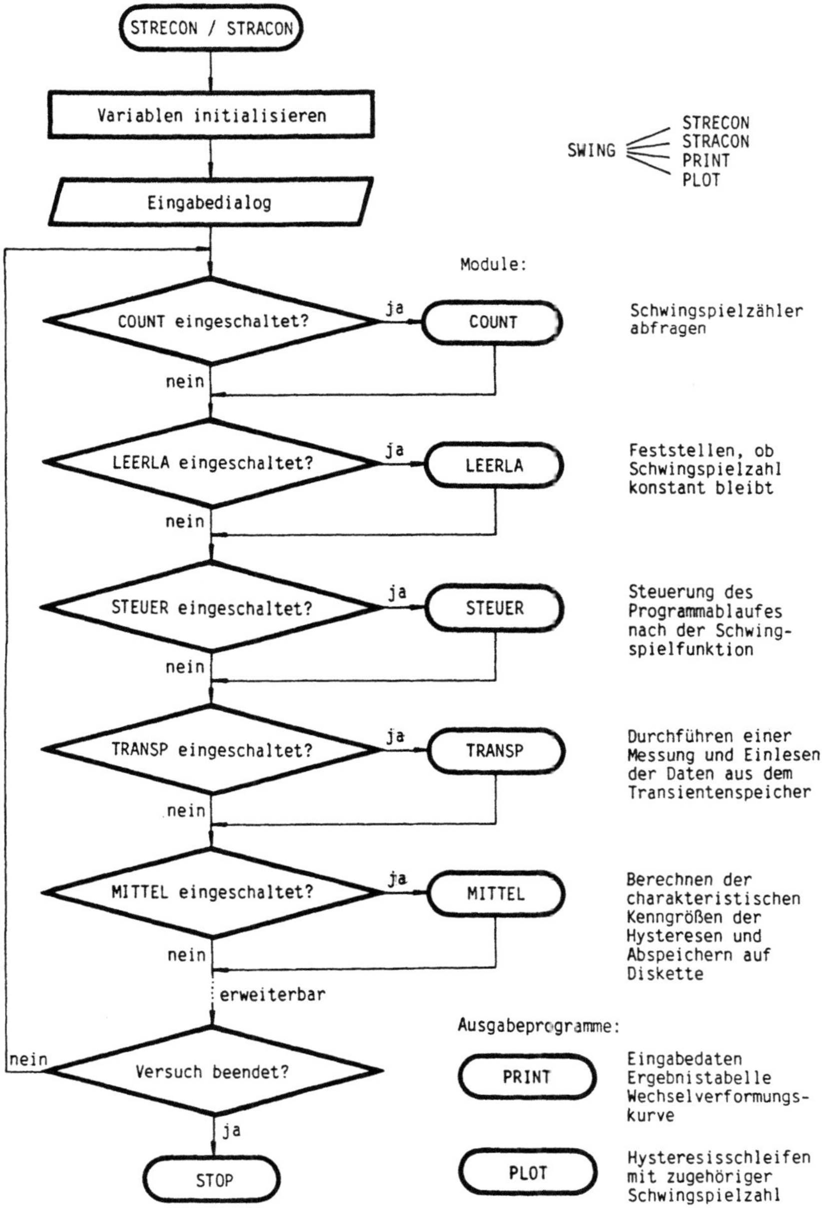

Bild 21: Programmssystem SWING.

brechung oder Frequenztransformation für die Messung, wie sie bei anderen Meßmethoden (z. B. Aufzeichung mit Hilfe eines x-y-Schreibers) erforderlich ist, entfällt bei den vorgesehenen Versuchsfrequenzen. Mit dem jeweiligen Programmaufruf wird die Initialisierung der Variablen durchgeführt, und es läuft anschließend der Eingabedialog mit dem Benutzer ab. Zuerst werden die Daten zur Kalibrierung des Transientenspeichers (TRC) eingegeben: Meßbereich am TRC in Volt und Zuordnung zwischen elektrischen und mechanischen Einheiten der aufzunehmenden Meßsignale (Kraft: 1V = ? kN; Längenänderung: 1V = ? mm). Die weiteren Angaben dienen zum Teil nur für das Versuchsprotokoll, z. B. die mechanischen Kennwerte aus dem Zugversuch, Versuchstemperatur, Schwingungsform, Beanspruchungsart, Belastungsamplitude, Mittelspannung bzw. Mitteldehnung. Aus den Angaben über die Messungsart (lokal oder integral) wird bei integraler Messung die Meßlänge L_0 abgefragt. Die Angabe des Prüfdurchmessers D_0 wird zur Berechnung der mechanischen Spannungen benötigt; aus der Versuchsfrequenz wird die Einstellung der Abtastrate am Transientenspeicher ermittelt und die Grenz-Schwingspielzahl N_G bestimmt das Programmende.

Die Programme sind aus überschaubaren Modulen aufgebaut und werden sequentiell abgearbeitet (Bild 21).

Den Modulen

- COUNT: Schwingspielzähler abfragen
- LEERLA: Feststellen, ob Schwingspielzähler konstant bleibt
- STEUER: Steuerung des Programmablaufs nach der Schwingspielfunktion
- TRANSP: Durchführung einer Messung und Übertragen der Daten vom Transientenspeicher zum Rechner
- MITTEL: Berechnen der charakteristischen Kenngrößen der Hysteresen und Abspeichern auf Diskette

ist je eine Steuervariable zugeordnet, die den Wert

- ON (Modul aktiv)
- OFF (Modul nicht aktiv)

annehmen kann.

Zu jedem Zeitpunkt hat genau eine dieser Steuervariablen den Wert ON. Die Module können sich selbst abschalten (OFF) und ein Nachfolge-Modul einschalten (ON). Damit kann jede beliebige Modul-Reihenfolge bei der Programmausführung ermöglicht werden. Außerdem ist das Programm so strukturiert, daß es um beliebig viele Module erweitert werden kann.

Im Arbeitsspeicher des Rechners ist ein Zwischenspeicherbereich für 30 Meßwertgruppen vorgesehen, wobei die charakteristischen Kennwerte (σ_{max}, σ_{min}, σ_m, ε_{max}, ε_{min}, ε_m, ε_{ar1} und ε_{ar2} der Hysteresis als eine Meßwertgruppe zusammengefaßt werden. Bei Überlauf wird der Zwischenspeicher automatisch auf den Diskettenspeicher (File: SAVE.DAT) ausgelagert, d. h. es steht ein Meßwertstack von der Kapazität der Diskette (600 kB) zur Verfügung.

5.2.2 Programmodule

Die Aufgabe des Moduls COUNT - Abfragen des Schwingspielzählers - ist aus dem vereinfachten Flußdiagramm in Bild 22 ersichtlich. Die Benutzung des Moduls bedarf keinerlei Voraussetzungen vom Programm her; nach jeder Schwingung wird die aktuelle Schwingspielzahl gelesen. Überschreiten der eingestellten Grenz-Schwingspielzahl N_G führt zum regulären Programmende. Zeigt der Zähler eine konstante Schwingspielzahl an, wird das Modul LEERLA aktiviert. Dies kann z. B. eintreten bei einem Probenbruch bzw. bei einem "Reset" am dynamischen Funktionsgenerator zum erforderlichen vor- bzw. zwischenzeitlichen Probenausbau für weitere Untersuchungen. Während der Schwingbeanspruchung wird kontinuierlich gemessen, die Abspeicherung der Meßwertgruppen erfolgt aber nach der Schwingspielfunktion (d. h. Bestimmung von 10 Meßwertgruppen pro Zehnerpotenz der Schwingspielzahl) und außerdem aufgrund gravierender Änderungen (innerhalb festgelegter Schranken) gegenüber der vorangegangenen Meßwertgruppe.

Mit Hilfe des Moduls LEERLA wird festgestellt, ob die Schwing-

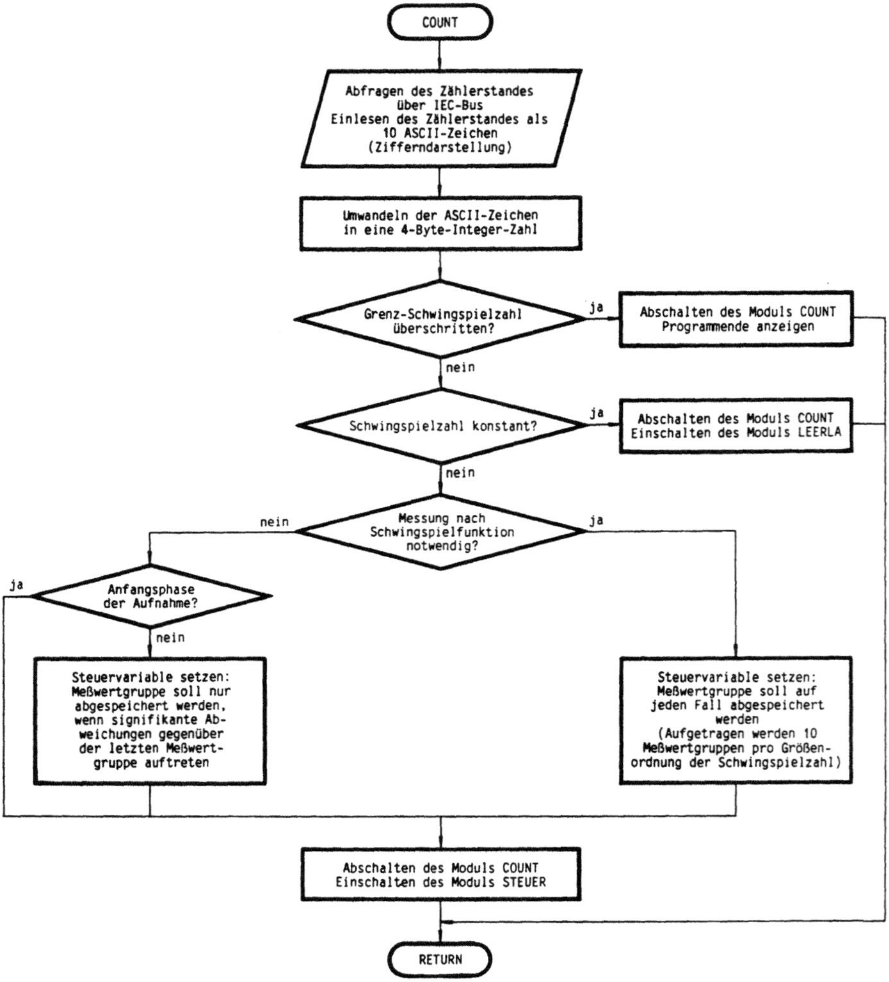

Bild 22: Vereinfachtes Flußdiagramm für den Modul COUNT.

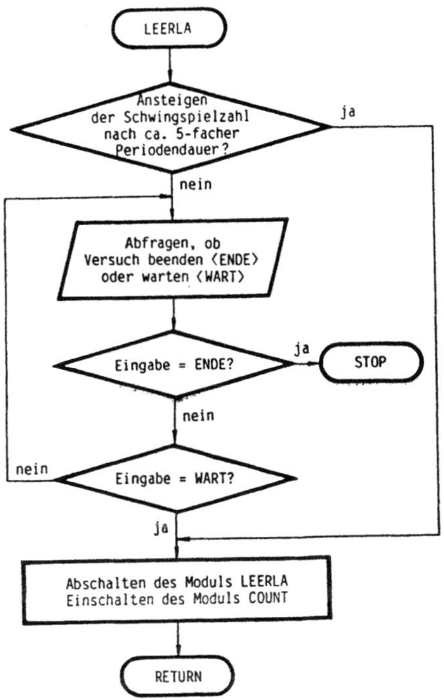

Bild 23: Vereinfachtes Flußdiagramm für den Modul LEERLA.

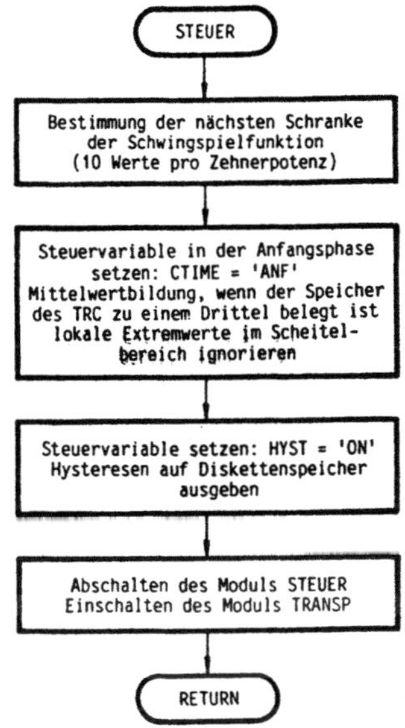
STEUER
Bestimmung der nächsten Schranke der Schwingspielfunktion (10 Werte pro Zehnerpotenz)
Steuervariable in der Anfangsphase setzen: CTIME = 'ANF'
Mittelwertbildung, wenn der Speicher des TRC zu einem Drittel belegt ist
lokale Extremwerte im Scheitelbereich ignorieren
Steuervariable setzen: HYST = 'ON'
Hysteresen auf Diskettenspeicher ausgeben
Abschalten des Moduls STEUER
Einschalten des Moduls TRANSP
RETURN

Bild 24: Vereinfachtes Flußdiagramm für den Modul STEUER.

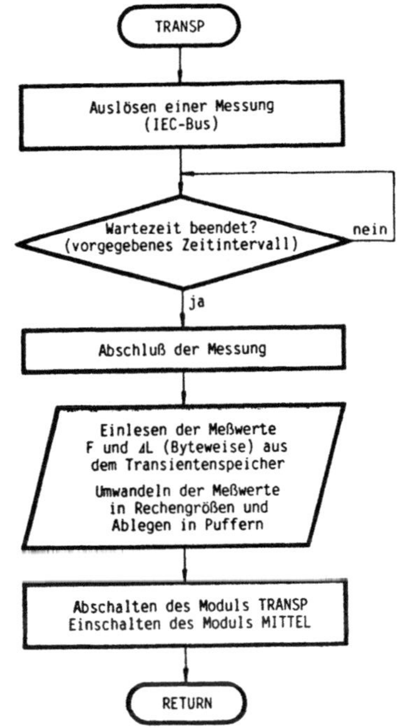

Bild 25: Vereinfachtes Flußdiagramm für den Modul TRANSP.

spielzahl konstant bleibt (siehe Bild 23). Steigt diese bzw. der Zählerstand innerhalb einer Zeit von ca. 5 Perioden der eingestellten Versuchsfrequenz weiter an, so wird der Modul LEERLA inaktiv und Modul COUNT aktiv. Bleibt die Schwingspielzahl konstant, wird über die Konsole abgefragt, ob der Versuch beendet oder gewartet werden soll, bis die Schwingspielzahl weiter ansteigt. Bei der Eingabe von "ENDE" wird das Programm regulär beendet. Die Eingabe von "WART" bewirkt Abwarten, bis die Schwingspielzahl weiter steigt sowie Aktivieren des Moduls COUNT.

Der Modul STEUER (Bild 24) übernimmt die Steuerung des Programmablaufs unter der Voraussetzung, daß die vorherige Messung abgeschlossen wurde (vor der ersten Messung Steuervariable auf 'ON' gesetzt). Der Modul liefert als Ergebnis die nächste Schranke der Schwingspielfunktion und aktiviert den Modul MITTEL. Meßwertgruppen die unbedingt zwischenzuspeichern sind, werden logarithmisch über der Schwingspielzahl aufgetragen. Soweit möglich werden 10 Meßwertgruppen pro Zehnerpotenz bestimmt. Über den Abstand in der Schwingspielfunktion werden die Steuervariablen CTIME und HYST beeinflußt. Hiermit wird der Rechenzeitbedarf für die Meßwertbildung variabel gehalten. In der Anfangsphase (Steuervariable CTIME = 'ANF') des Versuchs bzw. der Messung wird die Aufnahme abgebrochen, wenn der Speicher zu einem Drittel belegt ist, um in kürzeren Zeitabständen gemittelte F/ΔL-Wertepaare im Hinblick auf die logarithmische Auftragung der Ergebnisse zu erhalten.

Die Struktur des Moduls TRANSP ist im vereinfachten Flußdiagramm in Bild 25 dargestellt. Durch die vorgegebene Schwingspielfunktion wird eine Messung über den IEC-Bus angestoßen. Auch wenn der TRC eine leere Messung bei Probenbruch ausführt, kann es erforderlich sein, redundante Information zu ignorieren. Es liegen nach Abschluß der Messung je 2000 Meßwerte der F(t)- und ΔL(t)-Funktion als Rechengrößen vor. Nach Abschalten des Moduls TRANSP ist der Modul MITTEL aktiv.

Die Aufgabe des Moduls MITTEL geht aus dem vereinfachten Fluß-

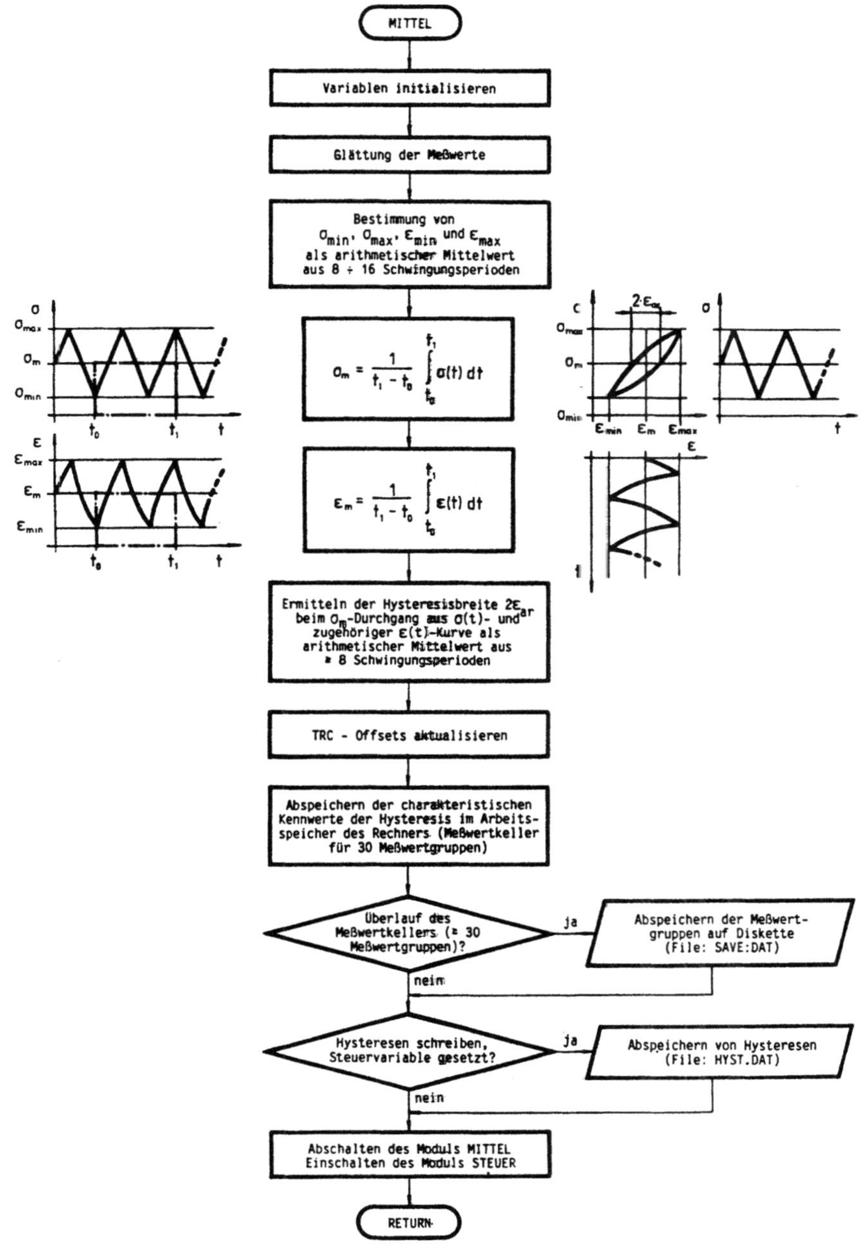

Bild 26: Vereinfachtes Flußdiagramm für den Modul MITTEL.

diagramm in Bild 26 hervor. Voraussetzung für den Ablauf in MITTEL sind die Ergebnisse aus TRANSP. Für die Meßwerte ist eine Glättung vorgesehen, die aber im Schweitelbereich der Meßwertfunktion sowie beim Mittelwertdurchgang wirkungslos ist. Die absoluten Meßwerte werden durch Addition der Offsets bestimmt. Abhängig von den Meßfunktionen wird versucht, die elektrische Spannung für die Mittelwerte an den beiden Kanälen in der Mitte des eingestellten Meßbereichs zu halten. Beispielsweise bei Versuchen mit Mittelspannungen ist das Nachführen des Meßbereichs sinnvoll, um mögliche Meßbereichsüberschreitungen aufgrund zyklischer Kriechvorgänge zu verhindern. Die Offsets werden vor dem Programmlauf grob voreingestellt und während des Schwingversuches vom Programm aus an der Frontplatte des TRC angezeigt.

Bestimmung der Extremwerte:
Mit relativ großer Schrittweite werden Intervalle gesucht, in denen Extremwerte für die F(t)- und $\Delta L(t)$-Funktion liegen. Durch binäres Suchen wird ein (lokales) Maximum bzw. (lokales) Minimum gefunden. Nach der Anfangsphase werden alle lokalen Maxima (Minima) im Scheitelbereich gemittelt. Die lokalen Extremwerte werden durch schrittweises Suchen gefunden. Dadurch können innerhalb gewisser Grenzen Meßfehler toleriert werden (z. B. bei einem kleinen "Brumm" auf dem Meßsignal). Lokale Extremwerte können - müssen aber nicht - auf Meßfehler zurückzuführen sein. Derartige Fehler sind im Bereich um die tatsächlichen Extremwerte zu erwarten, da hier die Steigungen der Meßfunktionen im Bereich der Meßfehler liegen können. Die Extremwerte werden über eine gewisse Anzahl der Schwingspiele gemittelt, und durch Multiplikation mit skalierenden Faktoren die Kennwerte σ_{min}, σ_{max}, ε_{min} und ε_{max} bestimmt.

Bestimmung der Mittelwerte:
Die Mittelwerte σ_m und ε_m der $\sigma(t)$- und $\varepsilon(t)$-Funktion werden in einem bestimmten Zeitintervall definiert und in der Regel vom ersten Minimum bis zum letzten Maximum innerhalb des Zeitintervalls integriert. Nach Bestimmung der Mittelwerte werden die Spannungsoffsets am TRC aktualisiert. Die Berechnung der halben

Schwingbreite der Hysteresis ε_{ar} - wird am Mittelwertdurchgang (negative Steigung - ε_{ar1} bzw. positive Steigung - ε_{ar2}) der Kraft- bzw. Spannungsfunktion berechnet. Durch binäres Suchen werden die zwei aufeinanderfolgenden Meßwerte der F(t)-Funktion bestimmt, zwischen denen der Mittelkraftdurchgang liegt. Außerdem wird der Zeitpunkt für den F_m-Durchgang und der plastische Längenänderungs- bzw. Dehnungwert auf diesen Zeitpunkt interpoliert. Meßfehler sind hier unbedeutend, da für die kontrollierte F(t)-Funktion im Bereich um den Mittelwertduchgang relativ zum Meßfehler große Steigungen zu erwarten sind. Die ermittelten Längenänderungswerte werden gemittelt, und durch Multiplikation mit skalierenden Faktoren die Kennwerte ε_{ar1} und ε_{ar2} bestimmt. Analoges Vorgehen erfolgt bei totaldehnungskontrollierter Versuchsführung.

5.2.3 Ausgabemöglichkeiten

Die Ergebnisse aus dem Einstufenversuch werden durch das Programm PRINT (Bild 27) ausgegeben. Hierbei wird neben den Daten

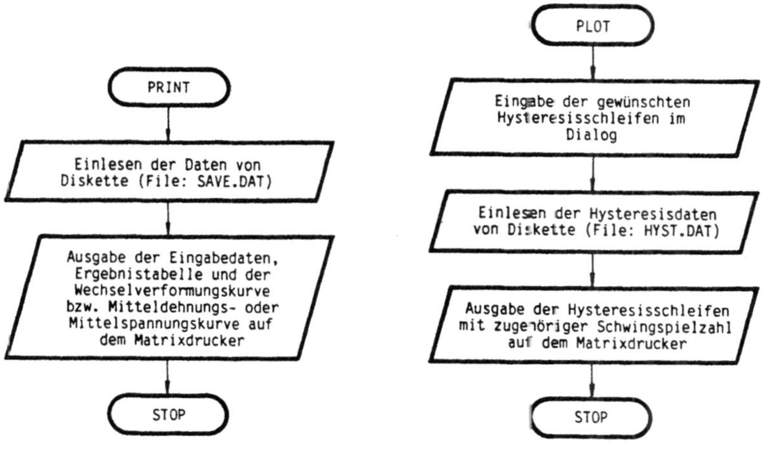

Bild 27: Vereinfachtes Flußdiagramm für die Ausgabediagramme PRINT und PLOT.

aus dem Eingabedialog eine Ergebnistabelle mit den charakteristischen Kennwerten der Hysteresis unter Zuordnung der Lebensdauer in Form der Schwingspielzahl aufgelistet. Weiterhin wird die vollständige Wechselverformungskurve bzw. bei Mittelspannung $\sigma_m \neq 0$ oder Mitteldehnung $\varepsilon_m \neq 0$ die Mitteldehnungs- oder Mittelspannungskurve graphisch dargestellt.

Ab ca. 300 Schwingspielen ist es möglich, mit dem Programm PLOT (Bild 27) verschiedene Stadien der Ermüdung (quasielastische Verformung, Rißinitiierung und Probenbruch) in Form von Hysteresisschleifen mit zugehöriger Schwingspielzahl auf dem Bildschirm und Matrixdrucker auszugeben. Durch einen Dialog ist ein gezielter Zugriff zum Datenspeicher gewährleistet.

6 EINFLUSSGRÖSSEN AUF DAS ERMÜDUNGSVERHALTEN

Im Vordergrund der Untersuchung standen die Auswirkung der beiden ausgewählten Umformverfahren auf das Ermüdungsverhalten der Werkstücke (Bild 28). Weiterhin wurde der Einfluß der Prüfbedingungen wie z. B. die Frequenz und die Art der Versuchsführung auf die Versuchsergebnisse behandelt.

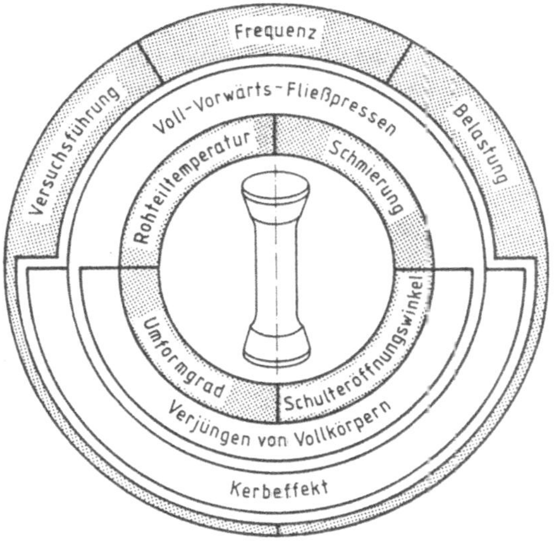

Bild 28: Einflüsse auf das Ermüdungsverhalten von massivumgeformten Werkstücken.

Zur Untersuchung der strukturmechanischen Änderungen im Werkstoff bei schwingender Beanspruchung eignen sich Hysteresismessungen (Registrierung von Spannung und zugehöriger Dehnung). Abgesehen von den ersten Schwingspielen stellt sich eine geschlossene Kurve ein, die als mechanische Hysteresisschleife bezeichnet wird. Die von ihr umschlossene Fläche ist ein Maß für die aufgebrachte Arbeit, die größtenteils in Wärme umgesetzt wird; der Rest wird als innere Energie in Form von Gitterfehlern in der Probe gespeichert. Die Hysteresiskurve hängt vom Werkstoff, seiner Vorbehandlung und der gewählten Spannungs- und Dehnungsamplitude ab /53/.

6.1 EINFLUSS DER VERSUCHSFÜHRUNG

In Bild 29 sind die beiden angewandten Arten der Versuchsführung gegenübergestellt. Alle Ermüdungsversuche wurden mit dreieckförmiger Schwingungsform, d. h. mit konstanter Spannungsanstiegsgeschwindigkeit, durchgeführt. Überwiegend wurden die Versuche kraftkontrolliert bzw. bei Annahme eines konstanten Prüfquerschnittes spannungsgeregelt gefahren, d. h. die Proben wurden während der gesamten Versuchsdauer zwischen zwei konstant gehaltenen Spannungsgrenzwerten schwingend beansprucht. Die beiden eingezeichneten Hysteresisschleifen geben dabei die Werkstoffreaktion zu zwei verschiedenen Zeitpunkten (t_A und t_B) wieder. Daraus ist auch zu ersehen, daß bei dieser Versuchsführung nur die Änderung der Hysteresisbreite beim Mittelspannungsdurchgang als relevante Kenngröße zur Beschreibung des Werkstoffverhaltens erfaßt werden muß.

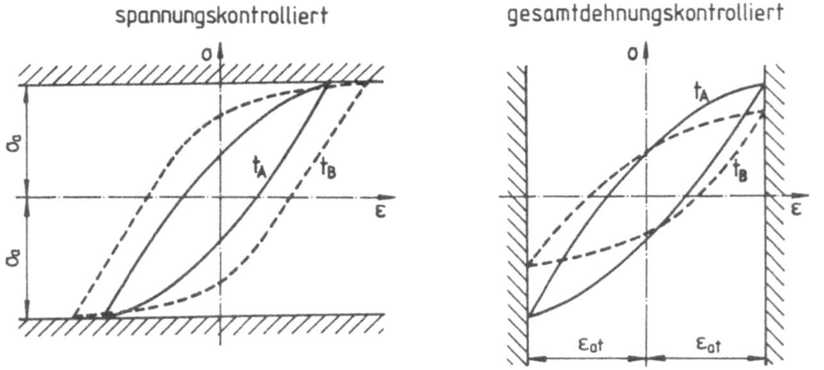

Bild 29: Versuchsführungen.

Im rechten Teilbild ist die gesamtdehnungskontrollierte Versuchsführung dargestellt, die in Einzelfällen zur Anwendung kam. Eine Änderung des Werkstoffverhaltens zeigt sich hier in einer Änderung der Spannungsamplitude und der irreversiblen plastischen Dehnungsamplitude in Form der halben Hysteresisbreite.

Die Auswertung eines spannungsgeregelten Versuches liefert die zu einem Schwingspiel gehörende irreversible plastische Dehnungsamplitude ε_{ar} als halbe Hysteresisbreite. Beim gesamtdehnungsgeregelten Versuch wird die Spannungsamplitude σ_a für die Auswertung verwendet. In beiden Fällen wird die die Meßpunkte ausmittelnde Kurve als Wechselverformungskurve bezeichnet.

In Bild 30 sind exemplarische Ergebnisse der beiden Versuchsarten vorgestellt. Im spannungskontrollierten Versuch zeigt die umgeformte Probe bei einem Spannungsausschlag von 470 N/mm^2 zyklische Wechselentfestigung mit der höchsten plastischen Dehnungsamplitude ε_{ar} = 3 ‰ und bei Spannungsamplituden im Bereich σ_a = 280 ÷ 300 N/mm^2 quasielastische Verformung bis zum Bruch. Bei Belastungsamplituden von 395 bzw. 430 N/mm^2 liegen im Lebensdauerbereich von 10^2 bis $8 \cdot 10^3$ bzw. $2 \cdot 10^3$ bis 10^4 Schwingspielen Sättigungsgebiete vor.

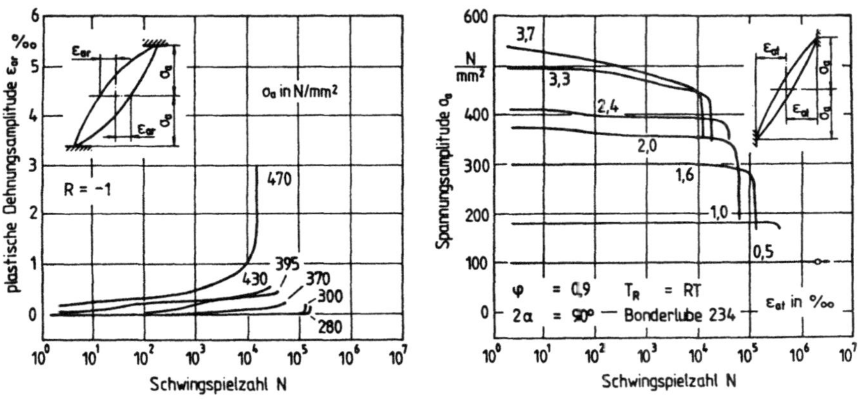

Bild 30: Wechselverformungskurven aus spannungs- und gesamtdehnungskontrollierten Versuchen (φ = 0,9 und 2α = 90°).

Beim gesamtdehnungskontrollierten Versuch bleiben für Beanspruchungen mit $\varepsilon_{at} \leq 1{,}6$ ‰ die Spannungsamplituden bis zum Auftreten eines makroskopischen Anrisses konstant. Gesamtdehnungen im Bereich $2{,}0 \leq \varepsilon_{at} \leq 3{,}3$ ‰ zeigen nach einer quasielastischen Initialphase eine in die Rißausbreitungsphase übergehende

Wechselentfestigung. Dagegen nimmt bei ε_{at} = 3,7 ‰ schon mit den ersten Schwingspielen die Spannungsamplitude ab, und der Werkstoff entfestigt.

Der Einfluß der Versuchführung wird in Bild 31 anhand eines zyklischen Spannungs-Dehnungs-Diagramms diskutiert. Da der über dem Querschnitt inhomogen verfestigte Werkstoff nur bei wenigen Werten der Beanspruchungsamplitude einen konstanten Kurvenbereich über hinreichend viele Schwingspiele aufweist, ist eine eindeutige Bestimmung der zyklischen Spannungs-Dehnungskurve schwierig. Deshalb wurde - wie von Morrow und Tuler /54/ vorgeschlagen - derjenige Dehnungswert ε_{ar} zugrundegelegt, der unter der aufgeprägten Beanspruchung bei der halben Bruch-Schwingspielzahl gemessen wurde. Die ermittelten Spannungs-Dehnungskurven lassen praktisch keinen Einfluß der Versuchsführung erkennen. Selbst die statische Spannungs-Dehnungskurve ($\dot{\varepsilon}$ in etwa wie bei 5 Hz) liegt nur geringfügig über der zyklischen; das Werkstück zeigt eine schwache Wechselentfestigung.

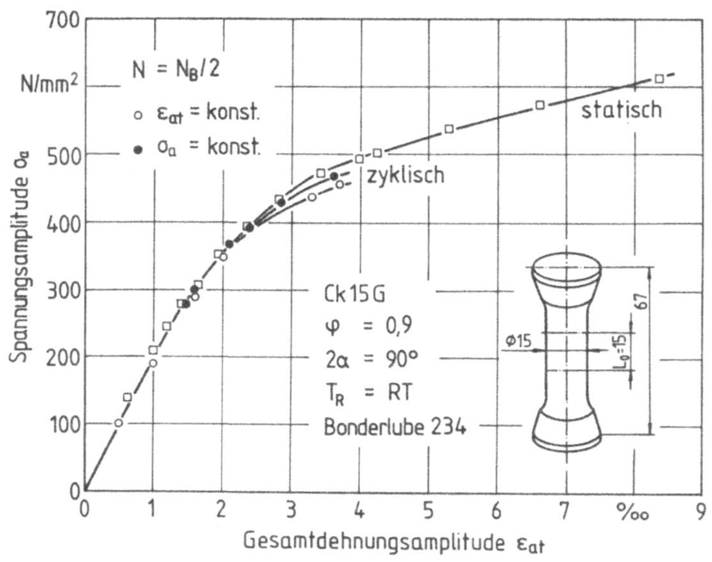

Bild 31: Vergleich der statischen und spannungs- bzw. gesamtdehnungskontrolliert ermittelten zyklischen σ/ε-Kurve.

6.2 FREQUENZEINFLUSS

Die Untersuchungen wurden mit einer Versuchsfrequenz im Bereich $1 \le f \le 10$ Hz, meistens mit 5 Hz durchgeführt. Bei höheren Beanspruchungsamplituden ($\sigma_a \le R_{p0,2}$) wurde, um eine Erwärmung der Probe zu unterdrücken, die Frequenz auf 1 Hz festgesetzt. Bei kleineren Belastungsamplituden im Bereich hoher Schwingspielzahlen ($N_B \ge 2\cdot10^6$) hat die Frequenz keinen signifikanten Einfluß auf das Wechselverformungsverhalten /55/; in diesen Fällen wurde sie zur Verringerung der Versuchsdauer auf 10 Hz festgelegt.

Im Schrifttum wird des öfteren über den Einfluß der Versuchsfrequenz auf die Dauerfestigkeit berichtet - teilweise mit widersprüchlichen Ergebnissen /56, 57/; aus dem Bereich der Zeitfestigkeit sind allerdings nur wenig Arbeiten bekannt. Heimbach /58/ wies an normalisierten und vergüteten Proben nach, daß der Abfall der Zeitfestigkeit bei Frequenzen über 33 Hz auf einer Probenerwärmung beruht.

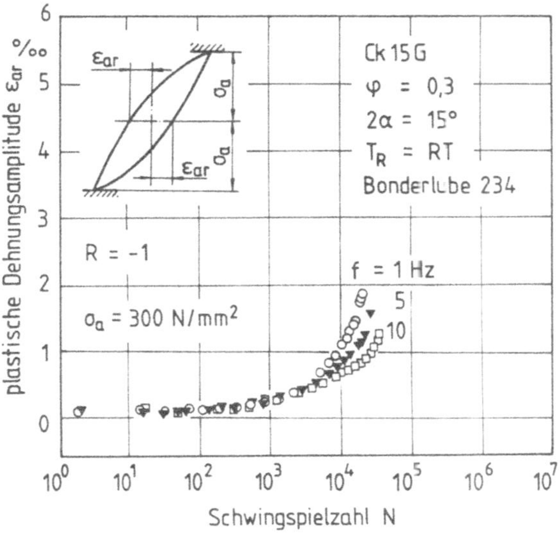

Bild 32: Frequenzeinfluß bei verjüngten Werkstücken.

Bild 32 zeigt Beispiele für das Frequenzverhalten bei verjüngten Schäften und belegt den relativ schwachen Frequenzeinfluß durch einzelne Meßpunkte in qualitativ vergleichbaren Wechselverformungskurven. Die zyklische Entfestigung ist umso ausgeprägter, je niedriger die Frequenz bzw. Verformungsgeschwindigkeit ist. Die plastische Dehnungsamplitude ($\varepsilon_{ar} = \varepsilon_{ar}^{(max)}(N_B)$) fällt mit zunehmender Frequenz linear ab; dabei liegen die sich einstellenden Bruchschwingspielzahlen in einem eng begrenzten Intervall ($2{,}0 \cdot 10^4 \leq N_B \leq 2{,}8 \cdot 10^4$).

6.3 WEICHGEGLÜHTER AUSGANGSZUSTAND

Bild 33 zeigt die Wechselverformungskurven für den weichgeglühten Stahl Ck15G; dies entspricht dem Ausgangszustand der Rohteile vor der Umformung. In der Anfangsphase tritt bei allen spannungskontrollierten Versuchen kein nennenswerter plastischer Deformationsanteil auf, da die Versetzungsbewegung unterhalb der Streckgrenze durch Verankerungen behindert wird /59/.

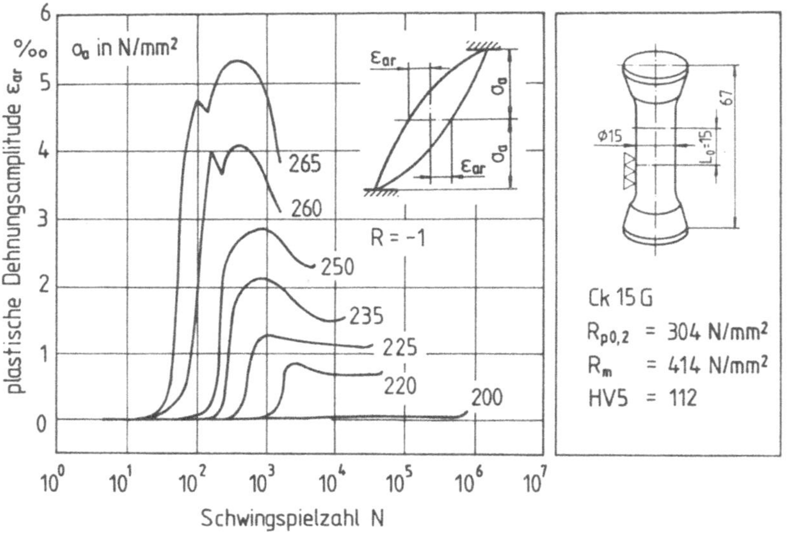

Bild 33: Wechselverformungsverhalten von weichgeglühtem Ck15.

An das von der gefahrenen Spannungsamplitude σ_a abhängige Inkubationsintervall (≈1% der Gesamtlebensdauer; $\varepsilon_{ar} \leq 0{,}05$ ‰) schließt sich eine Wechselentfestigung in Form einer allmählichen Zunahme der plastischen Dehnungsamplitude an. Diese primäre Entfestigung wird durch spannungsinduzierte Diffusion und eine damit verbundene Befreiung der Versetzungen von ihren Verankerungspunkten bewirkt /60/. Für Spannungsamplituden $\sigma_a > 250$ N/mm^2 wird nach einer schnell ablaufenden Entfestigung eine Entfestigungsspitze beobachtet, der eine Verfestigunsphase (primäre Verfestigung) und danach eine sekundäre Entfestigung folgt. Nach Erreichen eines zweiten Höchstwertes setzt sekundäre Verfestigung bis zum Ermüdungsbruch bei ca. $2 \cdot 10^3$ Schwingspielen ein. Bei mittleren Beanspruchungen ($225 \leq \sigma_a \leq 250$ N/mm^2) schließt sich an den Bereich der primären Entfestigung eine Verfestigungsphase (sekundäre Verfestigung) an, während sich bei $\sigma_a = 220$ N/mm^2 mit zunehmender Schwingspielzahl ($N > 10^4$) eine konstante plastische Dehnungsamplitude einstellt ("Sättigung").

Im Bereich der primären Verfestigung liegt gegenüber dem unverformten Werkstoffzustand eine erhöhte Versetzungsdichte vor, die nach /60/ die Gleitwege der Versetzungen innerhalb der Körner verringert und zu einer Abnahme der plastischen Dehnungsamplitude führt. Dagegen kann angenommen werden, daß sich im Bereich der sekundären Enfestigung die homogen vorliegenden Versetzungen mit fortschreitender Lebensdauer umorientieren und die Versetzungswege wieder größer werden. Während der sekundären Verfestigung nehmen bei großen Spannungsamplituden durch dreidimensionale Zellstrukturbildung und bei kleineren durch Enstehung von Versetzungsflecken und -clustern Anzahl und Laufweg der gleitfähigen Versetzungen ab. Dieses Wechselverformungsverhalten erweist sich als relevant für ungefähr 70 bis 95 % der Gesamtlebensdauer /60/.

Der Wiederanstieg der ε_{ar}/log N-Kurven in der Nähe der Bruch-Schwingspielzahl ist vermutlich auf eine zunehmende Nachgiebigkeit der glatten Proben zurückzuführen.

Zum Vergleich sind in Bild 34 die Wechselverformungskurven für den zweiten Versuchswerkstoff dargestellt. Das Ermüdungsverhalten des niedriglegierten Kohlenstoffstahls 16MnCr5G zeigt nach einigen Schwingspielen eine Anfangsentfestigung mit einer sich anschließenden verhältnismäßig schwach ausgeprägten Verfestigungsphase. Danach folgt wiederum zyklische Werkstoffentfestigung; im Beanspruchungsbereich $225 \leq \sigma_a \leq 260$ N/mm² bis zum Probenbruch und bei Spannungsamplituden $\sigma_a \geq 265$ N/mm² mit einer Verfestigung bis zum Versagen. Das Symbol o• kennzeichnet einen Durchläufer, d. h. die Probe hat nach quasielastischer Deformation die eingestellte Grenz-Schwingspielzahl $N_G = 2 \cdot 10^6$ ohne Bruch erreicht.

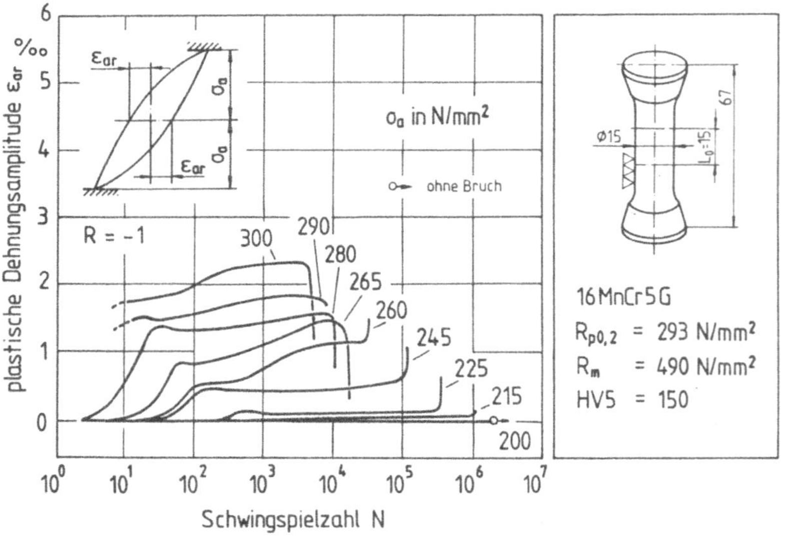

Bild 34: Wechselverformungskurven von weichgeglühtem 16MnCr5.

6.4 VERFAHRENSPARAMETER BEIM VOLL-VORWÄRTS-FLIESSPRESSEN

Plastische Deformationsvorgänge sind für die anrißfreie Phase der Ermüdung wesentlich und führen zum Aufbau charakteristischer Ermüdungsstrukturen im Werkstoff. Die folgenden Ergebnisse sollen in einer makroskopischen Betrachtung das Wechselverformungsverhalten in Abhängigkeit von den jeweiligen Verfahrensparametern beim Voll-Vorwärts-Fließpressen darstellen.

6.4.1 Umformgrad

6.4.1.1 Werkstoff Ck15G

Der Härteverlauf für $\varphi = 0{,}5$ im rechten oberen Teil von Bild 35 ist homogen in Längsrichtung des fließgepreßten Schaftes und zeigt eine deutlichen Anstieg zum Rand hin. Mit der Umformung ist eine Erhöhung der mechanischen Festigkeitskennwerte verbunden (siehe Tabelle 3 in Abschnitt 4.4). Zu Beginn der Schwingbeanspruchung wird in allen Fällen eine quasielastische Verformung bis zu ε_{ar} = 0,05 ‰ beobachtet. Die Initialphase nimmt mit zunehmender Spannungsamplitude ab. Daran schließt sich ein kontinuierlicher Anstieg der plastischen Dehnungsamplitude und somit eine Entfestigung mit steigender Schwingspielzahl an. Der Kurvenverlauf für σ_a = 430 N/mm² zeigt eine beschleunigte

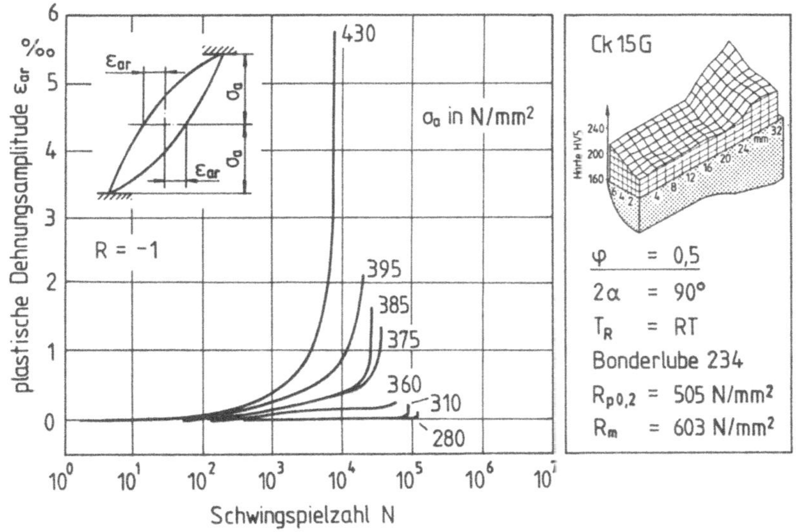

Bild 35: Wechselverformungsverhalten von Fließpreßteilen aus Ck15G (φ = 0,5 und 2α = 90°).

Entfestigung; die plastische Dehnungsamplitude wächst progressiv ohne erkennbare Unstetigkeit bis zur Anrißbildung bzw. bis zum Bruch. Bei kleineren Spannungsamplituden (σ_a = 280 und 310 N/mm^2 - jedoch oberhalb der Wechselfestigkeit - erfolgt bis zum Probenbruch eine quasielastische Verformung; es werden Bruch-Schwingspielzahlen von ca. 10^5 erreicht mit ε_{ar}-Werten in der Größenordnung unter 0,5 ‰. (siehe auch die Ergebnisse für φ = 0,9 in Bild 30).

Im Vergleich dazu sind in den Bildern 36 und 37 die Wechselverformungskurven für die Umformgrade φ = 1,2 und 1,6 dargestellt. Das Härteprofil weist in beiden Fällen einen nicht so hohen Gradienten über den Querschnitt auf wie für φ = 0,5. Bei diesen hohen Umformgraden zeigen sich selbst bei hohen Spannungsamplituden relativ kleine plastische Dehnungsamplituden ($\varepsilon_{ar} \leq$ 1,5 ‰). Es ist wiederum zyklische Wechselentfestigung festzustellen. Sättigungsgebiete (ε_{ar} = konst.) werden vornehmlich bei φ = 1,2 und Spannungsausschlägen von σ_a = 500 N/mm^2 sowie im

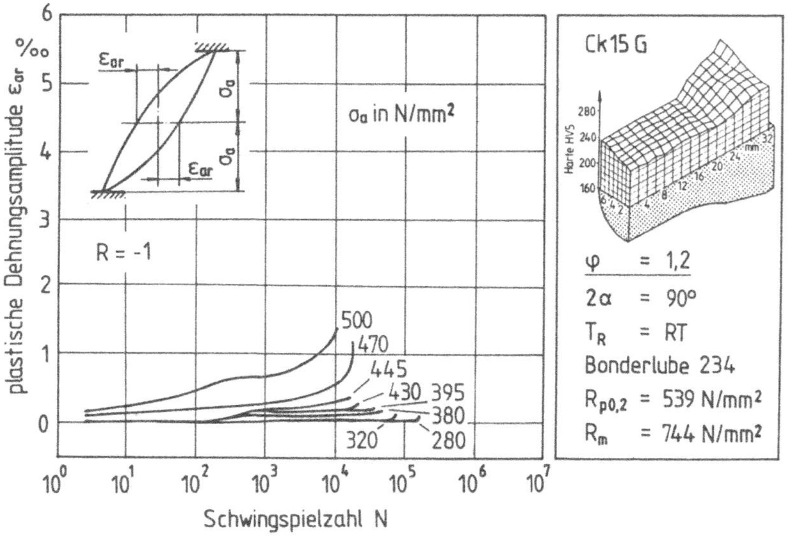

Bild 36: Wechselverformungsverhalten von Fließpreßteilen aus Ck15G (φ = 1,2 und 2α = 90°).

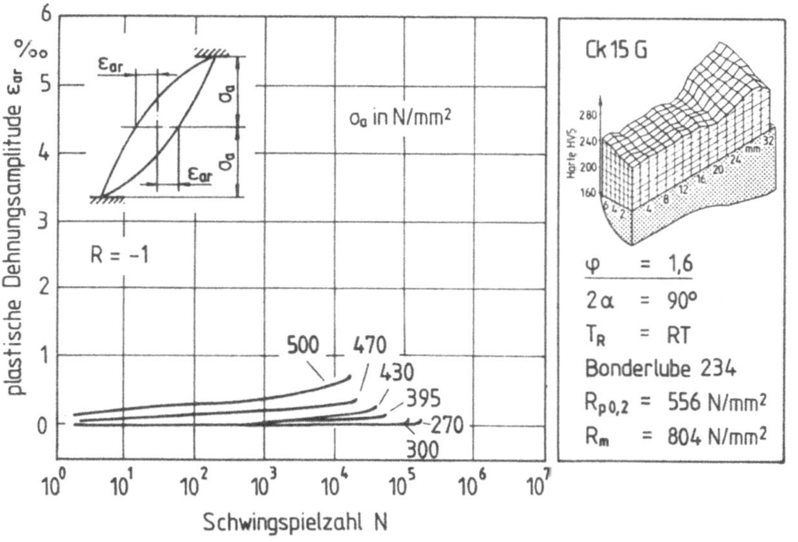

Bild 37: Wechselverformungsverhalten von Fließpreßteilen aus Ck15G (φ = 1,6 und 2α = 90°).

Bereich 380 ≤ σ_a ≤ 445 N/mm² beobachtet. Die Entfestigung liegt beim kaltumgeformten Werkstoffzustand im Bauschinger-Effekt begründet /17, 40/. Es wird vermutet, daß Eigenspannungen infolge von Gitterverzerrungen und aufgestauten Versetzungen das Fließen in die Gegenrichtung erleichtern. Allerdings ist der Bauschinger-Effekt bei kleinen Umformgraden (φ ≈ 0,05) am stärksten ausgeprägt und nimmt mit zunehmendem Umformgrad ab /61/. Kleine Beanspruchungsamplituden bewirken eine praktisch rein elastische Deformation bis zum Probenbruch.

In Bild 38 sind die sich aus den Wechselverformungskurven ergebenden zyklischen Spannungs-Dehnungskurven zusammengestellt. Da der unterschiedlich kaltverfestigte Werkstoff nicht bei allen gefahrenen Beanspruchungsamplituden einen ausgeprägten Sättigungsbereich (von der Schwingspielzahl unabhängiger konstanter Kurvenast des ε_{ar}-Verlaufs) über hinreichend viele Schwingspiele aufweist, wurde der Dehnungswert ε_{ar} bei der halben Lebensdauer zugrundegelegt. Diese Vorgehensweise er-

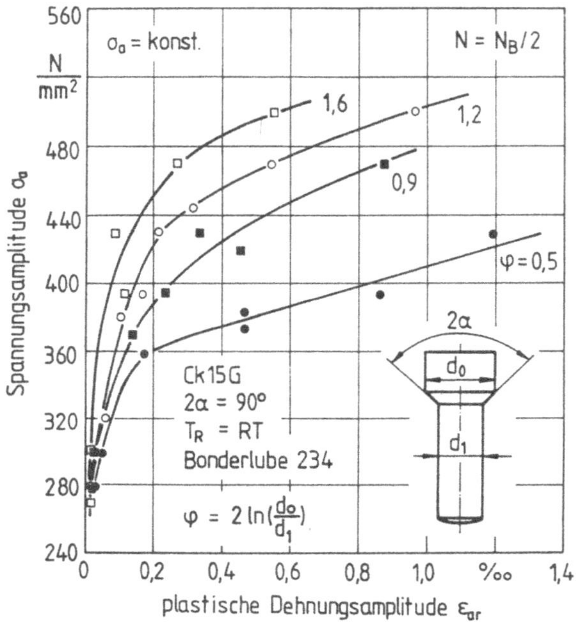

Bild 38: Zyklische Spannungs-Dehnungskurven als Funktion des Umformgrades.

scheint etwas willkürlich und nicht hinreichend metallphysikalisch fundiert. Eine Kontrollmöglichkeit für die Güte des Bestimmungsverfahrens ist die getrennte Ermittlung der zyklischen Fließkurve aus spannungs- und gesamtdehnungsgeregelten Versuchen /1/. Bild 31 zeigte, daß das Werkstoffverhalten der bauteilähnlichen Proben unter schwingender Beanspruchung durch eine zyklische Spannungs-Dehnungskurve beschrieben werden kann, da für beide Versuchsführungen die Kurvenverläufe quantitativ recht gut übereinstimmen.
Der Einfluß des Umformgrades auf die mechanischen Festigkeitseigenschaften unter schwingender Beanspruchung geht aus dem vorliegenden Diagramm hervor. Die zyklischen Spannungs-Dehnungskurven werden mit zunehmendem Umformgrad zu höheren Spannungswerten verschoben. Normiert man die Spannungamplituden σ_a auf die Zugfestigkeit R_m des sich durch die Kaltmassivumformung

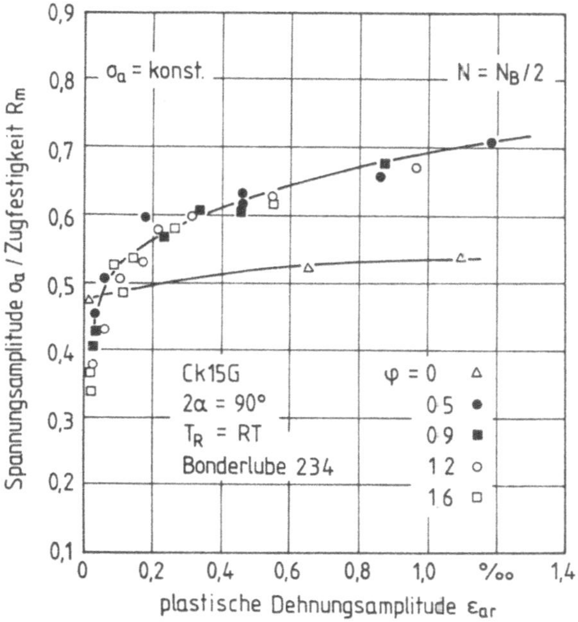

Bild 39: Normierte zyklische Spannungs-Dehnungskurven für unterschiedliche Werkstoffverfestiungen ($0 \le \varphi \le 1{,}6$).

einstellenden Werkstoffzustandes, so ergibt sich nach Bild 39 für die umgeformten Proben eine gemeinsame Ausgleichskurve, die gegenüber der Kurve des weichgeglühten Ausgangszustandes der Rohteile wesentlich höher liegt. Dies belegt die unter Wechselverformung unterschiedlich ablaufenden strukurmechanischen Vorgänge im weichgeglühten und kaltverfestigten Werkstoffzustand.

Im untersuchten Lebensdauerbereich verschiebt sich der Kurvenast der Wöhlerlinie (Bild 40) bei hohen Beanspruchungen mit zunehmendem Umformgrad (größere Steigung des Zeitfestigkeitsastes) zu höheren Lebensdauerwerten. Allerdings sagt das noch nichts darüber aus, wie sich der Umformgrad bei $N \ge 2 \cdot 10^6$ Schwingspielen auswirkt, denn mit höherer Zugfestigkeit sind nicht unbedingt auch höhere Wechsel- bzw. Dauerfestigkeiten verbunden (vgl. auch /62, 63/).

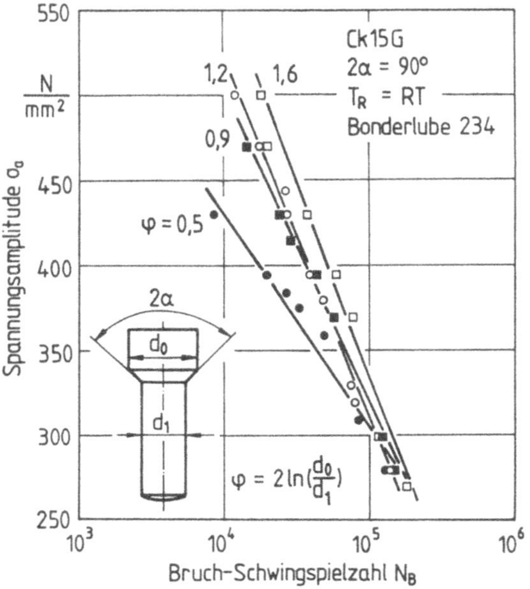

Bild 40: Wöhlerkurven als Funktion des Umformgrades.

6.4.1.2 Werkstoff 16MnCr5G

Der niedriglegierte Kohlenstoffstahl 16MnCr5G unterlag den gleichen Umformbedingungen ($2\alpha = 90^o$ = konst., Umformung bei Raumtemperatur mit beseiften Rohteilen) wie der Versuchswerkstoff Ck15G. Beispielhaft sind in den Bildern 41 und 42 die Wechselverformungskurven für φ = 0,5 und 1,2 zusammengestellt. Sie sind qualitativ ähnlich und von zyklischer Entfestigung geprägt. Die im vorigen Abschnitt erörterten makroskopischen Phänomene sind durchweg auch auf den Stahl 16MnCr5G übertragbar. Dieser Zusammenhang wird nochmals durch Bild 43 bestätigt. Die Unterschiede im Ermüdungsverhalten zwischen beiden Werkstoffen äußern sich überwiegend in der Höhe der akkumulierten Zustandsänderungen (aus Zug- und Druckverformung bestehender Verformungszyklus) und in der erreichten Lebensdauer. Unter der Annahme, daß sich qualitativ ähnliche Härteverteilungen über

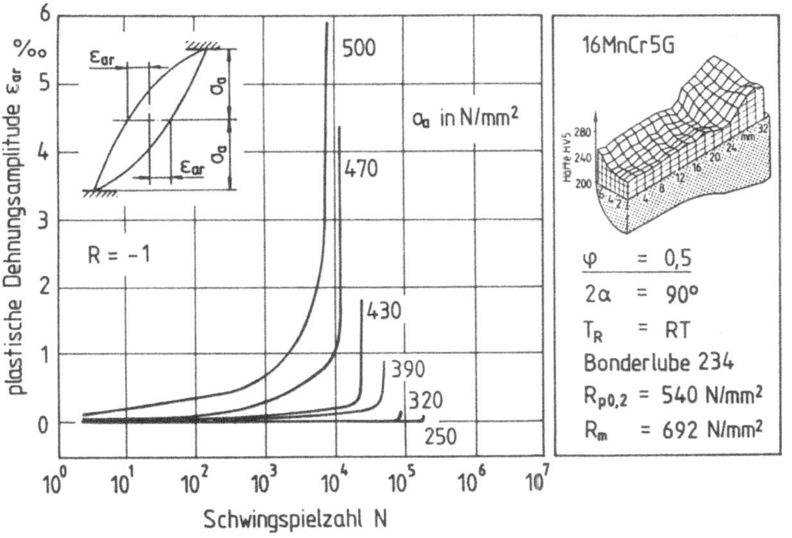

Bild 41: Wechselverformungskurven von Fließpreßteilen aus 16MnCr5G (φ = 0,5 und 2α = 90°).

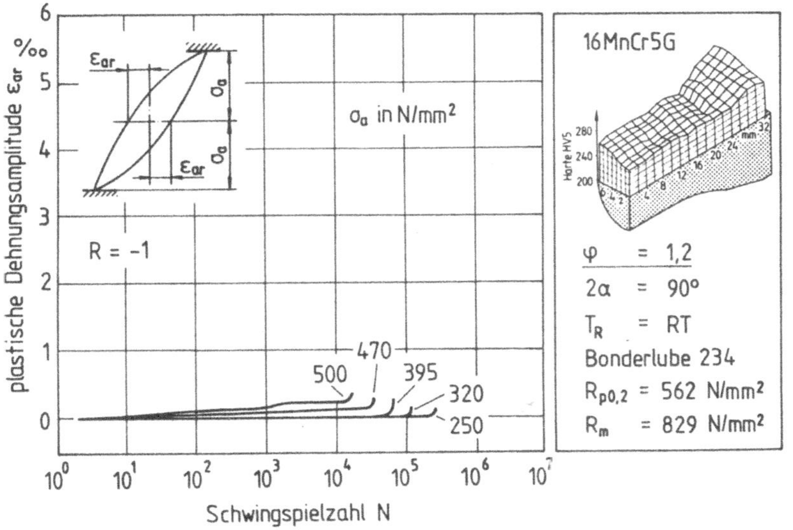

Bild 42: Wechselverformungskurven von Fließpreßteilen aus 16MnCr5G (φ = 1,2 und 2α = 90°).

dem Schaftquerschnitt einstellen wie bei Ck15G, liegen die Unterschiede in der höheren Ausgangsfestigkeit begründet.

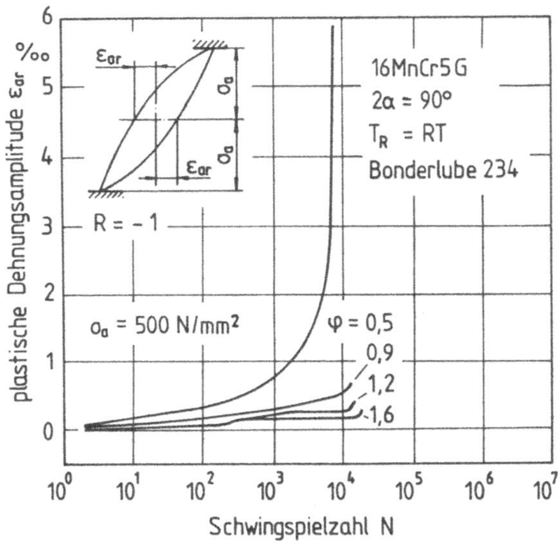

Bild 43: Wechselverformungskurven von Fließpreßteilen aus 16MnCr5G in Abhängigkeit vom Umformgrad.

6.4.2 Schulteröffnungswinkel

Bei konstantem Umformgrad φ = 1,2 und sonst gleichen Umformbedingungen wurde der Schulteröffnungswinkel 2α variiert (30°, 60°, 90°, 120° und 150°). Werden die bauteilähnlichen Proben mit einer spannungskontrollierten, mittelspannungsfreien Schwingbelastung und Spannungsamplituden $\sigma_a < R_{p0,2}$ beaufschlagt, so stellen sich für den jeweiligen Umformzustand charakteristische plastische Dehnungen in Abhängigkeit von der Schwingspielzahl ein. Die Ergebnisse sind in Form von Wechselverformungskurven in den Bildern 44 bis 47 zusammmengestellt (2α = 90°, siehe Bild 36). Der Einfluß des Schulteröffnungswinkels zeigt sich schon deutlich im unterschiedlichen Härteprofil: bei 2α = 30° nahezu konstanter HV5-Verlauf über dem

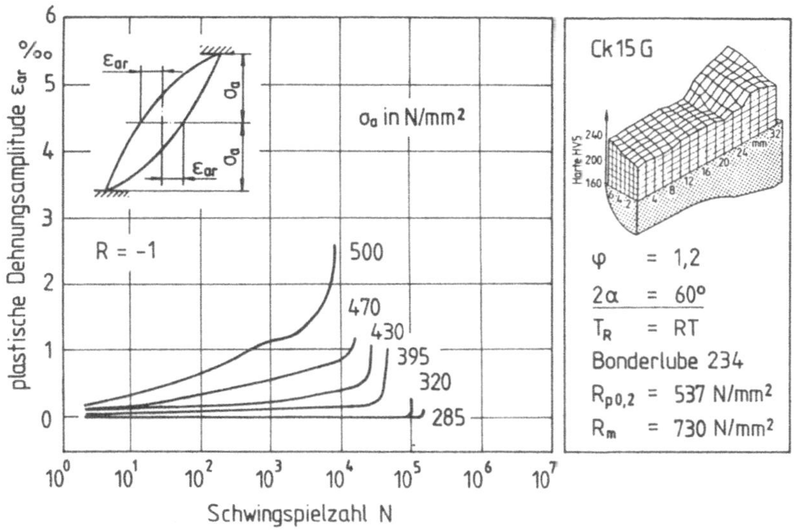

Bild 44: Wechselverformungskurven von Fließpreßteilen aus Ck15G ($2\alpha = 30^{\circ}$ und $\varphi = 1,2$).

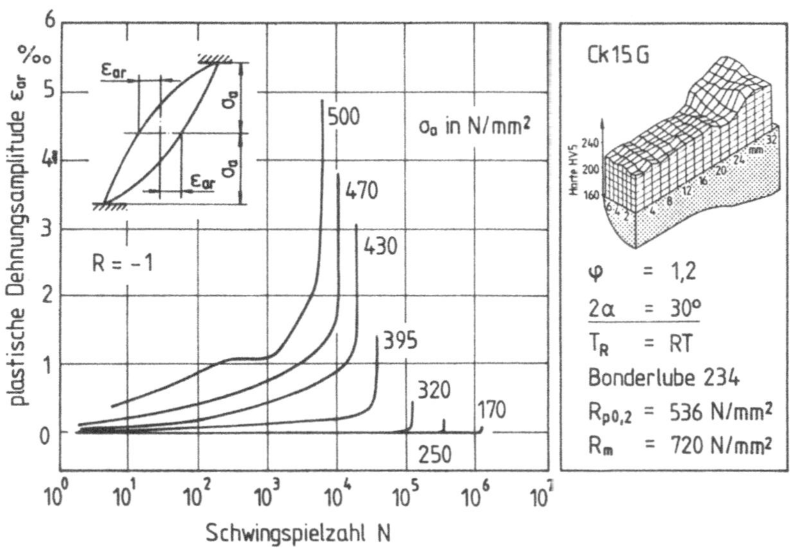

Bild 45: Wechselverformungskurven von Fließpreßteilen aus Ck15G ($2\alpha = 60^{\circ}$ und $\varphi = 1,2$).

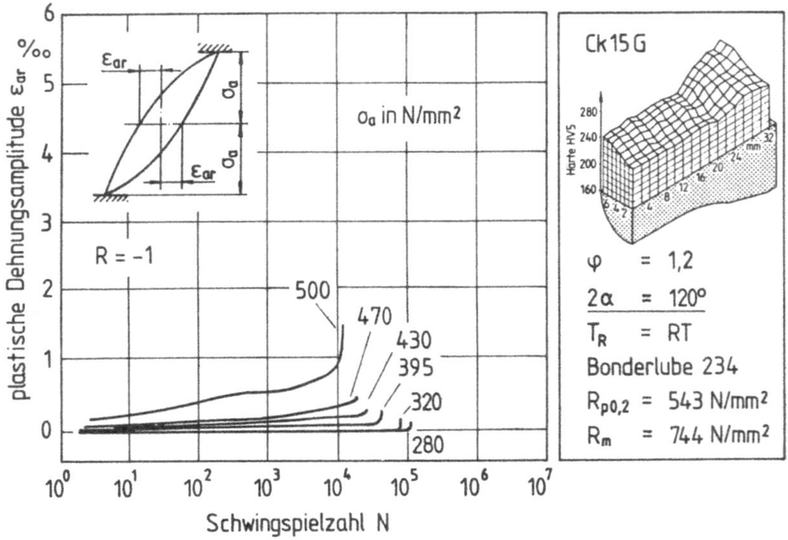

Bild 46: Wechselverformungskurven von Fließpreßteilen aus Ck15G ($2\alpha = 120^{\circ}$ und $\varphi = 1{,}2$).

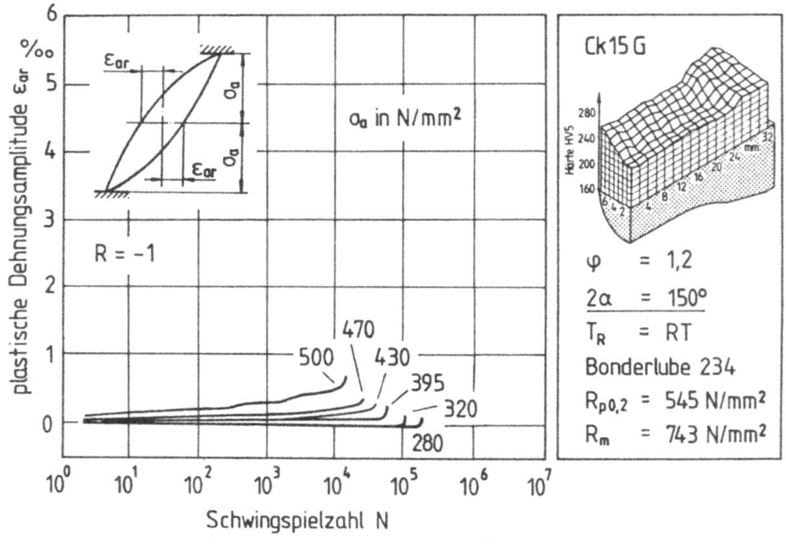

Bild 47: Wechselverformungskurven von Fließpreßteilen aus Ck15G ($2\alpha = 150^{\circ}$ und $\varphi = 1{,}2$).

Schaftquerschnitt, dagegen steiler Anstieg bei $2\alpha = 150^{o}$. Dieser Einfluß spiegelt sich auch in den gemessenen Wechselverformungskurven wieder. Auffallend ist bei der Spannungsamplitude $\sigma_a = 500\ N/mm^2$ und dem Schulteröffnungswinkel $2\alpha = 30^{o}$ das sich einstellende Sättigungsgebiet im Lebensdauerbereich $2 \cdot 10^2 \div 10^3$. Außerdem wird hierfür die höchste plastische Dehnungsamplitude (nahezu 5 ‰) beobachtet, während diese beim größten Schulteröffnungswinkel bei allen gefahrenen Belastungen unter 1 ‰ liegt. Die sich einstellenden Werkstoffzustände zeigen im allgemeinen makroskopische Wechselentfestigung, d. h. die plastischen Dehnungen nehmen kontinuierlich zu und gehen ohne erkennbare Unstetigkeit in die Rißausbreitungsphasen über. Spannungsamplituden von $170 \leq \sigma_a \leq 320\ N/mm^2$ führen praktisch ohne meßbare Verformung zum Probenbruch.

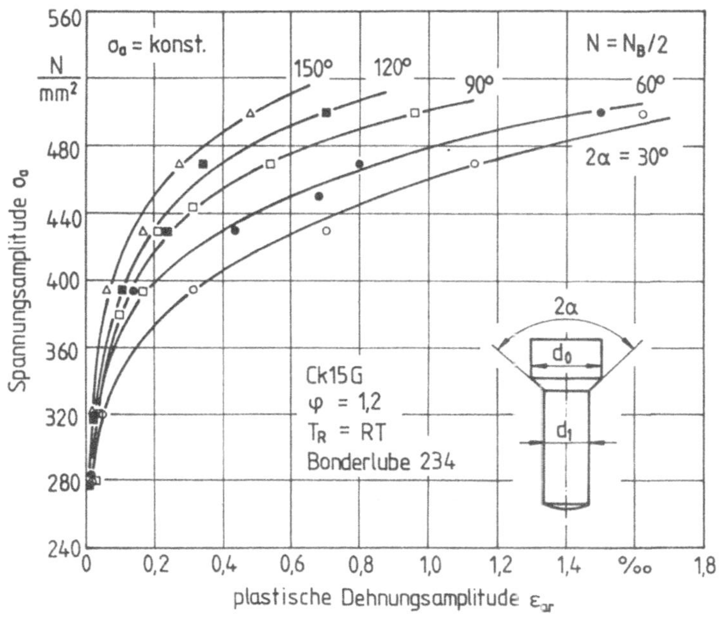

Bild 48: Zyklische Spannungs-Dehnungskurven als Funktion des Schulteröffnungswinkels.

In Bild 48 sind in Abhängigkeit vom Schulteröffnungswinkel die sich ergebenden zyklischen Spannungs-Dehnungskurven für N = $0{,}5 \cdot N_B$ zu sehen. Diese werden mit größer werdendem Schulteröffnungswinkel der Matrize zu höheren Spannungswerten verschoben und liegen wiederum auf einer gemeinsamen Ausgleichsgeraden, falls man die Spannungsamplitude auf die Zugfestigkeit (σ_a/R_m) bezieht (vgl. Bild 39).

Im untersuchten Lebensdauerbereich $10^3 \leq N_B \leq 2 \cdot 10^6$ liegen für alle Schulteröffnungswinkel die Meßpunkte in einem schmalen "Streuband" des Wöhlerdiagramms (Bild 49). Es erscheint deshalb schwierig, bei den einzelnen Schulteröffnungswinkeln Ausgleichskurven durch die Meßpunkte zu legen. Die Wechselfestigkeit der bauteilähnlichen Proben liegt aufgrund der inhomogenen Verfestigung beim Fließpressen (vgl. /36/) und der von der Umformung her beibehaltenen Oberflächentopographie nur bei ca. 140 N/mm²; eine präzisere Bestimmung würde eine statistische Versuchsplanung und Auswertung erfordern /64/.

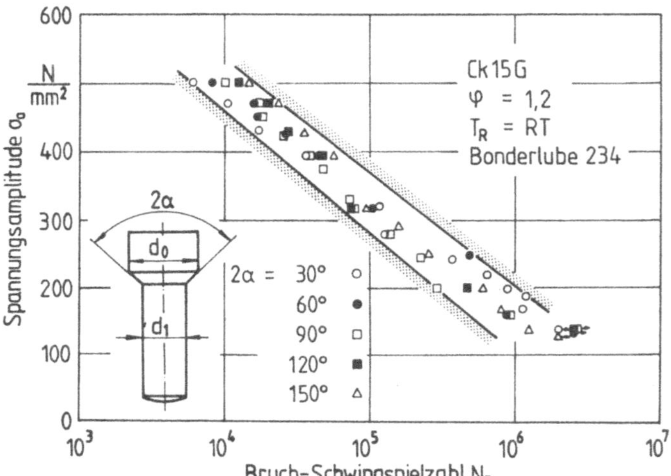

Bild 49: Wöhlerdiagramm in Abhängigkeit vom Schulteröffnungswinkel.

6.4.3 Schmierung

Eine Variation der Schmierungsbedingungen - bei sonst konstant gehaltenen Umformparametern (φ = 1,2 und 2α = 90°; Ck15G) - wurde ausschließlich für das Kaltfließpressen durchgeführt. Hierfür wurden die in Abschnitt 3.3.1 angegebenen Schmierstoffe Bonderlube 234 (Einsatztemperatur ca. 240 °C) und Molydag 15 (bis ca. 400 °C) eingesetzt. Für beide Schmierstoffe wurde als Schmierstoffträger eine ca. 10 ÷ 15 µm dicke Phosphatschicht aufgebracht, um auch unter hohem Druck einen zusammenhängenden Schmierfilm beim Gleiten des Werkstückes am Werkzeug zu erreichen. Der Einfluß der Schmierung läßt sich u. a. anhand einer Oberflächenmessung nachweisen. Dabei begünstigt - vermutlich infolge ihrer höheren Tragfähigkeit - die wässrige MoS_2-Suspension (Molydag 15) nicht in dem Maße wie die Metallseife den Glättungsvorgang und führt damit zu rauheren Schaftoberflächen (die Oberflächenmaßzahlen liegen ca. 25 % über denen beseifter Rohteile; vgl. Bild 14).

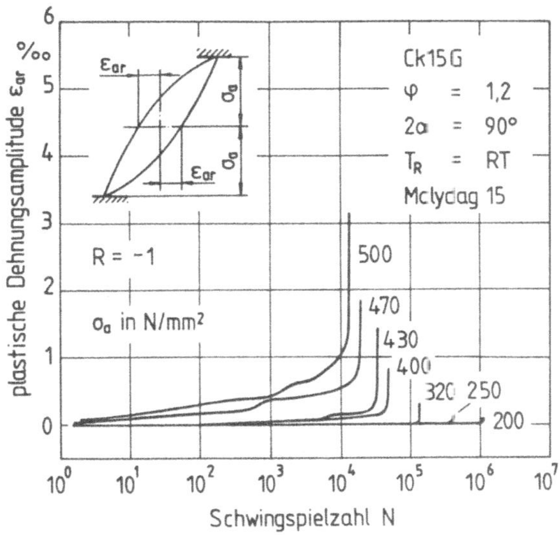

Bild 50: Wechselverformungskurven von Fließpreßteilen aus Ck15G (Molydag 15; φ = 1,2 und 2α = 90°).

In Bild 50 zeigen die Wechselverformungskurven der Werkstücke im Vergleich zu Bild 36 durchweg eine etwas höhere plastische Dehnungsamplitude ε_{ar} bei der Bruch-Schwingspielzahl N_B; über etwa 95 % der Lebensdauer liegen allerdings betragsmäßig ähnliche Werte vor. Insgesamt stellt sich gegenüber der Metallseife Bonderlube 234 kein signifikanter Einfluß des Schmierstoffes auf die erreichte Lebensdauer ein.

6.4.4 Umformtemperatur

Der Anwendungsbereich des Halbwarmfließpressens wird nach unten durch das Gebiet der Blausprödigkeit (niedriglegierte Kohlenstoffstähle und Einsatzstähle im Bereich $200 \leq T \leq 400$ °C) und nach oben durch das Gebiet der Rotsprödigkeit (ca. 800 °C) begrenzt. In dem dazwischenliegenden Intervall nimmt die Fließspannung der Stähle mit steigender Temperatur ab. In gleichem Maße reduziert sich auch die Werkzeugbelastung.

Zur Untersuchung der dynamischen Eigenschaften halbwarmfließgepreßter Werkstücke erschien es sinnvoll, die Rohteiltemperatur vor der Umformung auf 500 und 700 °C festzulegen. Die bauteilähnlichen Proben wurden mit der in Abschnitt 3.3.1 beschriebenen kombinierten Werkstück-/Werkzeugschmierung und einem geometrischen Umformgrad φ von 1,2 bzw. 1,6 sowie unverändertem Schulteröffnungswinkel $2\alpha = 90^\circ$ hergestellt.

Die Ergebnisse der Ermüdungsversuche sind aus den Bildern 51 bis 54 zu entnehmen. Halbwarmgefertigte Fließpreßschäfte zeigen teilweise ein verändertes Wechselverformungsverhalten. Bei beiden Umformgraden stellen sich nach dem Fließpressen mit einer Rohteiltemperatur von 500 °C noch qualitativ ähnliche Wechselverformungskurven wie nach einer Kaltmassivumformung ein. Dagegen erreicht die plastische Dehnungsamplitude ε_{ar} nach dem Halbwarmfließpressen mit $\varphi = 1{,}2$ und $T_R = 700$ °C zumindest bei den höheren Belastungen von 395 und 430 N/mm^2 nach einer allmählichen Zunahme - ohne auftretenden Sättigungszustand - ein Entfestigungsmaximum, dem sich eine Verfestigungsphase bis

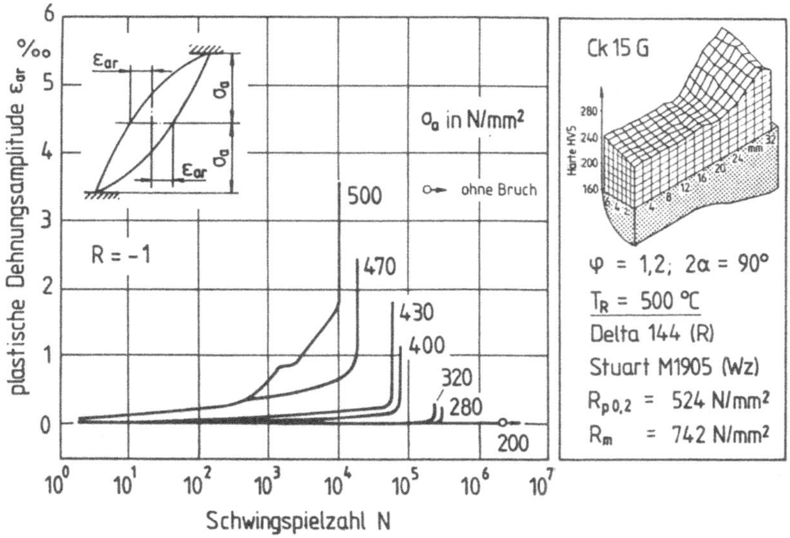

Bild 51: Wechselverformungskurven von halbwarmfließgepreßten Werkstücken aus Ck15G (T_R = 500 °C und φ = 1,2).

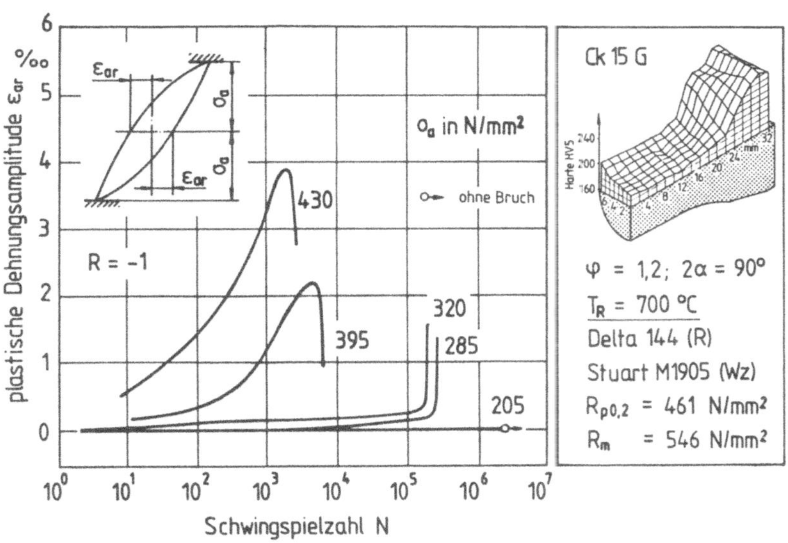

Bild 52: Wechselverformungskurven von halbwarmfließgepreßten Werkstücken aus Ck15G (T_R = 700 °C und φ = 1,2).

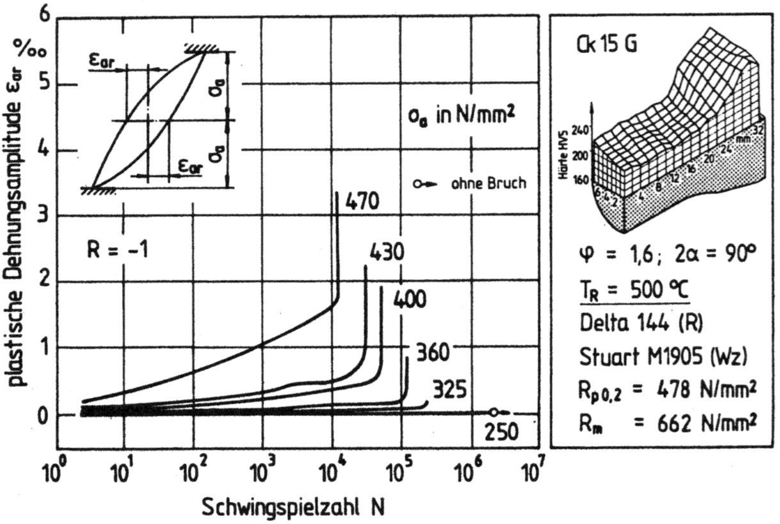

Bild 53: Wechselverformungskurven von halbwarmfließgepreßten Werkstücken aus Ck15G (T_R = 500 °C und φ = 1,6).

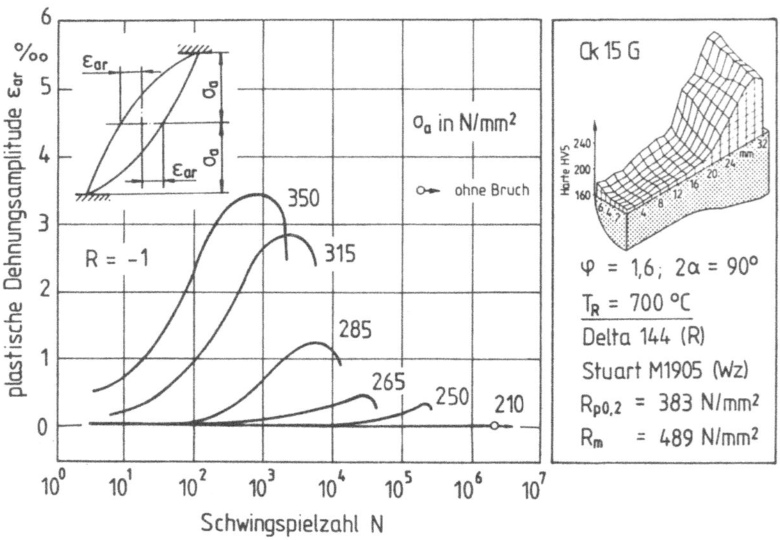

Bild 54: Wechselverformungskurven von halbwarmfließgepreßten Werkstücken aus Ck15G (T_R = 700 ° und φ = 1,6).

zum Probenbruch anschließt (Bild 52).

Deutlich wird dieses geänderte Verformungsverhalten unter mechanischer Beanspruchung beispielsweise erst nach $\varphi = 1{,}6$ und $T_R = 700\ ^{o}C$ sowie Spannungsamplituden im Bereich $250 \leq \sigma_a \leq 350$ N/mm^2 (Bild 54); bei allen ε_{ar}/log N-Kurven wird eine anfängliche Entfestigung mit zunehmender Schwingspielzahl bis zu einem Entfestigungspeak beobachtet. Daran schließt sich bei allen Spannungsamplituden ein Verfestigungsintervall mit abnehmenden ε_{ar}-Werten bis zum Bruch an. Tendenziell zeigen halbwarmfließgepreßte Werkstücke im Vergleich zu kaltfließgepreßten eine höhere Wechselfestigkeit. Dieses Phänomen ist vermutlich auf eine über dem Querschnitt homogenere Umformung zurückzuführen, denn ausgehend von der geringsten Härte der Preßteile in der Kernzone (kleinste örtliche Umformung, geringste Abkühlung auf dem Weg vom Ofen zur Matrize, verzögerte Abkühlung nach der Umformung) wird der Härteanstieg zum Randbereich hin mit zunehmender Temperatur geringer. Während beim Kaltfließpressen die Härte in der Schaftmitte mit dem Umformgrad steigt, ist dieser Zusammenhang beim Halbwarmfließpressen nicht gegeben (vgl. die Härteprofile in Kap. 6). Auffallend ist, daß nach dem Halbwarmfließpressen ($500 \leq T_R \leq 700\ ^{o}C$ mit dem Umformgrad $\varphi = 1{,}2$ eine höhere Härte erzielt wird als mit $\varphi = 1{,}6$ (siehe auch Bilder 51 bis 54). Denkbar wäre, daß beim Fließpressen mit der höheren relativen Querschnittsänderung auch die Temperaturerhöhung während der Umformung größer ist und somit Erholungs- sowie Rekristallisationsvorgänge die erwartete Festigkeitssteigerung mehr als nur kompensieren. Die Ergebnisse stimmen mit denen in /3/ überein.

Die bei der halben Lebensdauer $N/N_B = 0{,}5$ gemessenen Verformungen werden in Abhängigkeit von der Spannungsamplitude in ein zyklisches Spannungs-Dehnungsdiagramm eingetragen (Bild 55). Die $\sigma_a/\varepsilon_{ar}$-Kurven spiegeln in ihrer Lage genau die oben erörterten Ergebnisse aus den Härtemessungen wider; die zyklische Fließkurve ist bei beiden Temperaturen jeweils für den Umformgrad $\varphi = 1{,}2$ gegenüber $\varphi = 1{,}6$ zu höheren Spannungsausschlägen verschoben.

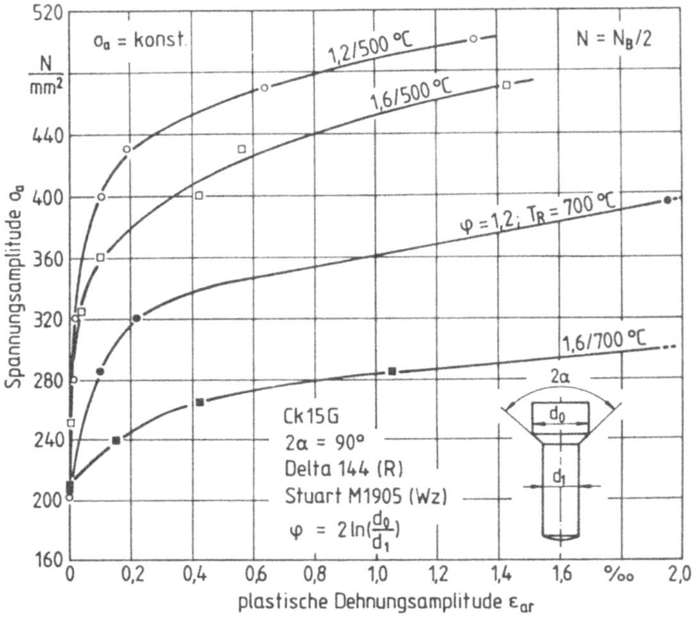

Bild 55: Zyklische Spannungs-Dehnungskurven in Abhängigkeit vom Umformgrad und der Rohteiltemperatur.

Zur lebensdauerorientierten Bewertung sind die Versuchsergebnisse in einem Wöhlerschaubild (Bild 56) zusammengefaßt. Im Zeitfestigkeitsgebiet nimmt bei gleichbleibendem Umformgrad (φ = 1,2 ÷ 1,6) mit zunehmender Temperatur T_R die Steigung des Kurvenastes ab, d. h. auf gleichem Spannungshorizont σ_a werden somit niedrigere Bruch-Schwingspielzahlen registriert. Weiterhin zeigt bei gleichbleibender Temperatur T_R der kleinere Umformgrad die größere Steigung der Zeitfestigkeitsgeraden.

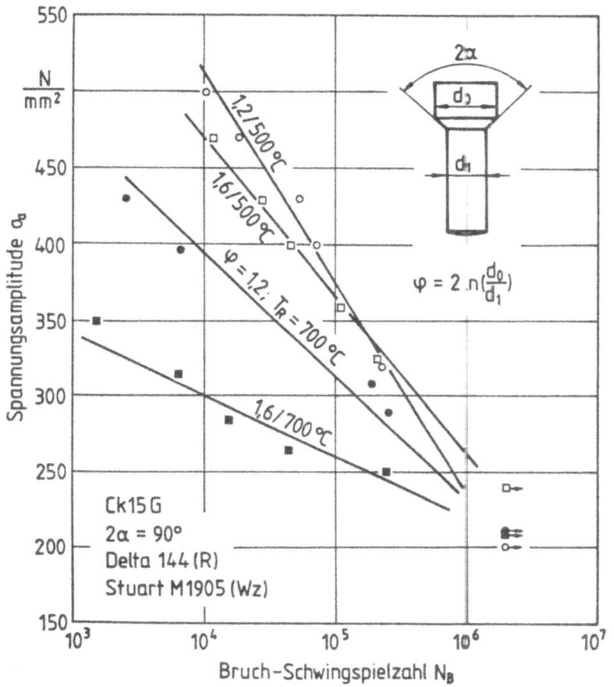

Bild 56: Wöhlerkurven in Abhängigkeit vom Umformgrad und der Rohteiltemperatur.

6.5 VERFAHRENSPARAMETER BEIM VERJÜNGEN

Das Verjüngen gehört gemäß der Krafteinleitung zu den Durchdrückverfahren. Hierbei wird das Rohteil mit kleinen Formänderungen durch eine formgebende Werkzeugöffnung (siehe Bild 1) gedrückt. Die Versuche in dieser Arbeit beschränkten sich auf das Verjüngen von Vollkörpern, das laut DIN 8583 wie folgt definiert wird:

> Verjüngen von Vollkörpern ist Reduzieren ohne Abstützung des nicht umgeformten Werkstückteils in einem Aufnehmer. Das freie, gedrückte Werkstückende darf sich dabei weder aufstauchen noch ausknicken.

Das Verjüngen eignet sich vornehmlich zur Kombination mit anderen Kaltfließpreßverfahren (z. B. Fließpressen, Stauchen, Abstreckgleitziehen) und findet eine Vielzahl von Anwendungsmöglichkeiten bei der Herstellung von Maschinenelementen (u. a. Schrauben, Nieten, Wellen).

6.5.1 Umformgrad

Die Auswirkungen des Umformgrades (φ = 0,1 und 0,3 bei jeweils $2\alpha = 15^o$) bei einer mittelspannungsfreien Schwingbeanspruchung sind den Bildern 57 und 58 zu entnehmen. Der durch Verjüngen verfestigte Werkstoffzustand weist ein ähnliches Wechselverformungsverhalten auf wie nach dem Voll-Vorwärts-Fließpressen; makroskopisch zeigt sich ausschließlich eine zyklische Entfestigung ohne jegliche Sättigungsphasen (mit Ausnahme des ε_{ar}/log N-Verlaufes für σ_a = 265 N/mm² bei φ = 0,3). Der ε_{ar}-Verlauf geht dabei ohne erkennbare Unstetigkeit in die Rißaus-

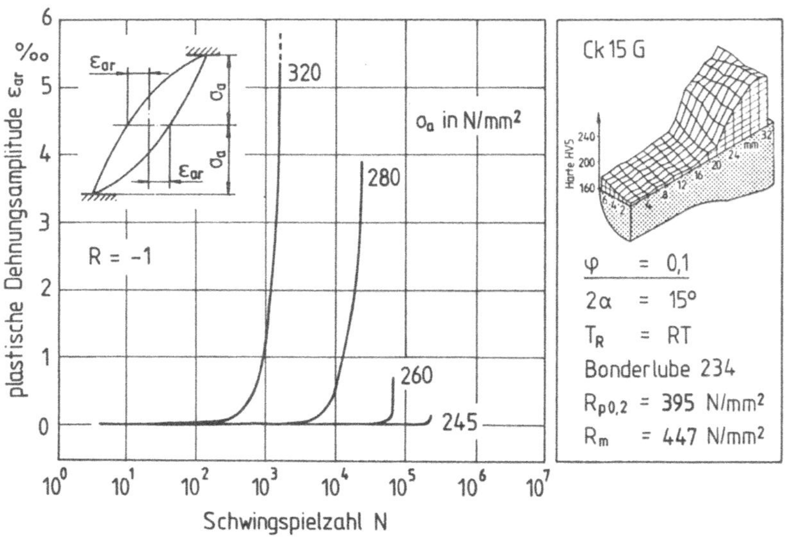

Bild 57: Wechselverformungskurven von verjüngten Werkstücken (φ = 0,1 und $2\alpha = 15^o$).

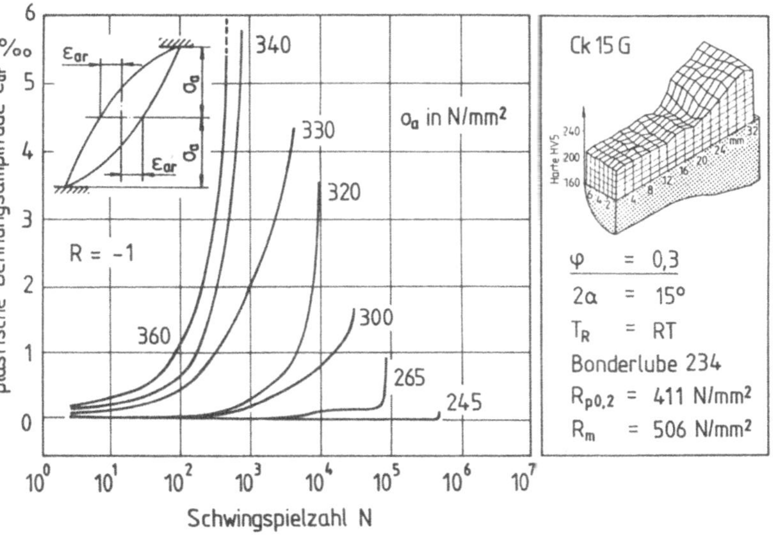

Bild 58: Wechselverformungskurven von verjüngten Werkstücken (φ = 0,3 und 2α = 15°).

breitungsphase über und führt zum Bruch. Mit dem größeren Umformgrad werden im sich einstellenden Lebensdauerbereich $10^2 \leq N_B \leq 10^6$ durchweg höhere Bruch-Schwingspielzahlen erreicht. Auffallend ist bei φ = 0,1 die mit wachsender Spannungsamplitude deutlich abnehmende Inkubationsphase quasielastischer Deformationen.

6.5.2 Schulteröffnungswinkel

Ein Reduzieren bei einem Schulteröffnungswinkel der Matrize von 2α = 30° bedeutet ein weniger sanftes Umlenken des Werkstoffes an der Einlaufdüse wie bei 15°. Dementsprechend verläuft der Härteanstieg zur Bauteiloberfläche etwas steiler (Bild 59); eine Umformung bei 2α = 15° zeigt nahezu keinen Gradienten. In Analogie zum Fließpressen zeichnet sich mit zunehmendem Schulteröffnungswinkel eine höhere Schwingspielzahl im Zeitfestigkeitsgebiet ($N_B \leq 8\cdot 10^4$) ab, während sich die Tendenz im Über-

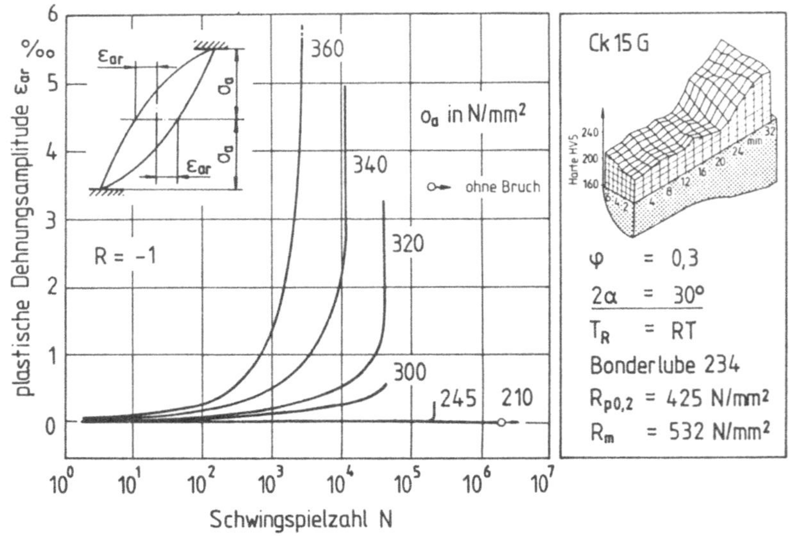

Bild 59: Wechselverformungskurven von verjüngten Werkstücken (φ = 0,3 und 2α = 30°).

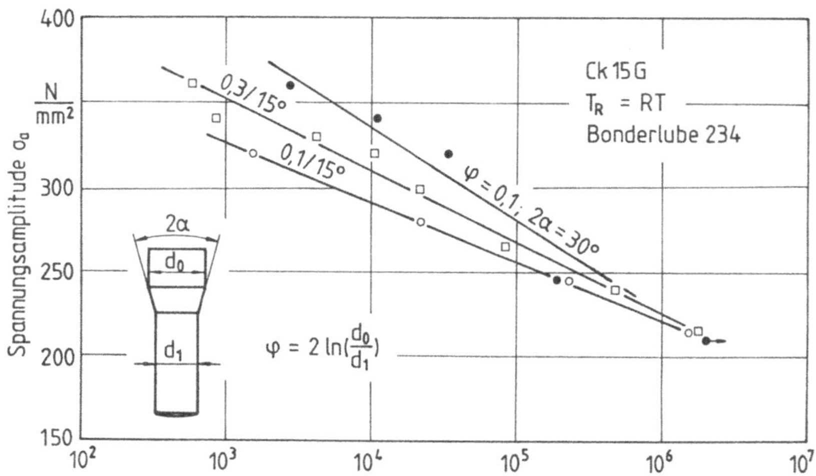

Bild 60: Wöhlerkurven von verjüngten Werkstücken in Abhängigkeit verschiedener $\varphi/2\alpha$-Kombinationen.

gangs- bzw. Dauerfestigkeitsgebiet umzukehren scheint. Im allgemeinen werden hohe ε_{ar}-Werte registriert, die sich allerdings durch eine progressiv verlaufende Entfestigung innerhalb weniger Schwingspiele ergeben.

Eine Analyse der Ergebnisse aus den Schwingversuchen mit dem Probenbruch als Versagenskriterium zeigt ein relativ enges Strahlenbündel für die untersuchten Verfahrensparameter Umformgrad und Schulteröffnungswinkel (Bild 60). Ein ausgesprochener Dauerfestigkeitsgewinn gegenüber dem weichgeglühten Ausgangszustand des Werkstoffs Ck15G scheint sich nicht abzuzeichnen. Eine genauere Aussage ist nicht möglich, da keine nach statistischen Kriterien ausgerichtete Versuchsführung erfolgte.

6.6 RANDZONENEINFLUSS

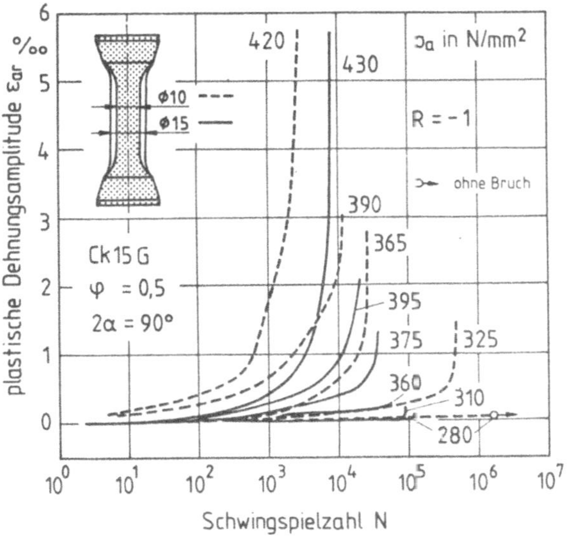

Bild 61: Wechselverformungskurven von Kaltfließpreßteilen aus Ck15G nach Abspanen der Randschicht (φ = 0,5 und 2α = 90°).

Um den Einfluß der Randzonenverfestigung und der Oberflächentopographie nachzuweisen, wurde die Randschicht der bauteilähnlichen Proben abgespant und der Prüfdurchmesser auf 10 mm reduziert. Im Restquerschnitt liegt der weitgehend homogen umgeformte Kern der Fließpreßteile. Am Beispiel des Umformgrades φ = 0,5 wird gezeigt (Bild 61), daß im Vergleich zu den ursprünglichen Werkstücken bei allen Spannungsamplituden größere plastische Dehnungsamplituden auftreten. Die Lebensdauer wird bei größeren Belastungen zu kleineren Werten verschoben, während bei kleineren Spannungsamplituden größere Schwingspielzahlen erreicht werden. Diese Beobachtungen wurden auch bei φ = 1,2 gemacht (Bild 62); sie sind vermutlich auf eine nach der Abspanung vorliegende nahezu über dem ganzen Probenquerschnitt homogene Umformung sowie auf eine veränderte Oberflächenstruktur zurückzuführen. Die Wechselverformungskurven zeigen einen qualitativ ähnlichen Verlauf wie die der bauteilähnlichen Proben.

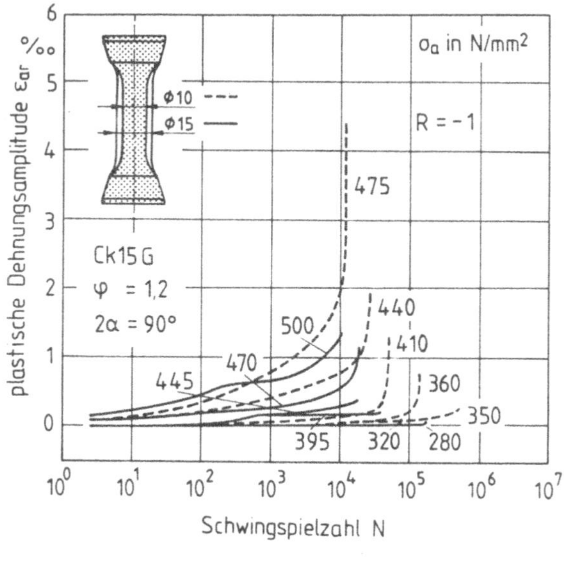

Bild 62: Wechselverformungskurven von Kaltfließpreßteilen aus Ck15G nach Abspanen der Randschicht (φ = 1,2 und 2α = 90°).

6.7 INHOMOGENE DEFORMATIONSERSCHEINUNGEN

Die während der Schwingbeanspruchung der Fließpreßteile stattfindenden Deformationsprozesse führen zu der Fragestellung, inwieweit der umgeformte Werkstoffzustand homogen oder inhomogen plastifiziert. Eine spannungsoptische Lokalisierug der Ermüdungszonen (Probenbereiche plastischer Verformung) wäre bei den rotationssymmetrischen Fließpreßteilen äußerst schwierig. Da nicht genau bekannt ist, wo die plastische Verformung initiiert, ist der Nachweis mit Hilfe lokaler Dehnungsmessungen nur bedingt einsetzbar.

Trotzdem wurden auf drei - in Bild 63 gekennzeichneten Meßebenen e_i ($i = 1...3$) jeweils vier Dehnungsmeßstreifen (Hottinger-Baldwin; Typ 0,6/120 LY11) DMS_j ($j = 1...4$) um 90° versetzt am zylindrischen Schaft appliziert. Zur Vermeidung von Axialitätsfehlern wurde größte Sorgfalt auf die Probenpräparation und die Einspannkonfiguration (Fluchtung der beiden Einspannköpfe) gelegt. Für die Meßwerterfassung wurden drei Meßwertverstärker (Hersteller Hottinger-Baldwin; Typ KWS 3082A) und zwei Transientenspeicher (Hersteller Krenz; Typ TRC 2010 sowie TRC 6010 und 6011) eingesetzt, um die insgesamt zwölf Dehnungen mit zugehöriger Kraftamplitude zeitsynchron messen zu können. Der konstante Spanungsausschlag wurde auf $\sigma_a = 430\ N/mm^2$ und die Versuchsfrequenz auf 1 Hz festgelegt.

Einige Meßstellen fielen schon vorzeitig aus, was vermutlich auf Haftungsprobleme zwischen Klebstoff und Probenoberfläche zurückzuführen war. Die Auswertung in Bild 63 deutet auf inhomogene Deformationserscheinungen bzw. auf inhomogen ablaufende Entfestigungsvorgänge hin. Teilweise liegen die lokal gemessenen Dehnungsamplituden $\varepsilon_{ar}^{(ij)}$ ($i = 1...3$ und $j = 1...4$; i - Meßebene und j - Lage des DMS) - was aber nicht unbedingt die höchsten sein müssen - betragsmäßig über der integral ermittelten Hysteresisbreite. Die lokalen Dehnungen $\varepsilon_{ar}^{(2j)}$ ($j = 1...4$) von Meßebene e_2 können durch den DMS-Ausfall im Lebensdauerbereich $2{,}7 \cdot 10^3 \leq N_B \leq 10^4$ nicht näher quantifiziert werden, lassen aber aufgrund der jeweiligen Steigung der $\varepsilon_{ar}^{(2j)}$-Kurve ($j =$

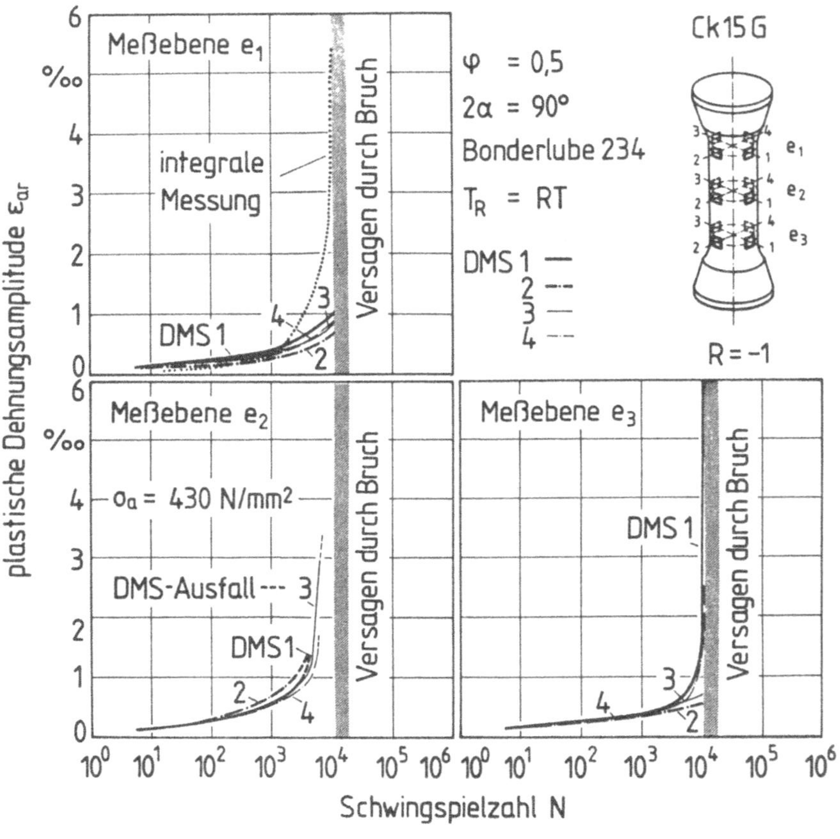

Bild 63: Inhomogene Wechselentfestigung eines kaltverfestigten Werkstoffzustandes (φ = 0,5 und 2α = 90°).

1...4) beim DMS-Ausfall und einer möglichen Extrapolation auf die Lebensdauergrenze von 10^4 Schwingspielen auf relativ hohe plastische Deformationen schließen. Die Werkstoffschädigung in dem mittleren zylindrischen Teilstück (Meßebene e_2 war infolge der vermutlich sehr hohen plastischen Deformation soweit fortgeschritten, daß sich hier auch der zum Versagen (durch Bruch) führende Ermüdungsriß bildete. Die Ergebnisse von Versuchen mit anderen Werkstoffzuständen (φ > 0,5) waren mit den erörterten kompatibel. Allerdings bewirkten die Versuche mit hohen Umformgraden kleinere plastische Dehnungen infolge geringerer Zähigkeit.

6.8 KERBWIRKUNG

Bei fließgepreßten Bauteilen wird manchmal die Endform erst durch eine spanende Nachbearbeitung (z. B. Nuten, Hinterschneidungen) erreicht. Dabei wird der Faserverlauf des Werkstückes unterbrochen und das dynamische Bauteilverhalten verändert.

Zur Untersuchung des Kerbeinflusses fließgepreßter Werkstücke wurden die bauteilähnlichen Proben (vgl. Bild 5) dahingehend modifiziert, daß nach dem Umformen in der Mitte des zylindrischen Schaftes eine umlaufende Kerbe (Kerbradius ρ = 2,5 mm und Kerbtiefe t = 2,5 mm) mit mechanisch polierter Oberfläche angebracht wurde.

Eine direkte Ermittlung der Dehnung im Kerbgrund (über der gesamten Lebensdauer) mit Hilfe von Dehnungsmeßstreifen erwies sich aufgrund der Geometrie bzw. durch Haftungsprobleme auf dem polierten Kerbgrund als unzweckmäßig. Daher wurde während der Schwingversuche die Kerbaufweitung mittels eines Längenänderungsaufnehmers (Clip-gauge nach ASTM E399 /65/) mit zugehörigem Meßverstärker (Hersteller Hottinger-Baldwin; Typ KWS 3082A) gemessen. Um einen entsprechend der Größe der Kerböffnung ausgelegten Clip-gauge mit seinen beiden Meßschneiden definiert befestigen zu könnnen, wurden in den Kerbauslauf gegenüberliegende Fixierungen gefräst. Unter Verwendung der in Kap. 5 beschriebenen Versuchseinrichtung einschließlich des Programms zur Meßwerterfassung und Datenverarbeitung konnte die Kerbaufweitungsamplitude u_{ka} in Abhängigkeit von der Schwingspielzahl N (Kerbaufweitungsamplituden-Schwingspielzahlkurve) bestimmt werden.

Im nächsten Schritt wurden mit dem auf einer VAX 11/780 (Rechenzentrum der Universität Stuttgart) installierten FE-Programm ANSYS (Engineering Analysis System /66/) für vier unterschiedlich ausgeprägte Entfestigungszustände eines Zeitschwingversuchs die den vier diskreten Kerbaufweitungsamplituden zugehörigen Gesamtdehnungsamplituden im Kerbgrund berechnet.

Wegen der gegebenen Axialsymmetrie und der Symmetrie zur Kerbgrundebene konnte ein zweidimensionales FE-Modell mit einem Probenviertel zugrundegelegt werden. Plastische Verformung im kerbnahen Bereich bedingt das Auftreten von Nichtlinearitäten bei der Darstellung des Werkstoffzustandes und somit eine iterative Lösungsfindung. Die Verwendung eines einfachen Vier-Knotenelementes erschien in diesem Falle sinnvoll /66/. Vorversuche mit verschiedenen Probeneinspannungen (z. B. Krafteinleitung über die kegeligen Spannschalen bzw. Probenköpfe) rechtfertigten die Reduzierung des FE-Modells ausschließlich auf den zylindrischen Fließpreßschaft. Außerdem wurde bei der Bestimmung der Kerbgrundspannung σ_{max} bei rein elastischer Verformung durch unterschiedliche Netzverfeinerungen im Kerbbereich (Variation der Elementanzahl in r-Richtung) das Konvergenzverhalten überprüft. Die Formzahl α_k wurde unter Verwendung des in Bild 64 dargestellten FE-Netzes mit 1,7 berechnet.

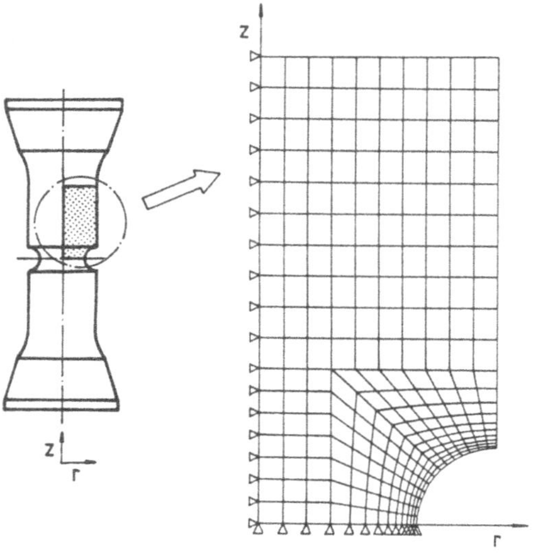

Bild 64: Netzidealisierung.

Bei der Festlegung der Eingabedaten zur Charakterisierung des Werkstoffverhaltens wurden mehrere Gesichtspunkte berücksichtigt:

- Fertigungsbedingte inhomogene Verfestigung über dem Querschnitt mit der Vergleichsspannung σ_V bzw. der Vergleichsformänderung ε_V (vgl. Abschnitt 4.1) als Maß. Dabei wurde für die Berechnung folgende Vereinfachung angenommen: Eine äußere Belastung erzeugt eine Spannungserhöhung im Kerbgrund (Bereich geringerer Verfestiung bzw. homogener Umformung), während im Randbereich der Probe (Zone stärkerer Verfestigung) nur niedrige Spannungen vorliegen. Dies bedeutet, daß der Werkstoff nur im nahezu homogenen Kernbereich fließt, während der Randbereich rein elastisch verformt wird. Der Verfestigungsgradient zum Rand hin hat somit wenig Einfluß auf das Festigkeitsverhalten des gekerbten Werkstückes. Für die FE-Berechnung kann das Werkstoffverhalten über den Kerbquerschnitt als homogen betrachtet werden.
- Durch die beim kaltverfestigten Werkstoff Ck15G unter schwingender Beanspruchung auftretende Entfestigung ändert sich das Spannungs-Dehnungsverhalten; Verwendung der an glatten Fließpreßschäften ermittelten zyklischen Spannungs-Dehnungskurven mit unterschiedlichen N/N_B-Verhältnissen.
- Zur Beschreibung des Bauschinger-Effektes wurde das Werkstoffmodell der kinematischen Verfestigung gewählt, das nach Untersuchungen von Stegmayer /67/ das reale Werkstoffverhalten am besten beschreibt.

Ein eventueller Frequenzeinfluß kann bei der niedrigen Frequenz von 1 Hz vernachlässigt werden. Die FE-Lösung hängt vom zeitlichen Belastungsverlauf ab, der mit einer sinnvollen Anzahl von Lastschritten möglichst genau nachgefahren werden muß (dreieckförmige Schwingungsform mit z. B. 25 Lastschritten für eineinviertel Schwingspiele). Als Folge der plastischen Verformung entstehen im Kerbgrund bei jeder Belastungsumkehr Eigenspannungen, die sich auf die Gesamtdehnungen auswirken.

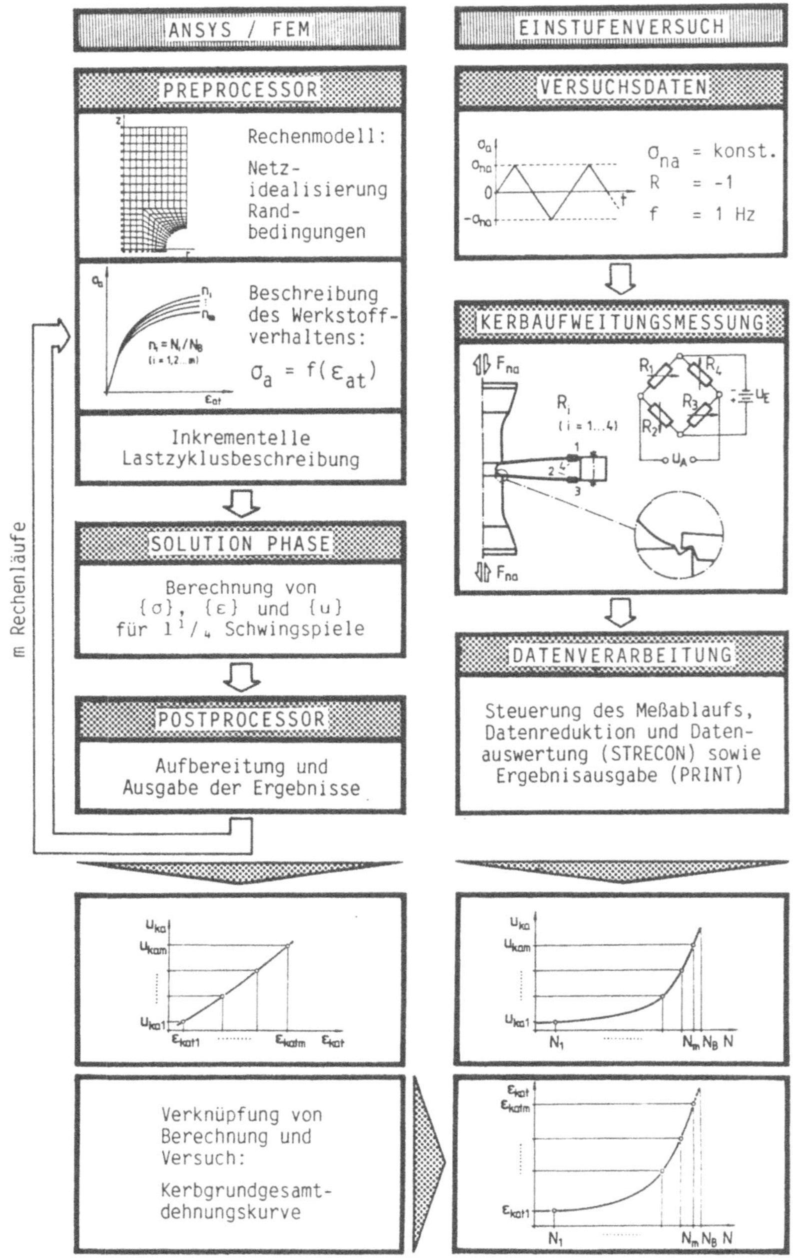

Bild 65: Ermittlung von ε_{kat}/log N-Kurven.

Bei der Bestimmung der Kerbgrundgesamtdehnungen werden diese Eigenspannungen berücksichtigt, indem für jeden Entfestigungszustand bzw. Rechenlauf eineinviertel Schwingspiele (ausreichend für f = 1 Hz) berechnet werden. Aus den für vier Entfestigungszustände erhaltenen Hysteresisschleifen in Form von Nennspannungs-Kerbgrundgesamtdehnungs- ($\sigma_n/\varepsilon_{kt}$-) und Kerbaufweitungs-Nennspannungskurven (u_k/σ_n-Kurven) wurden die Amplituden bestimmt. Daraus konnte für jede gefahrene Nennspannungsamplitude der Zusammenhang zwischen der Kerbaufweitungs- und Kerbgrundgesamtdehnungamplitude hergestellt werden. Durch Verknüpfung dieses Ergebnisses mit der Kerbaufweitungs-Schwingspielzahlkurve nach dem Nomogramm in Bild 65 läßt sich jeder berechnete Wert der Amplitude ε_{kat} einer Schwingspielzahl N zuordnen.

Die in Bild 66 beispielhaft dargestellten Wechselverformungskurven für gekerbte Fließpreßteile (φ = 1,2; 2α = 90°) aus Ck15G zeigen für alle Nennspannungsamplituden einen qualitativ

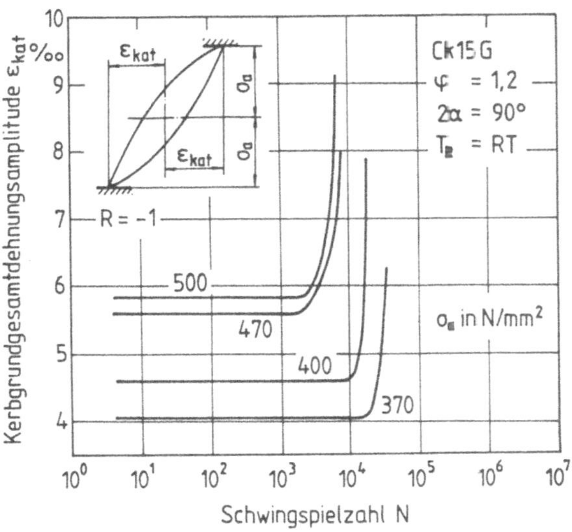

Bild 66: Kerbgrundgesamtdehnungskurven von Fließpreßteilen aus Ck15G (φ = 1,2 und 2α = 90°).

ähnlichen Verlauf. Bei Nennspannungsamplituden im Bereich $370 \le \sigma_{na} \le 400$ N/mm^2 stellt sich ein konstanter Kerbgrundgesamtdehnungsverlauf bis $N/N_B = 0{,}5$ ein. Dagegen setzt die zyklische Entfestigung bei σ_{na} im Bereich $470 \le \sigma_{na} \le 500$ N/mm^2 etwas früher bei $N/N_B = 0{,}3$ ein. Bis $N/N_B = 0{,}8$ nimmt die Wechselentfestigung des Werkstoffs langsam zu und setzt sich danach beschleunigt bis zum Bruch fort.

Vergleicht man die Wechselverformungskurven mit denen der glatten bauteilähnlichen Proben (Bild 36), so fällt neben der geringeren Lebensdauer der wesentlich ausgeprägtere Anstieg der ε_{kat}-Kurvenverläufe im letzten Viertel der Lebensdauer der gekerbten Werkstücke auf. Auch fehlt die Neigung zur Bildung von Plateaus (Sättigung; neutrales Werkstoffverhalten). Die Kerbgrundgesamtdehnung bleibt anfangs konstant, wobei es im Kerbgrund bei allen Nennspannungsamplituden σ_{na} aufgrund der Spannungserhöhung durch die Kerbe zu plastischen Deformationen kommmt. Die Unterbrechung des Faserverlaufs in der stärker verfestigten Randzone hat vermutlich keine gravierende Auswirkung auf die Lebensdauer im Zeitfestigkeitsgebiet. Eine Abschätzung der Gesamtdehnungen im Kerbgrund mit einer für schwingende Beanspruchung modifizierten Neuber-Formel /68, 69/:

$$\sigma_{ka} \cdot \varepsilon_{kat} = \alpha_k^2 \cdot \sigma_{na}^2 / E$$

ergibt für $N/N_B = 0{,}8$ (vermuteter Rißbeginn) eine gute Übereinstimmung mit den ermittelten ε_{kat}-Amplituden.

6.9 VARIATION DER MITTELSPANNUNG

Alle Versuche mit $\sigma_m \neq 0$ wurden ausschließlich mit kaltfließgepreßten Werkstücken ($\varphi = 1{,}2$ und $2\alpha = 90^\circ$) aus Ck15G durchgeführt. Nach Beaufschlagen mit der jeweiligen Mittelspannung wurde die Mitteldehnung bezügliche des elastischen Dehnungsanteils der statischen Vorspannung korrigiert.

Bei spannungskontrollierten Versuchen mit einem hinreichend

hohen Spannungsausschlag σ_a von 390 N/mm^2 und verschiedenen Mittelspannungen von $50 \leq \sigma_m \leq 150$ N/mm^2 wurden ähnliche Wechselverformungskurven registriert wie bei mittelspannungsfreier Beanspruchung (Bild 67). Die Größe der Mittelspannung beeinflußt analog zur maximal sich einstellenden plastischen Dehnungsamplitude die Mitteldehnungszunahme und verschiebt die Lebensdauer mit wachsender Mittelspannung zu kleineren Schwingspielzahlen. Außerdem weisen beide Kurventypen auf Phasen annähernder Sättigung ohne nennenswerte ε_{ar}- bzw. ε_m-Zunahme über größere Lebensdauerintervalle ($10^3 \leq N \leq 10^4$) hin. Obwohl die gewählten σ_a/σ_m-Kombinationen hinsichtlich ihrer Oberspannungen (σ_o = 490 und 440 N/mm^2) um 9 bis 18 % unterhalb der im Zugversuch ermittelten 0,2-Dehngrenze $R_{p0,2}$ = 539 N/mm^2 liegen, verlängert sich der Fließpreßschaft um 2,5 bis 7,5 ‰. Ein Vergleich von Wechselverformungs- und Mitteldehnungskurven zeigt, daß zyklische Entfestigung und Mittelspannungszunahme oft ungefähr in demselben Schwingspielzahlintervall einsetzen.

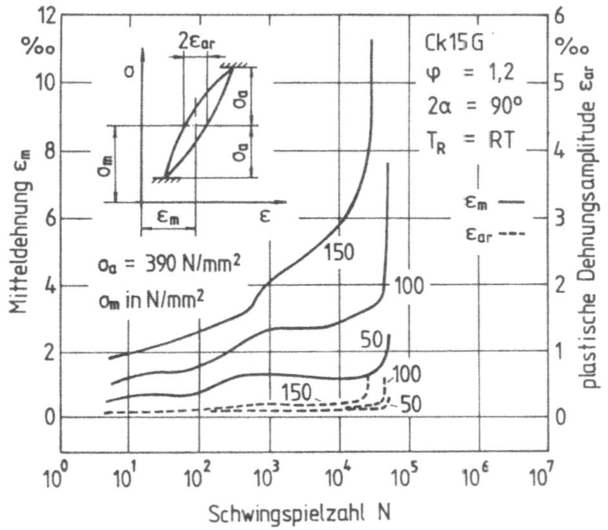

Bild 67: Einfluß der Mittelspannung auf die Wechselverformungs- und Mitteldehnungskurven (φ = 1,2 und 2α = 90°).

Versuche mit Druckmittelspannung führen (Bild 68) mit einsetzender Wechselentfestigung zu Schaftverkürzungen. Dieses Phänomen wurde auch für den vergüteten Werkstoffzustand beobachtet und von Eifler /70/ als Indiz gewertet, daß zunächst weder die plastischen Verformungen noch die Mitteldehnungen mit dem Ermüdungsrißfortschritt zusammenhängen. Als allgemein gültiges Ergebnis bleibt die Feststellung, daß bei Schwingbeanspruchung unter Raumtemperatur eine Mitteldehnungszunahme stets das gleiche Vorzeichen wie die Mittelspannung hat.

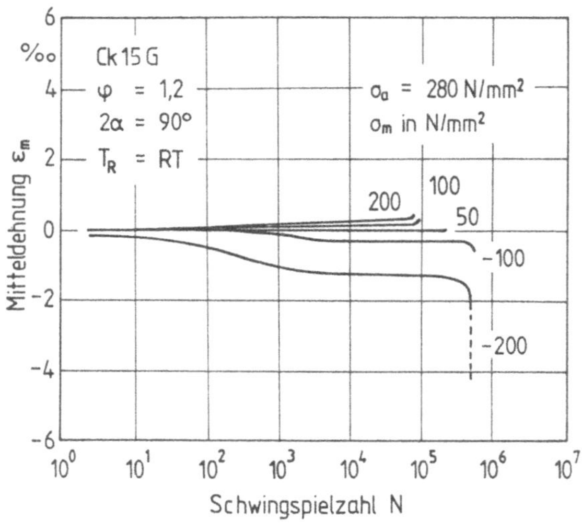

Bild 68: Einfluß von Zug- und Druckmittelspannung auf die Mitteldehnungskurven ($\varphi = 1{,}2$ und $2\alpha = 90^{\circ}$).

Während bei den bisher besprochenen Beanspruchungskombinationen stets mit einer makroskopischen Wechselentfestigung eine kumulierende Mitteldehnung verbunden war, konnten bei Versuchen mit $\sigma_m = 290$ N/mm^2 und überlagerten Spannungsamplituden ($90 \leq \sigma_a \leq 270$ N/mm^2) mit der verwendeten Meßtechnik keine plastischen Dehnungsamplituden nachgewiesen werden (Bild 69).

Denkbar wäre, daß sich geringe lokale Plastifizierungen konti-

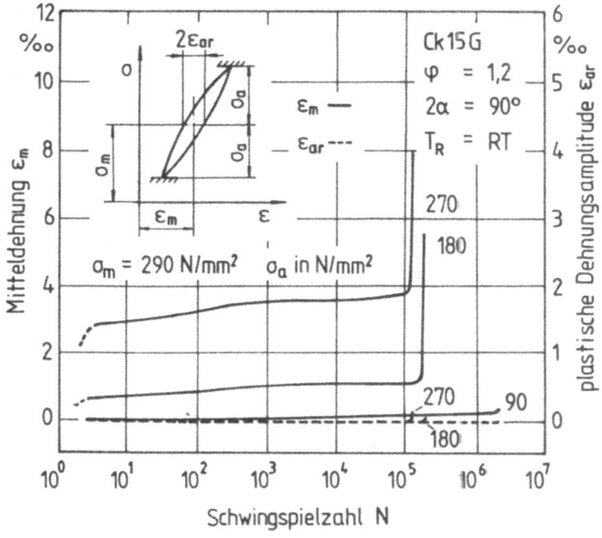

Bild 69: Einfluß der Spannungsamplitude auf die Wechselverformungs- und Mitteldehnungskurven ($\varphi = 1{,}2$ und $2\alpha = 90^{o}$).

nuierlich zu einer großen Mitteldehnung aufaddieren, ohne daß makroskopisch eine Wechselentfestigung beobachtet wird. Auffallend ist die zu Versuchsbeginn innerhalb weniger Schwingspiele ($\Delta N \approx 10$ Schwingspiele) auftretende relativ starke Mitteldehnungszunahme, die zu offenen Hysteresisschleifen führt und folglich keine genauen Angaben zuläßt (gestrichelter Verlauf der ε_m/log N-Kurven). Daran schließt eine Quasisättigungsphase an, mit ε_m-Zunahmen unter 0,1 % im Lebensdauerbereich $10^1 \leq N \leq 10^5$. Die erneute und sehr schnell verlaufende Mitteldehnungszunahme gegen Ende der Schwingbeanspruchung beruht auf einer Überlagerung von zyklischem Kriechen und makroskopischer Ermüdungsrißausbreitung. Trotz relativ hoher Oberspannungen von $470 \leq \sigma_o \leq 560$ N/mm^2 im Bereich der 0,2-Dehngrenze und einer erwarteten Lebensdauer im Kurzzeitfestigkeitsgebiet werden Bruch-Schwingspielzahlen von $N_B > 10^5$ erreicht (ähnliche Merkmale bei wechselentfestigendem Vergütungstahl /70/).

Die unterschiedlichen Mitteldehnungskurven können durch Differenzieren näher interpretiert werden. Dazu wird jeweils eine Beanspruchungskombination aus Bild 67 und 69 gewählt und die Mitteldehnungsänderung im Lebensdauerintervall $10^1 \leq N \leq 10^4$ betrachtet (Bild 70). Der Versuch mit der höheren Mittelspannung von 290 N/mm^2 ist durch permanent abnehmende Mitteldehnungsänderungen charakterisiert. Die $\Delta\varepsilon_m/\Delta N$-Werte sind hierbei aufgrund des langanhaltenden Quasisättigungsgebietes (vgl. Bild 69) für ca. 99 % der Lebensdauer kleiner als 10^{-6}/Schwingspiel und liegen damit unter dem Auflösungsvermögen des Längenänderungsmeßsystems. Folglich ergeben sich makroskopisch quasielastische Wechselverformungskurven. Dagegen zeigt die Beanspruchung mit σ_m = 100 N/mm^2 und σ_a = 390 N/mm^2 neben tendenziell abnehmenden $\Delta\varepsilon_m/\Delta N$-Werten auch zwei Unstetigkeiten ($\Delta\varepsilon_m/\Delta N \rightarrow 0$) gegen Anfang (≈ 10^2 Schwingspiele) und Ende (≈ 10^4 Schwingspiele) des Lebensdauerintervalls jeweils nach annähernd neutralem Werkstoffverhalten.

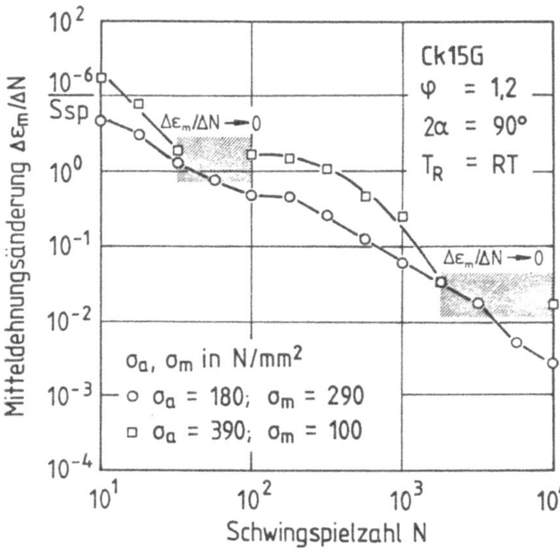

Bild 70: Mitteldehnungsänderung als Funktion der Schwingspielzahl (φ = 1,2 und 2α = 90°).

Bild 71 zeigt Versuchsergebnisse von überlagerten zeitlich konstanten mit determinierten zeitlich veränderlichen Beanspruchungen für drei Lebendauerbereiche in Form eines Haigh-Diagramms. Ersichtlich ist mit einer wachsenden Mittelspannung prinzipiell eine Reduzierung des ertragbaren Spannungsausschlages verbunden. Diese ist im Zeitfestigkeitsgebiet etwas stärker ausgeprägt als im Dauerfestigkeitsgebiet.

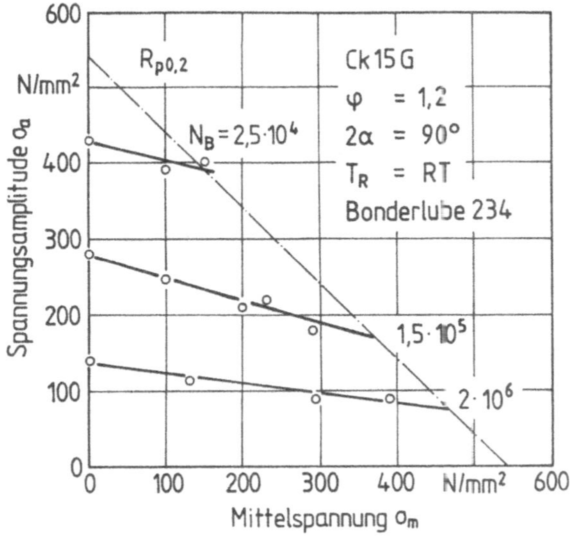

Bild 71: Haigh-Diagramm für kaltverfestigten Werkstoffzustand (Ck15G; $\varphi = 1{,}2$ und $2\alpha = 90^{\circ}$).

Die Untersuchung führte zu der Kenntnis, daß bei dem kaltverfestigten Werkstoffzustand auch irreversible Schaftverlängerungen über 0,2 % Dehnung hinaus auftreten können, obwohl die Oberspannung $(\sigma_m + \sigma_a)$ unterhalb von $R_{p0,2}$ des quasistatischen Zugversuchs liegt. Selbst bei dauerfest ertragenen Belastungen ($N \geq 2 \cdot 10^6$ Schwingspiele) kommt es zum zyklischen Kriechen mit der Ausbildung einer kumulierenden Mitteldehnung $\varepsilon_m \leq 0{,}05$ ‰. Zur Beurteilung des zyklischen Verformungsverhaltens sollten diese Probenverlängerungen - wie in /71/ vorgeschlagen - bei konstanten Schwingspielzahlen als Funktion der Spannungsamplitude σ_a und der Mittelspannung σ_m in einem erweiterten Haigh-Diagramm berücksichtigt werden (siehe Ausschnitt in Bild 72).

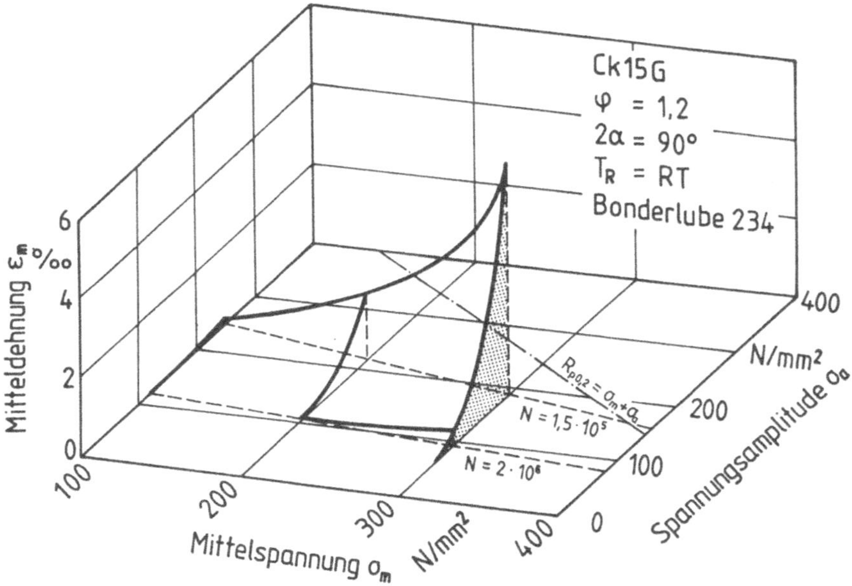

Bild 72: Ausschnitt aus einem erweiterten Haigh-Diagramm für kaltverfestigten Werkstoffzustand (Ck15G; φ = 1,2 und 2α = 90°).

7 ELEKTRONENMIKROSKOPISCHE UNTERSUCHUNGEN ALS ERGÄNZUNG ZUR MAKROSKOPISCHEN BETRACHTUNG DES WECHSELVERFORMUNGSVERHALTENS

Nach der makroskopischen Betrachtung des Einflusses von Herstellparametern der beiden Durchdrückverfahren auf das Ermüdungsverhalten (vgl. Kap. 6) wurde beim Fließpressen die Auswirkung ausgewählter Verfahrensparameter auf die Mikrostruktur und auf das Bruchverhalten untersucht. Als Hilfsmittel dienten die Transmissionselektronen- (TEM) und die Rasterelektronenmikroskopie (REM). Die Untersuchungen wurden am Max-Planck-Institut für Metallforschung in Stuttgart durchgeführt.

7.1 ERMÜDUNGSFEINSTRUKTUR

Aus den fließgepreßten Schäften (Werkstoffzustand vor der Schwingbeanspruchung) und den ermüdeten bauteilähnlichen Proben wurden aus der Werkstückmitte (Meßstrecke) bzw. in genügendem Abstand von der Bruchfläche und dem Übergang zum Einspannkopf Proben (Radial- und Längsschnitt) entnommen. Mit Hilfe einer wassergekühlten Diamantsäge wurden Scheiben von ca. 1 mm Dicke abgetrennt und durch beidseitiges vorsichtiges Naßschleifen (abschließend mit Körnung 600) planparallel auf eine Dicke von 0,1 ÷ 0,15 mm gebracht. Hieraus ausgeschnittene Scheibchen von 3 mm Durchmesser wurden in einem Folienpoliergerät (Hersteller Struers - Typ Tenupol; Düsenstrahlverfahren) elektrolytisch gedünnt bis in Probenmitte ein Loch entstand. Die Polierbedingungen (elektrische Spannung sowie Art, Temperatur und Strömungsgeschwindigkeit des Elektrolyten) wurden so gewählt, daß im randnahen Bereich des Loches ein weitgehend keilförmiger Werkstoffabtrag erfolgte und somit Durchstrahlungspräparate von 0,05 ÷ 0,15 µm Dicke entstanden. Die Metallfolien wurden in einem Transmissionselektronenmikroskop (Hersteller JEOL; Typ JEM-200CX bzw. JEM-200A) mit einer Beschleunigungsspannung von 200 kV untersucht /72/.

Während des Fließpressens erhöht sich die Versetzungsdichte und führt zu einer Änderung der von der Versetzungsdichte (bzw. den Verfahrensparametern) abhängigen mittleren Länge des Versetzungsweges. Je größer dabei die Versetzungsdichte, um so mehr Hindernisse stellen sich den Versetzungsreaktionen entgegen und um so kürzer sind die Versetzungswege /73/. Mit der hierbei auftretenden fertigungsbedingten Kornstreckung sind Gleitverformungen und Versetzungserscheinungen verbunden.

Auf detallierte TEM-Untersuchungen wechselbeanspruchter Proben aus weichgeglühtem Ck15 wurde verzichtet, da die sich einstellenden Mikrostrukturen aus dem Schrifttum bekannt sind und schon in Abschnitt 6.3 im Zusammenhang mit dem Wechselverformungsverhalten diskutiert wurden /59, 60/.

In Bild 73 sind für verschiedene Umformbedingungen charakteristische Versetzungskonfigurationen zusammengestellt. Schon während der Kaltumformung laufen Erholungsvorgänge ab. Dabei entstehen Subkörner mit geringer Versetzungsdichte, wobei die Kleinwinkelkorngrenzen (Subkorngrenzen) mit Versetzungsnetzwerken hoher Dichte belegt sind (Bild 73A). Neben diesem als Polygonisation bezeichneten Vorgang ist vor allem die Zellbildung von Bedeutung. Durch die hohe Stapelfehlerenergie wird das zur Bildung der Zellwände erforderliche Klettern der Versetzungen erleichtert und führt zur Ausbildung einer Zellstruktur /74/. Das Innere dieser Zellen ist weitgehend versetzungsfrei (Bild 73C). Die Versetzungsdichte steigt u. a. durch hohe lokale Umformgrade so stark an, daß die Versetzungen nicht mehr auflösbar sind und nur noch als dunkle Knäuel die Ausscheidungen (wie z. B. globular eingeformtes Fe_3C; Bild 73B) umgeben.
Bei der Halbwarmumformung ($500 \leq T_R \leq 700$ °C) wird durch die Stapelfehlerenergie (Ck15 - hohe SFE) sowie insbesondere durch den Umformgrad beim Fließpressen ($\varphi = 1{,}6$ - hoher Umformgrad) das dynamische Erholungs- und Rekristallisationsverhalten und somit die resultierende Versetzungsstruktur beeinflußt. Während sich bei einer Rohteiltemperatur T_R von 500 °C teilweise noch ähnliche Versetzungsanordnungen wie nach einer vorangegangenen Kaltumformung einstellen (Bild 73D), ist bei 700 °C keine so

ausgeprägte Zellstruktur (Quasizellstruktur) zu verzeichnen. Außerdem bewirkt die thermische Aktivierung eine Zunahme der Zellgröße und damit ein vermehrtes Auftreten von Versetzungen im Zellinnern (Bild 73E).

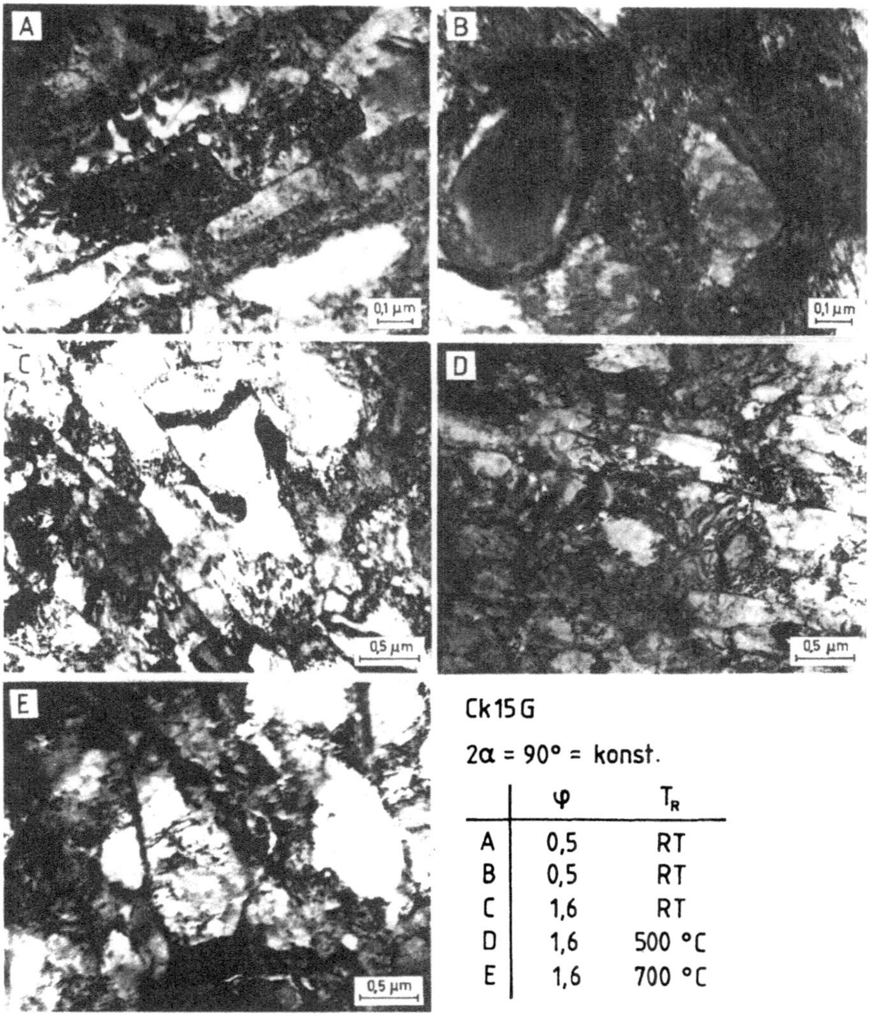

Ck15G

2α = 90° = konst.

	φ	T_R
A	0,5	RT
B	0,5	RT
C	1,6	RT
D	1,6	500 °C
E	1,6	700 °C

Bild 73: Versetzungsstrukturen nach unterschiedlichen Umformbedingungen.

Mit Hilfe der energiedispersiven Röntgenspektroskopie wurden im Durchstrahlungsbetrieb die nadelförmigen Ausscheidungen als Fe_3C-Karbide (Zementit) analysiert (Bild 74); bei den H-förmigen Einschlüssen handelt es sich vermutlich um Verunreinigungen (Schlackepartikel; Mn-Sulfide). Die gestreckte Form fällt mit der Probenlängsachse zusammen und ist durch die Vorbehandlung und das Umformverfahren Voll-Vorwärts-Fließpressen bedingt.

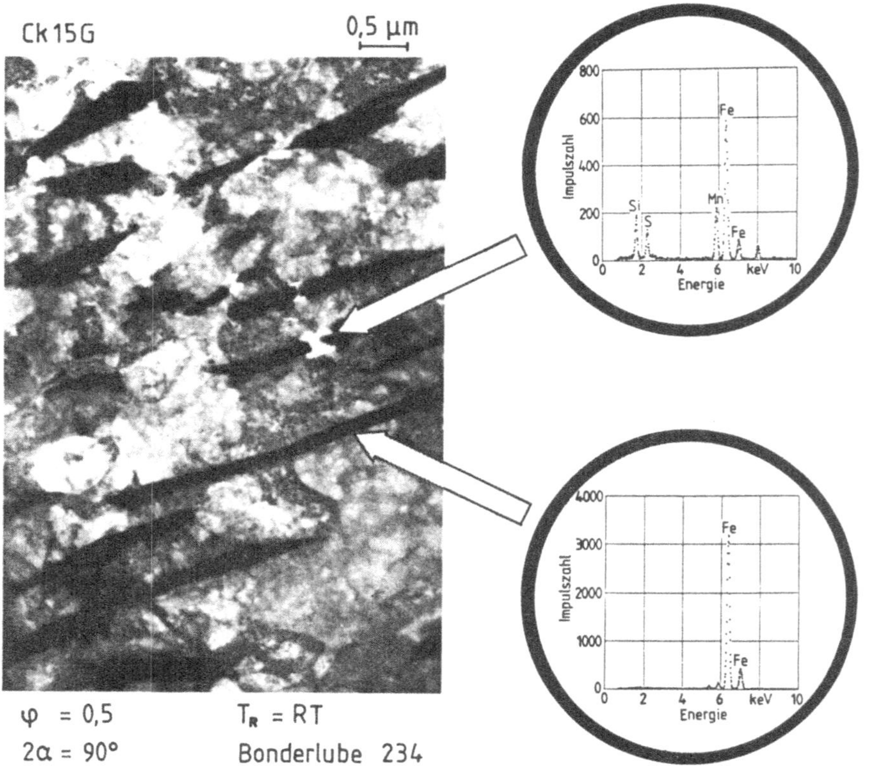

Bild 74: Mikroanalyse mittels energiedispersiver Röntgenspektroskopie (Ck15G; $\varphi = 0{,}5$ und $2\alpha = 90^{\circ}$).

Nach einer Schwingbeanspruchung (σ_a = konst.) bleibt die charakteristische Verformungszellstruktur erhalten. Beim kleinsten Umformgrad φ = 0,5 und der größten unterhalb der makroskopischen 0,2-Dehngrenze gefahrenen Spannungsamplitude σ_a = 430 N/mm^2 werden Zellen unterschiedlicher Größe mit nahezu verset-

	φ	σ_a	N_B
A	0,5	430	$8{,}7 \cdot 10^3$
B	0,5	360	$5{,}0 \cdot 10^4$
C	1,6	500	$1{,}8 \cdot 10^4$
D	1,6	270	$1{,}8 \cdot 10^5$

Ck15G

2α = 90° = konst.

T_R = RT = konst.

σ_a in N/mm^2

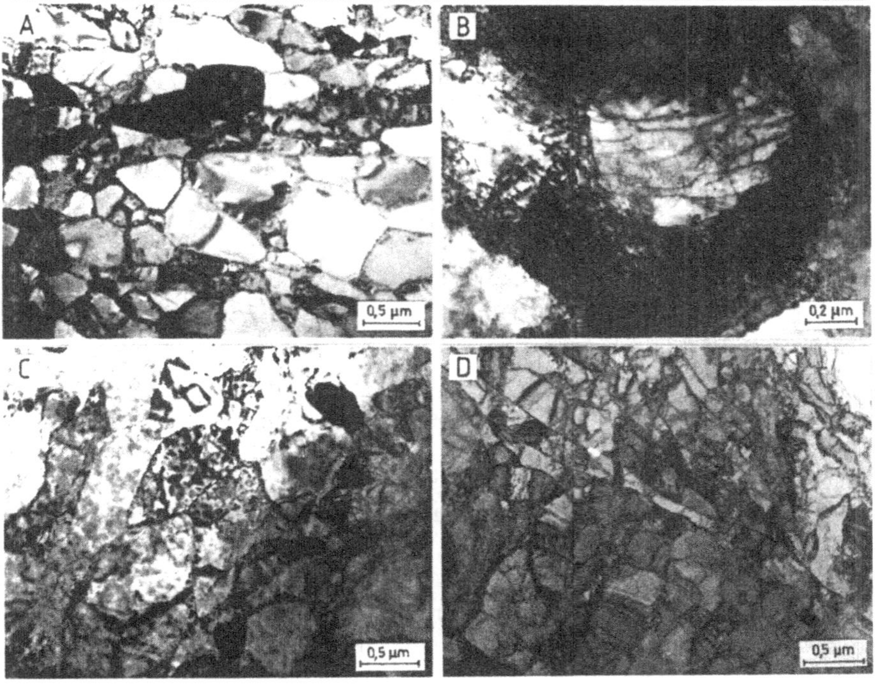

Bild 75: Versetzungsanordnung kaltfließgepreßter Werkstücke aus Ck15G nach unterschiedlichen Schwingbeanspruchungen (σ_a = konst.).

zungsfreiem Zellvolumen beobachtet (Bild 75A). Dies kann zu der relativ hohen irreversiblen plastischen Dehnungsamplitude der Wechselverformungskurve Anlaß geben. Selbst nach $5 \cdot 10^4$ Schwingspielen mit einem Spannungsausschlag von 360 N/mm^2 konnten die Knäuel hoher Versetzungsdichte nicht wesentlich verändert werden (Bild 75B). Zum Vergleich stellt sich beim größten Umformgrad von 1,6 und einer kleinen Schwingbeanspruchung (quasielastisches Wechselverformungsverhalten) eine qualitativ ähnliche Versetzungsanordnung wie bei kleinem φ und großem σ_a ein. Auffallend ist ein in Bild 75D diagonal verlaufendes und von dünnen Wänden begrenztes bandförmiges Subkorn von ungefähr 0,2 µm Breite; dieses Band ist ebenfalls noch in Zellen unterteilt. Eine hohe Belastung von σ_a = 500 N/mm^2 hingegen weist auf eine geringere Versetzungsdichte in den Zellwänden hin (Bild 75C), was möglicherweise auf stattfindende Annihilationsprozesse von Versetzungen schließen läßt /75/. Die Gesamtversetzungsdichte wird dabei reduziert und die Anzahl möglicher Laufwege von gleitfähigen Versetzungen erhöht. Ein lokalisiertes Anwachsen der plastischen Dehnungsamplitude ist die Folge.

Auch im gesamtdehnungskontrollierten Versuch bleibt die durch die Umformkombination $\varphi/2\alpha$ von $0{,}9/90^{\circ}$ bei Raumtemperatur erzeugte Mikrostruktur erhalten (Bild 76). Bei dem relativ breiten Band (Kontrastunterschied durch Orientierungsunterschied) in Teilbild 76B handelt es sich vermutlich wieder um eine Korn- oder Subkorngrenze. Ein Vergleich zu der Ermüdungszellstruktur im spannungskontrollierten Versuch läßt keinen signifikanten Unterschied erkennen.

Bei halbwarmumgeformten Werkstücken mit der niedrigsten Rohteiltemperatur (500 °C) stellen sich für die jeweilige Höhe der Schwingbeanspruchung ähnliche Versetzungsstrukturen ein wie nach einer Kaltumformung bei sonst gleichen Umformbedingungen (φ = 1,6 und $2\alpha = 90^{\circ}$; Bild 77A und 77B). Dementsprechend wurden tendenziell ähnliche Wechselverformungskurven wie nach dem Kaltfließpressen ermittelt. Großwinkelkorngrenzen, die vollständige Körner charakterisieren, sind in Proben mit hohem Umformgrad und hoher Rohteiltemperatur zu finden (siehe Bild

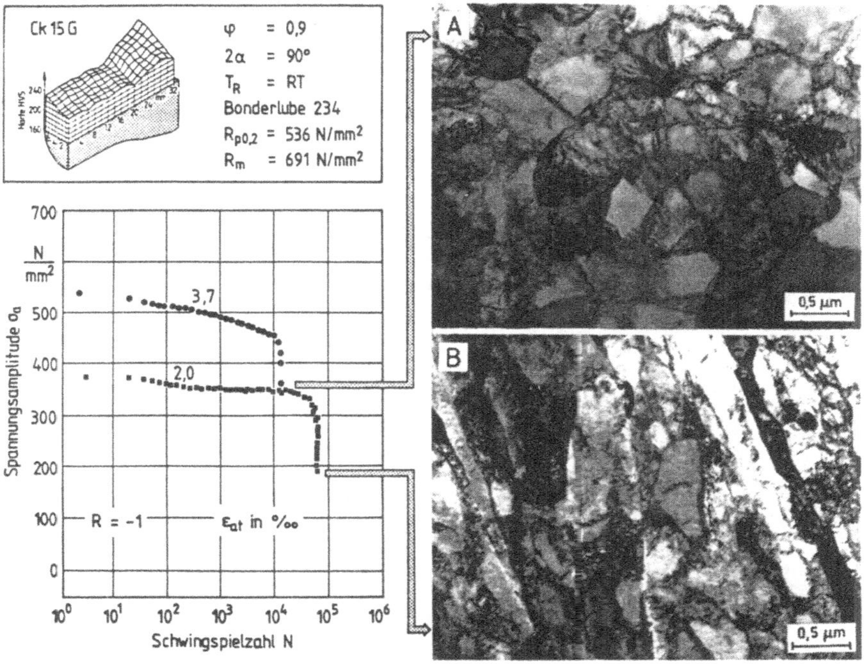

Bild 76: Versetzungsstrukturen kaltfließgepreßter Werkstücke aus Ck15G nach einer gesamtdehnungskontrollierten Schwingbeanspruchung (ε_{at} = konst.).

77D; Streifenkontrast durch Großwinkelkorngrenze). Denkbar wäre, daß es sich um eine beginnende primäre Rekristallisation handelt. Weiterhin sind etwas größere Zellen mit Wänden hoher Versetzungsdichte zu erkennen, die in Strukturen mit Versetzungswänden geringer Dichte unterteilt sind. Außerdem sind innerhalb des Korns regellose Versetzungen zu beobachten (Bild 77C), was mit der zyklischen Verfestigungsphase und dem damit verbundenen Abfall der plastischen Dehnungsamplitude vor dem Bruch übereinstimmt.

	T_R	σ_a	N_B
A	500	470	$1{,}2 \cdot 10^4$
B	500	325	$2{,}1 \cdot 10^5$
C	700	350	$1{,}7 \cdot 10^3$
D	700	240	$2{,}8\ 10^5$

Ck15G

φ = 1,6 = konst.

2α = 90° = konst.

T_R in °C und σ_a in N/mm²

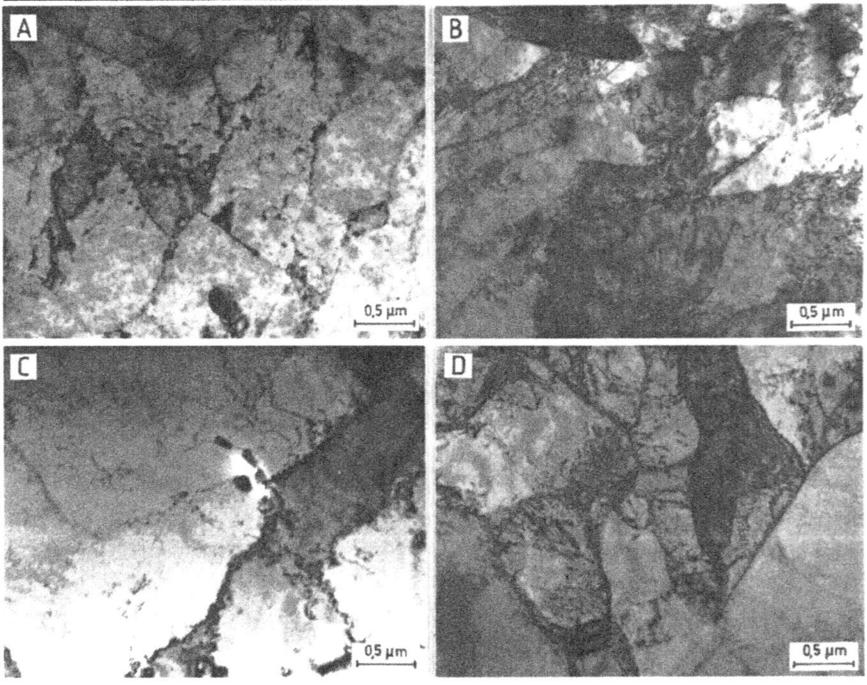

Bild 77: Versetzungsanordnung halbwarmfließgepreßter Werkstücke aus Ck15G nach unterschiedlichen Schwingbeanspruchungen (σ_a = konst.).

7.2 BRUCHAUSBILDUNG

Schwingungsbrüche initiieren bevorzugt an freien Oberflächen. Durch Wechselbeanspruchung entstehen Gleitbänder, die an der Oberfläche Aus- und Einwölbungen (Extrusionen und Intrusionen) bilden. Die nach Richtung und Dichte unterschiedlich verteilten Oberflächenveränderungen werden durch Gefügeinhomogenitäten verursacht /76/. Da die Oberflächenstruktur nach der Umformung unverändert blieb, war es nicht möglich, solche Oberflächenerscheinungen nachzuweisen. Die Rißeinleitung erfolgt häufig an Stellen mit hoher Spannungskonzentration - verbunden mit plastischen Deformationen; Ausgangspunkte sind u. a. Einschlüsse an der Oberfläche, eingedrückte Fremdkörper, fertigungsbedingte Riefen bzw. Risse (Formänderungsvermögen erschöpft). Ein Beispiel für die Rißauslösung durch eine lokale Spannungskonzentration an einer Werkstoffverunreinigung (Rißkeim in Form eines Schlackeneinschlusses) wird in Bild 78A und 78B gegeben. Die bauteilähnliche Probe (φ = 0,5 und 2α = 90°) wurde im

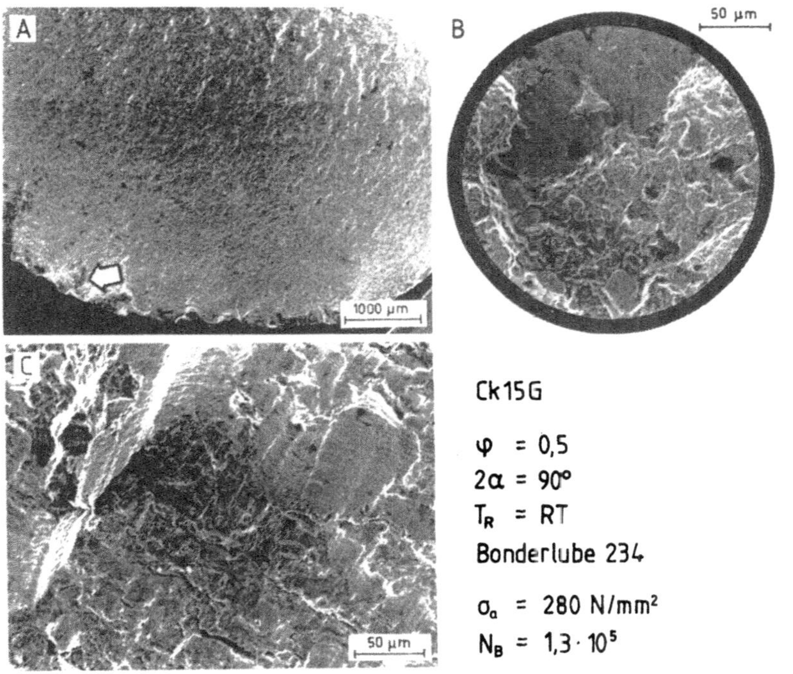

Bild 78: Ermüdungsbruchfläche (lokale Rißinitiierung; A, B) von einem Fließpreßteil aus Ck15G (φ = 0,5 und 2α = 90°).

spannungskontrollierten Versuch mit einer Spannungsamplitude von 280 N/mm^2 beaufschlagt und erreichte eine Lebensdauer von $1{,}3 \cdot 10^5$ Schwingspielen. Teilbild 78C weist auf Abgleitvorgänge unter 45° zur Rißausbreitungsrichtung hin. Außerdem ist ein typisches Merkmal eines Ermüdungsbruches - das Auftreten von zahlreichen, senkrecht zur Rißausbreitungsrichtung angeordneten Nebenrissen - zu erkennen. Diese Nebenrisse treten umso zahlreicher auf, je weiter die Entfernung zur Rißausgangsstelle ist.

Die freigelegte Bruchfläche wurde mit Hilfe eines Profilprojektors um den Faktor 10 vergrößert und durch Ausplanimetrieren das Verhältnis von Ermüdungsbruchfläche zur Ausgangsfläche ermittelt. Am Beispiel des Schulteröffnungswinkels ist zu erkennen, daß mit zunehmender Spannungsamplitude die Ermüdungsbruchfläche bei linearem Zusammenhang abnimmt (Bild 79). Weiterhin wird mit steigendem Schulteröffnungswinkel der Kurvenast zu höheren Spannungsamplituden verschoben. Äquivalente Zusammenhänge wurden auch bei den Verfahrensparametern Umformgrad

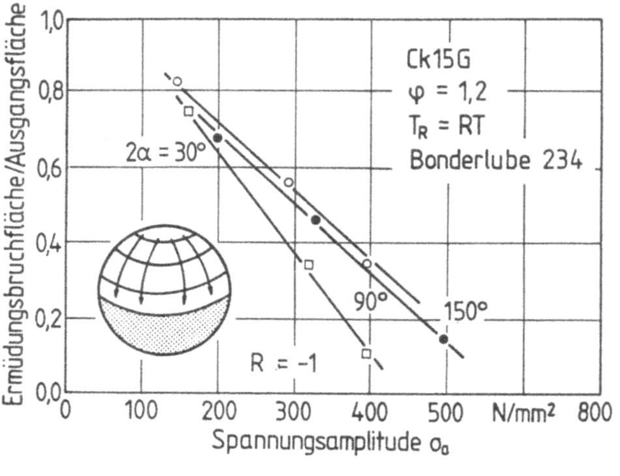

Bild 79: Zusammenhang zwischen Spannungsausschlag und der sich einstellenden Ermüdungsbruchfläche in Abhängigkeit vom Schulteröffnungswinkel.

und Rohteiltemperatur festgestellt. Eine visuelle Bestätigung der obengenannten quantitativen Zusammenhänge ist für halbwarmfließgepreßte Werkstücke (φ = 1,2 und T_R = 500 °C) aus den nachfolgenden REM-Aufnahmen zu entnehmen (Bild 80). Das makroskopische Aussehen von Schwingungsbrüchen ist oft dadurch gekennzeichnet, daß die Bruchfläche aus mehreren Bereichen mit verschiedenartiger Oberflächenstruktur besteht. Während die eigentliche Ermüdungsbruchfläche meist eben verläuft (senkrecht zur Belastungsrichtung), feinkörnig ausgebildet ist, matt und samtartig aussieht, zeigt die Restbruchfläche die Struktur eines mechanischen Gewaltbruches. Die Größe der Ermüdungsbruchfläche ist ein direktes Maß für die aufgeprägte Spannungsamplitude (Dehnungsamplitude) im Bruchquerschnitt; bei hoher Bean-

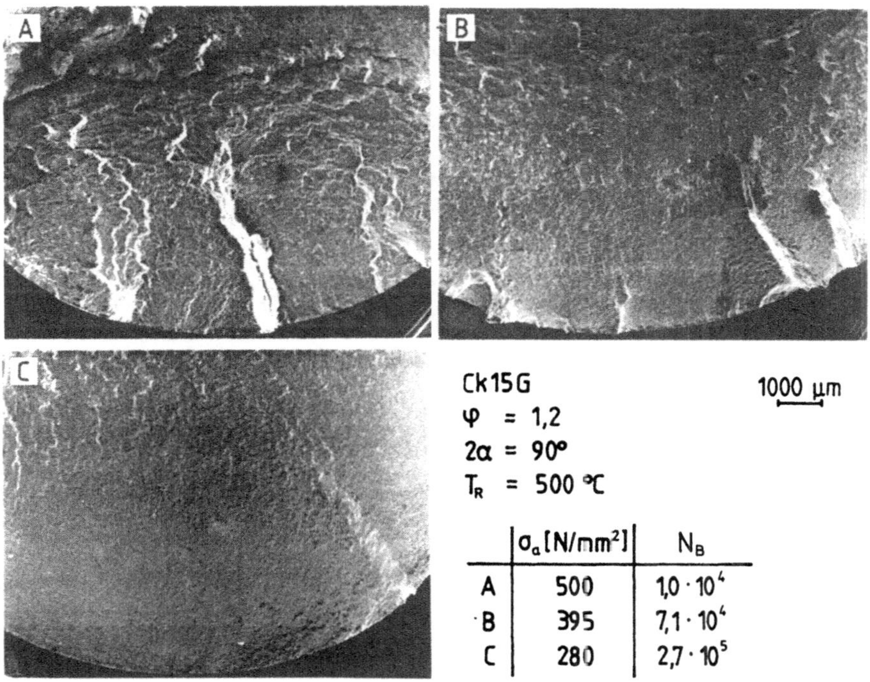

Bild 80: Ermüdungsbruchflächen von halbwarmfließgepreßten Werkstücken aus Ck15G (T_R = 500 °C und φ = 1,2).

spruchung ist der Restbruchanteil an der gesamten Bruchfläche groß und bei kleiner entsprechend gering /77/. Das am sichersten erkennbare Merkmal für einen duktilen Gewaltbruch ist die sog. Wabenstruktur; für den Umformgrad $\varphi = 0{,}9$ ist nach gesamtdehnungskontrolliertem Versuch ein Ausschnitt aus dem Übergangsbereich Ermüdungsbruch/Restgewaltbruch sowie aus dem Gewaltbruchbereich gezeigt (Bild 81A). Die Metallmatrix ist mit Löchern durchsetzt, in denen Fremdkörper bzw. Fremdphasen (u. a. Verunreinigungen) eingebettet sind. Nach fortschreitender plastischer Dehnung bleiben nur noch dünne Stege zwischen den Löchern zurück, die nach vollständiger Trennung der Verbindungen zu einer von "Halblöchern" bzw. Waben durchsetzten Bruchfläche führen (Bild 81B) /76, 78/.

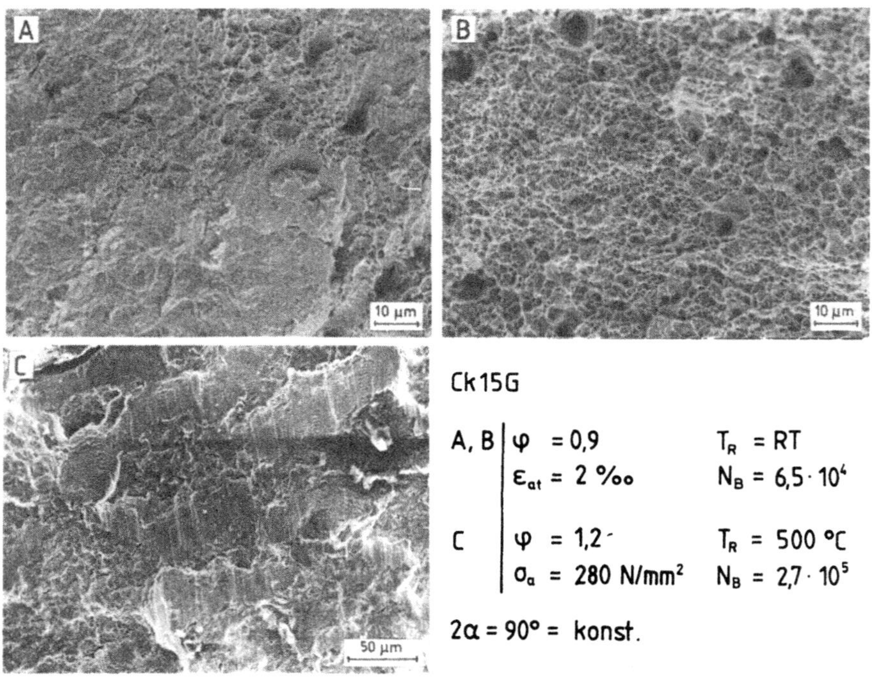

Bild 81: Charakteristische Bruchaufnahmen kaltfließgepreßter Werkstücke.

Neben den konzentrisch zur Bruchausgangsstelle verlaufenden Rastlinien (makroskopisches Merkmal) sind die mit Hilfe des Rasterelektronenmikroskops erfaßbaren Schwingungsstreifen ein eindeutiger Hinweis auf einen Schwingungsbruch. Diese Schwingungsstreifen bilden sich jeweils an der Rißspitze beim Durchlaufen eines Schwingspiels (Aufweiten und Zusammendrücken der Rißflanken). Der Abstand der Schwingungsstreifen ist ein Maß für die Rißfortschrittsgeschwindigkeit. Selbst bei hoher Auflösung im Rasterelektronenmikroskop waren keine charakteristischen Schwingungsstreifen zu beobachten. Allerdings muß ein Ermüdungsbruch nicht unbedingt mit der Ausbildung von Schwingungsstreifen in Verbindung stehen. Ein häufiges Merkmal von Schwingungsbrüchen sind auch Sekundäreffekte, die aus der Bruchfläche durch hervorstehende oder losgelöste harte Teilchen entstehen. Infolge der Relativbewegung der beiden Werkstückhälften beim Rißschließen entstehen riefenähnliche Spuren (Bild 81C) /79/.

8 HINWEISE FÜR DIE INDUSTRIELLE PRAXIS

Der Konstrukteur bewegt sich beispielsweise im Motoren- und Fahrzeugbau bei der Bauteilauslegung wegen immer neuen Forderungen nach höherer Zylinderleistung bei gleichzeitiger Massenreduktion in engen Grenzen. Da aber der Sicherheitsgedanke für jeden Produzenten absolute Priorität besitzt, wird es mehr denn je darauf ankommen, neben einer möglichst genauen Information über den Bauteileinsatz und einer detaillierten Beanspruchungsanalyse bei der Gestaltung der Bauteile die nötigen Entscheidungshilfen für die Wahl des Werkstoffes und der Fertigungs-, Nachbearbeitungs- und Wärmebehandlungsverfahren zu geben. Hierfür ist es unerläßlich, zunächst einmal in Grundlagenuntersuchungen fundierte Kenntnisse über Werkstoff- und Fertigungseinflüsse auf das dynamische Bauteilverhalten zu erarbeiten. Die Qualität der Bauteile und eventuell die Herstellkosten könnten dadurch verbessert bzw. gesenkt werden (Einsparung einer Fertigungsfolge - z. B. Abspanen der Randschicht -, wenn die Anforderungskriterien trotzdem erreicht werden).

Da die Werkstoff- und Bauteilprüfung zeit- und kostenintensiv ist, läßt sich die statistische Versuchsplanung und Auswertung zur Erfassung möglicher Streubreiten in vielen Bereichen der industriellen Praxis nur schwer einführen. Vermutlich wird auch weiter am einfachen Bruchkonzept der Wöhlerlinie (DIN 50100) festgehalten; eine strenge Separation von Ermüdungs- und Schädigungsphasen bereitet hierbei Schwierigkeiten. Zumindest sollten einfach zugängliche Merkmale (z. B. Oberflächenveränderungen, die Temperatur oder - wie in dieser Arbeit - die Deformation) sorgfältig verfolgt und dokumentiert werden, um in Zukunft eine breitere Informationgrundlage zu bekommen /80/. Für die Lösung konkreter Probleme ist die enge Zusammenarbeit zwischen Konstruktion, Versuchsfeld und Werkstofflabor erforderlich. Diese beginnt beim Problem der Übertragbarkeit von Versuchsergebnissen auf Bauteile, das sich im allgemeinen auf das Zusammenwirken der drei Grundgegebenheiten Werkstoff, geometrische Gestalt und Belastung zurückführen läßt /81/ (siehe hierzu auch /82/).

Für die funktionsgerechte Bauteilauslegung genügen unter Ausnutzung der verfahrensbedingten Werkstoffverfestigung häufig kostengünstigere Werkstoffe. In diesem Zusammenhang werden in der Massivumformung unter wirtschaftlichen Aspekten hohe Umformgrade angestrebt. Bei den Werkstückeigenschaften hat das neben einer höheren Verfestigung (Zugfestigkeit, Härte) eine abnehmende Duktilität zur Folge. Außerdem liegen beim Kalt- und Halbwarmfließpressen je nach Gestalt des Werkstückes, Größe des Umformgrades, Umformfolge, Rohteilzustand etc. am Rand Bereiche mit unterschiedlich hohen Formänderungen vor. Ob und in welchem Umfang diese Bereiche von Einfluß sind, muß im jeweiligen Anwendungsfall beurteilt werden. So bewirkt eine lokale Verfestigung (inhomogene Härteverteilung über dem Querschnitt mit Härtegradient zum Rand hin) zumindest im Zeitfestigkeitsgebiet ($N_B < 10^5$) höhere Lebensdauerwerte bei konstant ertragenen Spannungsamplituden. Dagegen ist mit einem Abspanen der Randschicht aufgrund des verbleibenden weitgehend homogen umgeformten Kernbereiches und durch eine veränderte Oberflächentopographie ein Schwingfestigkeitsgewinn im Bereich der Dauerfestigkeit verbunden. Das gleiche Phänomen - höhere ertragbare Beanspruchungen im Intervall größerer Schwingspielzahlen ($5 \cdot 10^5 \le N \le 2 \cdot 10^6$) durch eine mit zunehmender Temperatur homogeneren Umformung über dem Querschnitt - ist auch nach einer Halbwarmumformung zu verzeichnen. Während bei einer Kaltumformung noch vorwiegend zyklische Wechselentfestigung (mit Ausnahme von Sättigungsgebieten) dominiert, treten zumindest bei hohem Umformgrad und hoher Rohteiltemperatur (z. B. $\varphi = 1{,}6$ und $T_R = 700\ ^oC$) Verfestigungsphasen auf.

Oft bringt die Kombination von Wärmebehandlung und Kaltumformung eine günstige Voraussetzung für die Verbesserung der Dauerfestigkeit von gekerbten Bauteilen (z. B. Schrauben). Liegt beispielsweise zwischen dem Fließpressen und dem Gewindewalzen eine Glühbehandlung, so kann die Dauerfestigkeit um mehr als 35 % gesteigert werden /17/.

Gerade das Verbindungselement Maschinenschraube bietet sich als Beispiel für ein Bauteil unter Zugschwellbeanspruchung an. Wie gezeigt werden konnte, führen mittelspannungsbehaftete Beanspruchungen (mit überlagerter Belastungs-Zeitfunktion) im Zeit- und Dauerfestigkeitsgebiet zu irreversiblen Probenverlängerungen ($\sigma_m > 0$) bzw. -verkürzungen ($\sigma_m < 0$). Der Einfluß des zyklischen Kriechens auf die Abmessungsstabilität der Bauteile ist beispielsweise aus einem modifizierten Haigh-Diagramm (Mitteldehnung ε_m steht senkrecht auf der durch σ_a und σ_m aufgespannten Ebene) ersichtlich.

Die zyklischen Spannungs-Dehnungskurven - für den Anfangsbereich der plastischen Verformung bestimmt - dienen als Berechnungsgrundlage von elastisch-plastischen Verformungsvorgängen an technischen Bauteilen mit Einsatzbereich im Zeitfestigkeitsgebiet. In diesem Zusammenhang kann durch Finite-Elemente-Berechnung (z. B. Bestimmung bzw. Quantifizierung lokal am höchsten beanspruchter Stellen) unter Anwendung einer geeigneten Schadensakkumulationshypothese (mit Hilfe der zyklischen Fließkurve und der Wöhlerlinie) die Lebensdauer komplexer Bauteile mit unterschiedlichem Beanspruchungszeitverlauf abgeschätzt werden /83/.

9 ZUSAMMENFASSUNG

Über den Einfluß von Verfahrensparametern bei den Durchdrückverfahren Voll-Vorwärts-Fließpressen und Verjüngen auf das Ermüdungsverhalten liegen noch keine fundierten Kenntnisse vor. Die durchgeführten Untersuchungen unter Variation des Umformgrades, Schulteröffnungswinkels, der Schmierung und Rohteiltemperatur sind als Beitrag zu dieser Thematik zu verstehen.

Zu diesem Zweck wurde ein Schwingprüfstand mit einer rechnergestützen Meßwerterfassung und Datenverarbeitung aufgebaut und ein Computerprogramm zur Steuerung des Meßablaufs, der Datenreduktion und Datenauswertung erstellt.

Ausgehend von der Herstellung bauteilähnlicher Proben (gebunden umgeformte Oberfläche bleibt erhalten) werden die Werkstücke durch eine Berechnung des lokalen Umformgrades mit der Finite-Elemente-Methode, der experimentellen Ermittlung der Umformeigenspannungen und der mechanischen Kennwerte, Messung des Härteprofils und der Oberflächenbeschaffenheit sowie begleitenden metallographischen Untersuchungen näher charakterisiert.

Das Ermüdungsverhalten des Werkstoffs Ck15G (für Stichversuche 16MnCr5G) vor und nach der Umformung wird - ausgehend von rechnergestützten Hysteresismessungen - anhand von Wechselverformungskurven diskutiert. Nach einer Kaltmassivumformung ist durchweg zyklische Wechselentfestigung zu beobachten. Bei kleineren Spannungsamplituden - wenig oberhalb der Wechselfestigkeit - kommt es nach quasielastischer Verformung zum Bruch. Ein zunehmender Umformgrad ($\varphi = 0{,}5 \div 1{,}6$) und ein steigender Schulteröffnungswinkel ($2\alpha = 30 \div 150^{o}$) liefern in der Tendenz ähnliche Wechselverformungskurven; bei mittleren und höheren Spannungsausschlägen - stets unterhalb der statischen 0,2-Dehngrenze - werden teilweise Sättigungsgebiete im spannungskontrollierten Einstufenversuch registriert. Der Vergleich der Schmierstoffe - wässrige Graphitdispersion mit Metallseife - zeigt bis ca. 95 % der Lebensdauer keinen signifikanten Einfluß auf die ε_{ar}/log N-Kurven (danach stellt sich eine etwas höhere plastische Dehnungsamplitude bei N_B nach einer Graphitschmierung ein).

Bei einer Halbwarmumformung schließt sich zumindest bei einem hohen Umformgrad (φ = 1,6) und hoher Temperatur (T_R = 700 °C) nach Durchlaufen eines Entfestigungsmaximums eine Verfestigungsphase bis zum Probenbruch an. Im Vergleich zu kaltfließgepreßten Werkstücken werden von halbwarmumgeformten Proben im Bereich hoher Schwingspielzahlen ($N > 10^6$) höhere Spannungsausschläge ertragen. Dies ist vermutlich auf eine mit zunehmender Temperatur homogenere Umformung (geringerer Härtegradient über dem Querschnitt) zurückzuführen. Der gleiche Effekt einer höheren Wechselfestigkeit läßt sich durch Abspanen der Randzone kaltfließgepreßter Werkstücke erzielen. Durch Verjüngen verfestigte Schäfte zeigen hingegen qualitativ ähnliche Wechselverformungskurven wie die nach dem Kaltfließpressen. Die Ergebnisse der Wechselverformungskurven sind für die einzelnen Verfahrensparameter in zyklischen Spannungs-Dehnungskurven und zur lebensdauerorientierten Bewertung in Wöhlerkurven zusammengefaßt.

Weiterhin ist der Einfluß verschiedener Versuchsführungen (spannungs- und gesamtdehnungskontrolliert), der Versuchsfrequenz und unterschiedlicher Mittelspannungen von Interesse. Der Nachweis eventueller inhomogener Deformationserscheinungen wird mit Hilfe lokaler Dehnungsmessungen versucht und der Einfluß äußerer Kerben auf das Ermüdungsverhalten mit einer numerisch/experimentellen Untersuchung erfaßt.

Für die ermüdeten Schwingproben wird eine mikroskopische Betrachtung der Feinstruktur durchgeführt. Anhand der Versetzungskonfigurationen erscheint eine Zuordnung zu den einzelnen Verfahrensparametern und Beanspruchungsamplituden (Vorgeschichte) möglich. Ähnlich verhält es sich bei den Folgerungen aus den fraktographischen Aufnahmen.

Schrifttum

/1/ Mayr, P.: Grundlagen zum Verhalten bei schwingender Beanspruchung. In: Verhalten von Stahl bei schwingender Beanspruchung. Dahl, W. (Hrsg.). Düsseldorf: Verlag Stahleisen m. b. H. 1978, S. 82-99.

/2/ Burgdorf, M.: Das Kaltfließpressen von Stahl. Z. Metallkde. 61 (1970) 11, S. 787-791.

/3/ Diether, U.: Fließpressen von Stahl im Temperaturbereich 773 K (500 °C) bis 1073 K (800 °C). Berichte aus dem Institut für Umformtechnik, Universität Stuttgart, Nr. 54. Berlin, Heidelberg, New York: Springer 1980.

/4/ Binder, H.: Untersuchungen über das Verjüngen von zylindrischen Vollkörpern. Berichte aus dem Institut für Umformtechnik, Universität Stuttgart, Nr. 58. Berlin, Heidelberg, New York: Springer 1980.

/5/ Hertel, H.: Ermüdungsfestigkeit der Konstruktionen. Berlin, Heidelberg, New York: Springer 1969.

/6/ MBB WF-Information 5/82. Erhöhung der Schwingfestigkeit metallischer Werkstoffe durch Kugelstrahlen.

/7/ Starker, P.; Macherauch, E.: Kugelstrahlen und Schwingfestigkeit. Z. Werkstofftechn. 14 (1983), S. 109-115.

/8/ Strigens, P.: Zum Einfluß der Oberflächenverfestigung auf die Dauerfestigkeit von Stählen. Dr.-Ing. Diss., TH Darmstadt 1971.

/9/ Wiegand, H.; Illgner, K. H.: Über den Einfluß der Oberflächenkaltverformung auf die Wechselfestigkeit glatter Probestäbe. Draht 16 (1965) 10, S. 703-714.

/10/ Berstein, G.; Fuchsbauer, B.: Festwalzen und Schwingfestigkeit. Z. Werkstofftechn. 13 (1982), S. 103-109.

/11/ Hempel, M.: Das Dauerschwingverhalten der Werkstoffe. VDI-Z. 104 (1962) 27, S. 1362-1377.

/12/ Gill, E. T.; Goodacre, R.: Some aspects of the fatigue properties of patented steel wires. II. Note on the effect of low-temperature heat treatment. J. Iron Steel Inst. 132 (1935) 2, S. 143-177.

/13/ Maier, H.-J.: Über den Einfluß einer Kaltverformung auf die Zeitfestigkeit biegewechselbeanspruchter glatter Proben. Techn.-wiss. Ber. MPA Stuttgart (1975), Heft 75-02.

/14/ Radhakrishnan, V. M.; Baburamani, P. S.: An investigation of the effect of pre-straining on fatigue crack growth. Materials Science and Engineering 17 (1975), S. 283-288.

/15/ Sonsino, C. M.; Hagedorn, K. E.: Einfluß einer Kaltumformung auf das Zeit- und Kurzzeitschwingfestigkeitsverhalten der Stähle StE47 und StE70. Arch. Eisenhüttenwes. 51 (1980) 8, S. 341-345.

/16/ Parker, T. E.; Montgomery, G. L.: Effect of balanced biaxial stretching on the low cycle fatigue behaviour of SAE 1008 hot rolled low carbon steel. SAE Automotive Engineering Congress and Exposition, Paper Nr. 750048, Detroit 1975.

/17/ Flemming, G.: Mechanische Eigenschaften von Stahl bei statischer und wechselnder Beanspruchung nach einer Massivumformung. Dr.-Ing. Diss., TH Darmstadt 1972.

/18/ Bilý, M.: Einfluß der plastischen Verformung auf die Dauerfestigkeit von Metallen. Materialprüf. 12 (1970) 8, S. 275-279.

/19/ Černjak, N. I.: Mechaniceskije svojstva stali v oblasti malych plasticeskich deformacij (Mechanische Eigenschaften von Stahl im Bereich kleiner plastischer Verformung). Kijev: Izdatelstvo AN USSR 1962.

/20/ Woodward, A. R.: Dauerfestigkeit unbearbeiteter stranggepreßter und gewalzter Proben aus verschiedenen Aluminiumlegierungen. Metall 22 (1968) 3, S. 219-223.

/21/ Feldmann, H. D.: Fließpressen von Leichtmetallen, Teil 1. TZ f. prakt. Metallbearb. 66 (1972) 3, S. 105-110.

/22/ Bauer, C. O.: Höhere Leistungsfähigkeit durch kaltumgeformte Sonderteile aus austenitischen Chrom-Nickel-Stählen. KEM 8 (1976), S. 71-74 u. KEM 10 (1976), S. 119-123.

/23/ Wiegand, H.; Illgner, K. H.; Beelich, K. H.: Festigkeit und Formänderungsverhalten von Schraubenverbindungen, insbesondere aus austenitischen Stählen. Draht 18 (1967) 8, S. 517-526.

/24/ Thomala, W.: Beitrag zur Dauerhaltbarkeit von Schraubenverbindungen. Dr.-Ing. Diss., TH Darmstadt 1978.

/25/ Pugh, H. Ll. D.; Ashcroft, K.: Das hydrostatische Strang- und Fließpressen von Metallen. Industrie-Anzeiger 86 (1964), S. 605-612.

/26/ Kerspe, J. H.: Hydrostatisches Fließpressen - Verfahrensparameter und Werkstückeigenschaften. Berichte aus dem Institut für Umformtechnik, Universität Stuttgart, Nr. 69. Berlin, Heidelberg, New York, Tokyo: Springer 1983.

/27/ Lange, K.: Neuere Möglichkeiten der Werkstückherstellung durch Massivumformen. Fertigungstechnisches Kolloquium, Stuttgart 1976.

/28/ Schaub, W.: Mechanische Eigenschaften halbwarmfließgepreßter Sintermetalle auf Eisenbasis. In: Seminarband "Neuere Entwicklungen in der Massivumformung", Stuttgart 1971, S. 5/1-5/20.

/29/ Zapf, G.; Hoffmann, G.; Dalal, K.: Entwicklung mit Hilfe des Warmfließpreßverfahrens hergestellter Sinterstähle mit optimaler Warmstreckgrenze, Dauerfestigkeit und Kerbschlagarbeit, Teil 2. Z. f. Werkstofftechn. (1975) 12, S. 424-432.

/30/ Doege, E.; Rupp, D. M.: Einflußgrößen auf die Dauerschwingfestigkeit bei der Herstellung von Schmiedeteilen. Ind.-Anz. 104 (1982) 5, S. 27-28 u. 30-31.

/31/ Knolle, B.: Dauerschwingfestigkeit von Gesenkschmiedestücken. HFF-Bericht Nr. 9 (1977), S. 19-26.

/32/ Herbst, P.: Zum Einfluß des Oberflächen- und Randzonenzustandes auf die Dauerfestigkeit von Schmiedeteilen aus Stahl. Fortschr.-Ber. VDI-Z., Reihe 5, Nr. 75 (1983).

/33/ Schumann, H.: Metallographie. Leipzig: VEB Deutscher Verlag für Grundstoffindustrie 1983.

/34/ Adler, A.; Walter, K.: Berechnung von einfachen und mehrfachen Preßpassungen. Ind.-Anz. 89 (1967), S. 805-809 u. 967-971.

/35/ Roll, K.: Einsatz numerischer Näherungsverfahren bei der Berechnung von Verfahren der Kaltmassivumformung. Berichte aus dem Institut für Umformtechnik, Universität Stuttgart, Nr. 66. Berlin, Heidelberg, New York: Springer 1982.

/36/ Lange, K. (Hrsg.): Lehrbuch der Umformtechnik, Band 2 Massivumformung. Springer-Verlag, Berlin Heidelberg, New York: Springer 1972.

/37/ Wilhelm, H.: Untersuchungen über den Zusammenhang zwischen Vickershärte und Vergleichsformänderung bei Kaltumformvorgängen. Berichte aus dem Institut für Umformtechnik, Universität Stuttgart, Nr. 9. Essen: Girardet 1969.

/38/ Geiger, R.; Dannenmann, E.; Stefanakis, J.: Untersuchungen zum Halbwarmfließpressen von Stahl. Berichte aus dem Institut für Umformtechnik, Universität Stuttgart, Nr. 41. Essen: Girardet 1976.

/39/ Stüwe, H. P.: Einfluß von Wechseln der Beanspruchungsrichtung auf die Fließspannung von Metallen. In: Grundlagen der Umformtechnik, Symposium Stuttgart 1983, Berichte aus dem Institut für Umformtechnik, Universität Stuttgart, Nr. 74. Berlin, Heidelberg, New York, Tokyo: Springer 1983.

/40/ Dietmann, H.: Werkstofftechnik I. Vorlesungsumdruck, Lehrstuhl für Materialprüfung, Werkstoffkunde und Festigkeitslehre, Universität Stuttgart.

/41/ Dannenmann, E.: Die Veränderung der Oberflächenbeschaffenheit beim Voll-Vorwärts-Fließpressen von Stahl. Annals of the CIRP 17 (1969), S. 353-365.

/42/ Macherauch, E.; Wohlfahrt, H.; Wolfstieg, U.: Zur zweckmäßigen Definition von Eigenspannungen. HTM 28 (1973) 3, S. 201-211.

/43/ Tekkaya, A. E.; Lange, K.: Determination of residual stresses in industrial extrusions. In: Proc. NAMRC-XII, Houghton/Michigan 1984, S. 103-110.

/44/ Peiter, A. (Hrsg.): Eigenspannungen I. Art, Ermittlung und Bewertung. Düsseldorf: Michael Triltsch Verlag 1966.

/45/ Bühler, H.; Schreiber, W.: Zur lückenlosen Bestimmung eines Eigenspannungszustandes in metallischen Vollzylindern. Metall 8 (1954) 17/18, S. 687-691.

/46/ Moore, M. G.; Evans, W. P.: Mathematical correction for stress in removed layers in x-ray diffraction residual stress analysis. SAE Transactions 66 (1958), S. 340-345.

/47/ Miaha, P. S.; Modlen, G. F.: Residual stresses in cold extruded rods. Metals Technology (1976) 4, S. 202-207.

/48/ Dorfschmidt, E.: Eigenspannungsuntersuchungen beim Voll-Vorwärts-Fließpressen. Dr.-Ing. Diss., Universität Hannover 1982.

/49/ Tekkaya, A. E.: Ermittlung von Eigenspannungen in der Kaltmassivumformung. Institut für Umformtechnik, Universität Stuttgart, Nr. 83. Berlin, Heidelberg, New York, Tokyo: Springer 1986.

/50/ Vöhringer, O.; Wohlfahrt, H.: Abbau von Eigenspannungen. In: Eigenspannungen und Lastspannungen (HTM-Beiheft; hrsgg. von Hauk, V. u. Macherauch, E.). München, Wien: Hanser 1982, S. 144-156.

/51/ Instron-Handbook for Model 1343 (servohydraulische Zug-Druck-Schwingprüfmaschine).

/52/ Gottlob, M. P.: IEC-Bus Handbuch. München: Ingenieur W. Hofacker G. m. b. H. Verlag 1980.

/53/ Munz, D.; Schwalbe, K.; Mayer, P.: Dauerschwingverhalben metallischer Werkstoffe. Braunschweig: Vieweg 1971.

/54/ Morrow, J.; Tuler, F. R.: Low cycle fatigue evaluation of Inconel 713 and Waspaloy. Trans. ASME, Ser. D, J. of basic Engng. 87 (1965), S. 275-289.

/55/ Dietmann, H.: Werkstofftechnik II. Vorlesungsumdruck, Lehrstuhl für Materialprüfung, Werkstoffkunde und Festigkeitslehre, Universität Stuttgart.

/56/ Körber, F.; Hempel, M.: Abhängigkeit der Wechselfestigkeit von der Lastwechselfrequenz. Mitt. Kais.-Wilh. Inst. Eisenforsch. 18 (1936), S. 15-19.

/57/ Wyss, T.: Influence of testing frequency on the fatigue strength of steels and light alloys. Bull. ASTM (1953) 188, S. 31-33.

/58/ Heimbach, H.: Zum Einfluß der Belastungsfrequenz auf die Zeit- und Dauerfestigkeit von Stahl. Materialprüf. 12 (1970) 11, S. 377-380.

/59/ Aurich, D.: Bruchvorgänge in metallischen Werkstoffen (hrsgg. von Macherauch, E.u. Gerold, V.). Karlsruhe: Werkstofftechnische Verlagsgesellschaft m. b. H. 1978.

/60/ Pilo, D.: Zum Wechselverformungsverhalten normalisierter unlegierter Stähle mit Kohlenstoffgehalten von 0,01 bis 1,02 Gew.-%. Dr.-Ing. Diss., Universität Karlsruhe 1979.

/61/ Sonsino, C. M.: Einfluß von Kaltverformungen bis 5 % auf das Kurzzeitschwingfestigkeitsverhalten metallischer Werkstoffe. Dr.-Ing. Diss., TH Darmstadt 1982.

/62/ Autorenkollektiv (Hrsg. Schott, G.): Werkstoffermüdung. Leipzig: VEB Deutscher Verlag für Grundstoffindustrie 1985.

/63/ VDI 2227 (Entwurf/1974). Festigkeit bei wiederholter Beanspruchung - Zeit- und Dauerfestigkeit metallischer Werkstoffe, insbesondere von Stählen.

/64/ Dengel, D.: Einige grundlegende Gesichtspunkte für die Planung und Auswertung von Dauerschwingversuchen. Materialprüf. 13 (1971) 5, S. 145-151.

/65/ ASTM E399-83. Standard test method for plane-strain fracture toughness of metallic materials.

/66/ DeSalvo, G.; Swanson, J.: ANSYS, Engineering Analysis Systems; user's manual, revision 4.1. Control Data Corporation, Minneapolis 1984.

/67/ Stegmayer, R.: Experimentelle und numerische Simualation des Bauteilverhaltens unter Wärmewechselbeanspruchung. Techn.-wiss. Ber. MPA Stuttgart (1985), Heft 85-01.

/68/ Neuber, H.: Kerbspannungslehre. Berlin, Heidelberg, New York, Tokyo: Springer 1985.

/69/ Zenner, H.: Niedrig-Lastwechsel-Ermüdung (low cycle fatigue). In: VDI-Jahrbuch 1979; VDI-Gesellschaft Werkstofftechnik. Düsseldorf: VDI-Verlag 1980.

/70/ Eifler, D.: Inhomogene Deformationserscheinungen bei Schwingbeanspruchung eines unterschiedlich wärmebehandelten Stahles des Typs 42CrMo4. Dr.-Ing. Diss., Universität Karlsruhe 1983.

/71/ Reik, W.; Mayr, P.; Macherauch, E.: Eine notwendige Änderung der Dauerfestigkeitsschaubilder bei Schwingfestigkeitsuntersuchungen. Arch. Eisenhüttenwes. 52 (1981) 8, S. 325-328.

/72/ von Heimendahl, M.: Einführung in die Elektronenmikroskopie. Braunschweig: Vieweg 1970.

/73/ Hempel, M.: Dauerschwingverhalten kaltverformter Stahlproben. Arch. Eisenhüttenwes. 43 (1972) 4, S. 337-344.

/74/ Böhm, H.: Einführung in die Metallkunde. B. I. Hochschultaschenbuch Bd. 196. Mannheim, Zürich: Bibliograph. Institut 1968.

/75/ Gil Sevillano, J.; van Houtte, P.; Aernoudt, E.: Large strain hardening and textures. In: Progress in Material Science, Vol. 25. Christian, J. W. et al. (eds.). Oxford, New York, Toronto, Sydney, Paris, Frankfurt: Pergamon Press 1982.

/76/ Engel; Klingele: Rasterelektronenmikroskopische Untersuchungen von Metallschäden. Köln: Gerling Institut für Schadensforschung und Schadensverhütung G. m. b. H. 1974.

/77/ Broichhausen, J.: Schadenskunde. München, Wien: Hanser 1985.

/78/ Müller, H.: Exemplarische Schadensfälle. In: Verhalten von Stahl bei schwingender Beanspruchung. Dahl, W. (Hrsg.). Düsseldorf: Verlag Stahleisen m. b. H. 1978, S. 195-207.

/79/ SEM/TEM Fractography Handbook. Metals and Ceramics Information Center, Battelle Columbus Laboratories. Columbus/ Ohio 1975.

/80/ Dengel, D.: Schwingfestigkeit heute - einige wichtige Aspekte. In: Tagungband "Werkstoffprüfung 1985", Deutscher Verband für Materialprüfung e. V., Bad Nauheim 1985, S. 26-52.

/81/ Razim, C.: Über den Stand, die künftigen Möglichkeiten und die Grenzen der Übertragbarkeit des an Proben ermittelten Werkstoffverhaltens auf Bauteile. In: VDI-Berichte 354; Übertragbarkeit von Versuchs- und Prüfergebnissen auf Bauteile. Düsseldorf: VDI-Verlag 1979.

/82/ Kloos, K. H.; Fuchsbauer, B.; Magin, W.; Zankov, D.: Übertragbarkeit von Probestab-Schwingfestigkeitseigenschaften auf Bauteile. In: VDI-Berichte 354; Übertragbarkeit von Versuchs- und Prüfergebnissen auf Bauteile. Düsseldorf: VDI-Verlag 1979.

/83/ Sander, W.; Schoeckle, S.: Design and fatigue life evaluation of pistons for high bmep diesel engines. SAE-Paper 790857.

Unveröffentlichte Studienarbeiten am Institut für Umformtechnik: R. Mürder und M. Knörr.

Berichte aus dem Institut für Umformtechnik der Universität Stuttgart

Herausgeber Professor Dr.-Ing. Kurt Lange

1 **Untersuchung über den Einfluß der Belastungszeit auf die Streuung der Rückfederung von Biegeteilen**
Von Dipl.-Ing. Klaus Tafel. 70 Seiten Text u. 64 Seiten mit 49 Bildern u. 15 Tafeln. Vergriffen

2/3 **Untersuchungen über das freie Napfen**
Von Dipl.-Ing. Gerhard Schmitt und Dipl.-Ing. Dieter Schmoeckel.
Untersuchungen über den Kraft- und Arbeitsbedarf sowie den Umformwirkungsgrad beim Vorwärts-Vollfließpressen von Stahl
Von Dipl.-Ing. Dieter Kast. 40 Seiten Text u. 43 Seiten mit 47 Bildern u. 5 Tafeln. 28,— DM

4 **Untersuchungen über die Werkzeuggestaltung beim Vorwärts-Hohlfließpressen von Stahl und Nichteisenmetallen**
Von Dipl.-Ing. Dieter Schmoeckel. 72 Seiten Text u. 117 Seiten mit 179 Bildern. 39,— DM

5 **Untersuchungen über das Stauchen und Zapfenpressen**
Von Dipl.-Ing. Märten Burgdorf. 126 Seiten Text u. 58 Seiten mit 138 Bildern u. 4 Tafeln. 55,— DM

6 **Untersuchungen über die Streuung der Kräfte und Arbeiten beim Fließpressen in der laufenden Fertigung und den Einfluß der Phosphatschichtdicke und des Schmiermittels**
Von Dipl.-Ing. Hans-Dietrich Witte. 38 Seiten Text u. 48 Seiten mit 49 Bildern 30,— DM

7 **Untersuchungen über das Rückwärts-Napffließpressen von Stahl bei Raumtemperatur**
Von Dipl.-Ing. Gerhard Schmitt. 132 Seiten Text u. 93 Seiten mit 130 Bildern u. 5 Tafeln. 34,— DM

8 **Die Abbildegenauigkeit beim Biegen im 90°-V-Gesenk und ihre Beeinflussung durch Nachdrücken im Gesenk**
Von Dipl.-Ing. Eckart Dannenmann. 50 Seiten Text u. 31 Seiten mit 28 Bildern u. 1 Tafel. Vergriffen

9 **Untersuchungen über den Zusammenhang zwischen Vickershärte und Vergleichsformänderung bei Kaltumformvorgängen**
Von Dipl.-Ing. Hans Wilhelm. 50 Seiten Text u. 35 Seiten mit 37 Bildern u. 2 Tafeln. Vergriffen

10 **Untersuchungen über das Abstreckziehen von zylindrischen Hohlkörpern bei Raumtemperatur**
Von Dipl.-Ing. Rolf K. Busch. 86 Seiten Text u. 92 Seiten mit 97 Bildern. Vergriffen

11 **Vorgänge beim elektromagnetischen und elektrohydraulischen Umformen von metallischen Werkstücken**
Von Dipl.-Ing. Herbert Müller. 90 Seiten Text u. 110 Seiten mit 93 Bildern u. 10 Tafeln. 22,— DM

12 **Ein Verfahren zur näherungsweisen Berechnung des Spannungs- und Formänderungszustandes beim Fließen starrplastischer Werkstoffe**
Von Dipl.-Ing. Gerhard Adler. 124 Seiten Text u. 76 Seiten mit 72 Bildern. Vergriffen

13 **Modellgesetzmäßigkeiten beim Rückwärtsfließpressen geometrisch ähnlicher Näpfe**
Von Dipl.-Ing. Dieter Kast. 101 Seiten Text u. 73 Seiten mit 60 Bildern u. 6 Tafeln. Vergriffen

14 **Untersuchungen über das Genauschneiden von Stahl und Nichteisenmetallen**
Von Dipl.-Ing. Wilfried Krämer. 96 Seiten Text u. 132 Seiten mit 128 Bildern u. 10 Tafeln. Vergriffen

15 **Entwicklung und Erprobung eines Simulators zur reproduzierbaren Nachahmung der Kraft-Weg-Verläufe von Umformvorgängen**
Von Dipl.-Ing. Kurt Schmid. 88 Seiten Text u. 38 Seiten mit 35 Bildern u. 2 Tafeln. 17,— DM

16 **Walzrichten von Metallbändern mit symmetrisch angestellter Fünf-Walzen-Richtmaschine**
Von Dipl.-Ing. Hans-Dietrich Witte. 108 Seiten Text u. 63 Seiten mit 60 Bildern u. 8 Tafeln. 22,— DM

17/18 **Erzeugung räumlicher Blechgebilde mittels Flächenbiegung**
Konstruktion, Abwicklung und Herstellung von Schraubtorsen aus Blech
Von Prof. Dr.-Ing. E. h. Dr. techn. h. c. Otto Kienzle.
120 Seiten Text u. 55 Seiten mit 86 Bildern u. 3 Tafeln. 22,— DM

19 **Einfluß der Alterung auf die mechanischen Eigenschaften von Stählen zum Kaltfließpressen**
Von Dipl.-Ing. Vladimir Hasek, CSc. 43 Seiten Text u. 54 Seiten mit 50 Bildern u. 3 Tafeln. 16,— DM

20 **Beitrag zur Frage der Spannungen, Formänderungen und Temperaturen beim axialsymmetrischen Strangpressen**
Von Dipl.-Ing. Rolf Dalheimer. 118 Seiten Text u. 76 Seiten mit 79 Bildern u. 3 Tafeln. Vergriffen

21 **Über den Einfluß der Werkzeuggeschwindigkeit auf den Stauchvorgang**
Von Dipl.-Ing. H.-J. Metzler. 127 Seiten Text u. 100 Seiten mit 94 Bildern u. 6 Tafeln. 25,— DM

22 **Numerische Behandlung von Verfahren der Umformtechnik**
Von Dr.-Ing. Elmar Steck. 67 Seiten Text u. 22 Seiten mit 43 Bildern. 16,— DM

23 **Ein Verfahren zur näherungsweisen Berechnung der Wärmeentwicklung und der Temperaturverteilung beim Kaltstauchen von Metallen**
Von Dipl.-Ing. Walther Pohl. 78 Seiten Text u. 51 Seiten mit 61 Bildern u. 4 Tafeln. 21,— DM

24 **Untersuchungen über das Drückwalzen zylindrischer Hohlkörper und Beitrag zur Berechnung der gedrückten Fläche und der Kräfte**
Von Dipl.-Ing. Hans-Jürgen Dreikandt. 161 Seiten Text u. 79 Seiten mit 73 Bildern u. 6 Tafeln. Vergriffen

25 **Über den Formänderungs- und Spannungszustand beim Ziehen von großen unregelmäßigen Blechteilen**
Von Dipl.-Ing. Vladimir Hasek, CSc. 129 Seiten Text u. 106 Seiten mit 109 Bildern u. 9 Tafeln. 35,— DM

26 **Über die Anisotropie des plastischen Verhaltens stranggepreßter Stäbe aus hexagonalen Metallen**
Von Dipl.-Ing. Günther Schröder. 129 Seiten Text u. 75 Seiten mit 97 Bildern u. 2 Tafeln. Vergriffen

27 **Die Messung der mechanischen Kontaktspannung in der Wirkfuge Werkzeug — Werkstück bei Umformverfahren**
Von Dipl.-Ing. Fritz Dohmann. 99 Seiten Text u. 82 Seiten mit 93 Bildern u. 4 Tafeln. Vergriffen

52 **Untersuchung der Verfahrensgrenzen beim 180°-Biegen von Fein- und Mittelblechen**
Von Dipl.-Phys. Wolfgang Schaub. ISBN 3-540-09881-X.
65 Seiten mit 24 Abbildungen. 38.– DM

53 **Abstreckgleitziehen von nichtrostenden austenitischen Stählen**
Von Dipl.-Ing. Jobst-H. Kerspe. ISBN 3-540-09882-8.
109 Seiten mit 36 Abbildungen. 43,– DM

54 **Fließpressen von Stahl im Temperaturbereich 773 K (500°C) bis 1073 K (800°C)**
Von Dipl.-Ing. Ulrich Diether. ISBN 3-540-09959-X.
165 Seiten mit 80 Abbildungen. 48,– DM

55 **Die numerisch gesteuerte Radial-Umformmaschine und ihr Einsatz im Rahmen einer flexiblen Fertigung**
Von Dipl.-Ing. Peter Metzger. ISBN 3-540-10073-3.
158 Seiten mit 65 Abbildungen. 43,– DM

56 **Möglichkeiten zur Steuerung des Stoffflusses beim Ziehen großer unregelmäßiger Blechteile**
Von Dr.-Ing. Vladimir V. Hasek. ISBN 3-540-10074-1.
193 Seiten mit 96 Abbildungen. 48,– DM

57 **Beitrag zur Arbeitsgenauigkeit des Kaltmassivumformens**
Von Dipl.-Ing. Herbert Leykamm. ISBN 3-540-10363-5.
165 Seiten mit 84 Abbildungen und 5 Tabellen.. 48,– DM

58 **Untersuchungen über das Verjüngen von zylindrischen Vollkörpern**
Von Dipl.-Ing. Helmut Binder. ISBN 3-540-10466-6.
146 Seiten mit 50 Abbildungen und 3 Tabellen. 43,– DM

59 **Umformverhalten legierter Sintereisen**
Von Dipl.-Ing. Manfred Stilz. ISBN 3-540-11051-8.
170 Seiten mit 75 Abbildungen und 5 Tabellen. 48,– DM

60 **Interaktives Programmsystem zur Erstellung von Fertigungsunterlagen für die Kaltmassivumformung**
Von Dipl.-Ing. Michael Rebholz. ISBN 3-540-11052-6.
121 Seiten mit 46 Abbildungen. 43,– DM

61 **Beitrag zum Ziehen von Blechteilen aus Aluminiumlegierungen**
Von Dipl.-Ing. Michael Blaich. ISBN 3-540-11067-4.
141 Seiten mit 64 Abbildungen und 5 Tabellen. 43,– DM

62 **Auslegung von rotationssymmetrischen Fließpreßwerkzeugen im Bereich elastisch-plastischen Werkstoffverhaltens**
Von Dipl.-Ing. Thomas Neitzert. ISBN 3-540-11623-0.
159 Seiten mit 51 Abbildungen. 53,– DM

63 **Fließpressen von Sintermetall im Temperaturbereich zwischen 873 K (600°C) und 1173 K (900°C)**
Von Dipl.-Ing. Wolfgang Schaub. ISBN 3-540-11678-8.
160 Seiten mit 85 Abbildungen und 9 Tabellen. 53,– DM

64 **Rechnerunterstützte Konstruktion von Umformwerkzeugen und die Fertigungsplanung von Werkzeugelementen**
Von Dipl.-Ing. Dieter Steuss. ISBN 3-540-11856-X.
178 Seiten mit 87 Abbildungen und 6 Tabellen. 53,– DM

65 **Möglichkeiten und Grenzen des Kaltgesenkschmiedens als eine fertigungstechnische Alternative für kleine, genaue Formteile**
Von Dipl.-Ing. Khang Hoang-Vu. ISBN 3-540-11876-4.
156 Seiten mit 62 Abbildungen und 5 Tabellen. 53,– DM

66 **Einsatz numerischer Näherungsverfahren bei der Berechnung von Verfahren der Kaltmassivumformung.**
Von Dipl.-Ing. Karl Roll. ISBN 3-540-11910-8.
166 Seiten mit 49 Abbildungen und 2 Tabellen. 53,– DM

67 **Untersuchung über das Verjüngen von dickwandigen, zylindrischen Hohlkörpern**
Von Dipl.-Ing. Knut Haarscheidt. ISBN 3-540-12229-X.
124 Seiten mit 58 Abbildungen und 6 Tabellen. Vergriffen

68 **Rechnerunterstützte Optimierung des Tiefziehens unregelmäßiger Blechteile**
Von Dipl.-Ing. Hans Glöckl. ISBN 3-540-12522-1.
143 Seiten mit 60 Abbildungen. Vergriffen

69 **Hydrostatisches Fließpressen: Verfahrensparameter und Werkstückeigenschaften**
Von Dipl.-Ing. Jobst H. Kerspe. ISBN 3-540-12537-X.
123 Seiten mit 69 Abbildungen und 5 Tabellen. 58,– DM

70 **Untersuchungen zum Halbwarmfließpressen von Automatenstählen**
Von Dipl.-Ing. Eberhard Nehl. ISBN 3-540-12568-X.
145 Seiten mit 104 Abbildungen. 58,– DM

71 **Entwicklung und Anwendung neuer Schmierstoffprüfverfahren für die Kaltmassivumformung**
Von Dipl.-Ing. Thomas Gräbener. ISBN 3-540-12836-0.
140 Seiten mit 65 Abbildungen. 58,– DM

72 **Einfluß der Blechoberfläche beim Ziehen von Blechteilen aus Aluminiumlegierungen**
Von Dipl.-Ing. Erhard Mössle. ISBN 3-540-12837-9.
142 Seiten mit 62 Abbildungen und 6 Tabellen. 58,– DM

73 **Werkzeugverschleiß in der Massivumformung**
Von Dipl.-Ing. Matthias Weiergräber. ISBN 3-540-13033-0.
72 Seiten mit 36 Abbildungen und 2 Tabellen. 58,– DM

74 **Grundlagen der Umformtechnik I · Fundamentals of Metal Forming Technique I**
298 Seiten. ISBN 3-540-13039-X. 58,– DM

75 **Grundlagen der Umformtechnik II · Fundamentals of Metal Forming Technique II**
280 Seiten. ISBN 3-540-13040-3. 58,– DM

76 **Herstellung und Versteifungswirkung von geschlossenen Halbrundsicken**
Von Dipl.-Ing. Michael Widmann. ISBN 3-540-13172-8.
150 Seiten mit 63 Abbildungen. 63,– DM

77 **Kostenoptimierter Einsatz der Radialumformmaschine in gemischten, flexiblen Fertigungssystemen**
Von Dipl.-Ing. Michael Dostal. ISBN 3-540-13286-4.
121 Seiten mit 61 Abbildungen. 63,– DM

78 **Rechnerische Ermittlung von Zustandsgrößen beim Radialumformen**
Von Dipl.-Ing. Roland Paukert. ISBN 3-540-13287-2.
131 Seiten mit 57 Abbildungen und 1 Tabelle. 63,– DM

79 **Numerische Steuerung einer flexiblen Bearbeitungseinheit zum Radialumformen**
Von Dipl.-Ing. Helmut Noller. ISBN 3-540-13550-2.
120 Seiten mit 41 Abbildungen und 2 Tabellen. 63,– DM

80 **Vergleichende Betrachtung der Verfahren zur Prüfung der plastischen Eigenschaften metallischer Werkstoffe**
Von Dr.-Ing. Klaus Pöhlandt. ISBN 3-540-13578-2.
178 Seiten mit 43 Abbildungen und 11 Tabellen. 63,– DM

81 **Aufweitung von Fließpreßmatrizen mit überlagerter thermischer und mechanischer Beanspruchung**
Von Dipl.-Ing. Ewald Kling. ISBN 3-540-15755-7.
139 Seiten mit 61 Abbildungen und 1 Tabelle. 63,– DM

82 **Messung des Werkzeugverschleißes bei der Kalt- und Halbwarmumformung mit Radionukliden**
Von Dipl.-Ing. Eberhard Nehl. ISBN 3-540-16497-9.
131 Seiten mit 55 Abbildungen und 11 Tabellen. 68,– DM

83 **Ermittlung von Eigenspannungen in der Kaltmassivumformung**
Von A. Erman Tekkaya. ISBN 3-540-16498-7.
162 Seiten mit 60 Abbildungen und 2 Tabellen. 68,– DM

84 **Korrosionsbeständigkeit tiefgezogener rotationssymmetrischer Werkstücke aus austenitischen Stählen**
Von Dipl.-Ing. Matthias Weiergräber. ISBN 3-540-16560-6.
137 Seiten mit 63 Abbildungen und 4 Tabellen. 68,– DM

85 **Simulation of Metal Forming Processes by the Finite Element Method (SIMOP-I)**
Workshop Stuttgart 1985. ISBN 3-540-16592-4.
316 Seiten mit 147 Abbildungen und 3 Tabellen. 68,– DM

86 **Beanspruchung von Napf-Rückwärts-Fließpreßmatrizen aus Keramik infolge mechanischer Belastung und Temperatureinwirkung**
Von Dipl.-Ing. Winfried Nester. ISBN 3-540-16845-1.
148 Seiten mit 66 Abbildungen und 2 Tabellen. 68,– DM

87 **Einfluß von Oberflächenbeschichtungen auf den Werkzeugverschleiß bei der Massivumformung**
Von Dipl.-Ing. Harald Westheide. ISBN 3-540-16846-X.
146 Seiten mit 84 Abbildungen und 9 Tabellen. 68,– DM

88 **Hydrostatisches Fließpressen von Profilen unter Verwendung von Matrizen mit stetigem Übergang**
Von Dipl.-Ing. Suwandi Sugondo. ISBN 3-540-16847-8.
130 Seiten mit 59 Abbildungen und 7 Tabellen. 68,– DM

89 **Untersuchungen über das kombinierte Quer-Napf-Vorwärts-Fließpressen**
Von Dipl.-Ing. Walter Osen. ISBN 3-540-17349-8.
153 Seiten mit 66 Abbildungen. 68,– DM

90 **Werkstoff und Umformung**
1. Workshop Stuttgart, 1986. ISBN 3-540-17370-6.
224 Seiten. 68,– DM

91 **Beanspruchungsgerechte Auslegung von Fließpreßwerkzeugen mit numerischen Berechnungsmethoden**
Von Dipl.-Ing. Vu The Cuong. ISBN 3-540-17472-9.
169 Seiten mit 80 Abbildungen und 12 Tabellen. 68,– DM

92 **Der Kerbzugversuch als Einfachprüfverfahren für das richtungsabhängige Umformvermögen von Blechwerkstoffen**
Von Dipl.-Phys. Christian Weist. ISBN 3-540-17666-7.
96 Seiten mit 48 Abbildungen und 5 Tabellen. 68,– DM

93 **Querfließpressen eines Flansches oder Bundes an zylindrischen Vollkörpern aus Stahl**
Von Dipl.-Ing. Winfried Schätzle. ISBN 3-540-17929-1.
129 Seiten mit 67 Abbildungen und 3 Tabellen. 68,– DM

94 **Untersuchung des Werkzeugbruches beim Voll-Vorwärts-Fließpressen**
Von Dipl.-Ing. Willi Reiss. ISBN 3-540-18376-0.
159 Seiten mit 69 Abbildungen und 3 Tabellen. 68,– DM

95 **Grundlagen für das Kaltwalzen von Voll- und Hohlkörpern nach dem Grob-Verfahren**
Von Dipl.-Ing. Norbert Kurz. ISBN 3-540-18509-7.
163 Seiten mit 72 Abbildungen und 5 Tabellen. 68,– DM

96 **Rechnergestützte Fertigung von Sonderprofilen auf der Radialumformmaschine**
Von Dipl.-Ing. Andreas Wöhr. ISBN 3-540-19161-5.
141 Seiten mit 80 Abbildungen. 73,– DM

97 **Optimierung der Oberflächenmikrogeometrie von Aluminiumfeinblech für das Karosserieziehen**
Von Dipl.-Ing. Rainer Balbach. ISBN 3-540-50168-1.
161 Seiten mit 86 Abbildungen. 73,– DM

98 **Ermüdungsverhalten von massivumgeformten bauteilähnlichen Proben aus Stahl**
Von Dipl.-Ing. Wolfgang Schwab. ISBN 3-540-50805-8.
142 Seiten mit 81 Abbildungen und 3 Tabellen. 73,– DM

99 **Optimaler Energieeinsatz bei der Fertigung durch Massivumformung**
Von Dipl.-Ing. Thomas Herlan. ISBN 3-540-50876-7.
204 Seiten mit 63 Abbildungen und 3 Tabellen. 73,– DM

GPSR Compliance

The European Union's (EU) General Product Safety Regulation (GPSR) is a set of rules that requires consumer products to be safe and our obligations to ensure this.

If you have any concerns about our products, you can contact us on ProductSafety@springernature.com

In case Publisher is established outside the EU, the EU authorized representative is:

Springer Nature Customer Service Center GmbH
Europaplatz 3
69115 Heidelberg, Germany

Batch number: 10682421

Printed by Printforce, the Netherlands